# Brain Calipers 2nd Ed.

## Descriptive Psychopathology and the
## Psychiatric Mental Status Examination

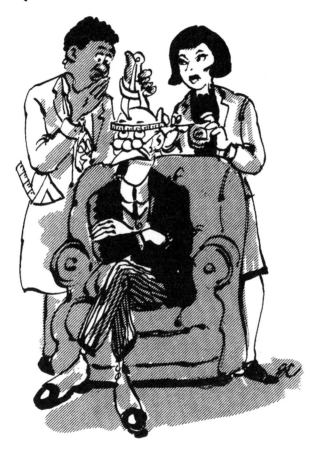

## David J. Robinson, M.D., F.R.C.P.C

### Diplomate of the American Board
### of Psychiatry and Neurology

# Rapid Psychler Press ðÖ

Suite 374
3560 Pine Grove Ave.
Port Huron, Michigan
**USA** 48060

Suite 203
1673 Richmond St.
London, Ontario
**Canada** N6G 2N3

*Toll Free Phone*  888-PSY-CHLE (888-779-2453)
*Toll Free Fax*  888-PSY-CHLR (888-779-2457)
Outside the U.S. & Canada – Fax  519-675-0610

*website*  www.psychler.com
*email*  rapid@psychler.com

ISBN 1-894328-02-7
Printed in the United States of America
© 2001, Rapid Psychler Press
Second Edition, First Printing

All caricatures are purely fictitious. Any resemblance to real people, either living or deceased, is entirely coincidental (and unfortunate). The author assumes no responsibility for the consequences of diagnoses made, or treatment instituted, as a result of the contents of this book – such determinations should be made by qualified mental health professionals. Every effort was made to ensure the information in this book was accurate at the time of publication. However, due to the changing nature of the field of psychiatry, the reader is encouraged to consult additional, and more recent, sources of information.

# Dedication

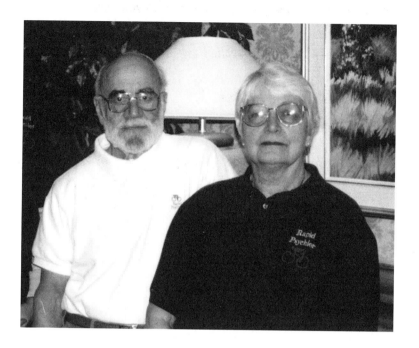

To my godparents, Brian and Fanny Chapman, for giving me my first transitional object (a teddy bear), and for all of the support and kindness you've shown me ever since.

# Rapid Psychler Press

produces books and presentation media that are:

- Comprehensively researched
- Well organized
- Formatted for ease of use
- Reasonably priced
- Clinically oriented, and
- Include humor that enhances education, and that neither demeans patients nor the efforts of those who treat them

# Table of Contents

## 1. Principles of the Mental Status Exam
### 3

## 2. Appearance
### 30

# 5. Speech                                      116

# 6. Thought Process                             148

# 11. Insight & Judgment   **310**

# 12. Sensorium & Cognitive Functioning   **332**

# Author's Foreword

The first edition of **Brain Calipers** was released in May, 1997. It was a departure from the other texts I had written. Prior to its release, I published a book of psychiatric mnemonics (now called **Mnemonics & More for Psychiatry**) and a primer on personality disorders (**Disordered Personalities**). These books are comprehensive in their scope, but not depth. In other words, they are good introductory books, but not authoritative. I developed **Brain Calipers** to be the opposite – a comprehensive presentation of a relatively compact area of psychiatry.

To me, a competent psychiatrist is one who has facility with the mental status exam (MSE). Too often, the MSE is squished into the last few minutes of an interview and globally reported as "within normal limits." This occurs because student interviewers are dubious about the relevance of the MSE, and do not understand the significance of the questions they are required to ask. On page 16, in presenting the findings of paper that looks at the least performed tasks in "medically clearing" patients, I make the subtle point that conducting the MSE is about as popular as performing a rectal exam. My sister, a marvelously thorough primary care physician, tells me there are two excuses for not conducting a rectal exam – no finger, and no rectum. I think that a similarly robust attitude is needed in training students and residents. The value of a rectal exam becomes apparent when a tumor is detected. Similarly, the value of the MSE is never questioned once a psychiatric disorder is detected that was not obvious from the patient's history. To this end, I hope that **Brain Calipers** is a useful guide and that I have broken some of the barriers to learning about the MSE.

Keep Psychling!

*Dave Robinson*

London, Ontario, Canada
March, 2001

# Teaching With Humor

Sigmund Freud, the pioneer of psychoanalysis and argu-
ably psychiatry's most prominent historical figure, developed many theories about behavior and emotional response.
Freud had a sense of humor and used it liberally in *Jokes
and their Relation to the Unconscious.* Freud had many theories about humor, but it appears that it is the "hidden, aggressive wish" proposal that most people remember from
his work. He had a good deal more to say about it, is aptly
summed up by Elliott Oring, *"Humor is one of the basic languages of intimacy and affection. Those who would reduce
humor to disguised expressions of hostility and aggression
might well ponder whether humor might not serve to mask
expressions of love and tenderness as well."* Humor is a
healthy mechanism that has such as potent influence that
omitting it from medical education is a travesty.

Few people would want to be thought of as being humorless. It is the rare speaker, medical or otherwise, who does
not include at least some levity in a presentation, whether
this is as a cartoon, wry observation, or witticism. However,
few medical educators make the effort to include humor in
printed teaching material.

At its most basic level, humor increases interest. Laughter
is stimulating and starts a cascade of beneficial psychological and physiological responses. Humorous material
sprinkled throughout a text encourages readers to continue
on, wondering where the next comment or caricature will
be found. The inclusion of humor also conveys that the author cared about enhancing the readability of the material.
Furthermore, humor enhances retention. Students who
enjoy a book will return to it more frequently and retain the
material more fully.

Humor conveys a sense of flexibility. If one can keep one's
mind open to the possibility of humor, many other connections become apparent.

Humor conveys a sense of perspective. The human brain and emotional responses are so complex that we have at best rudimentary ways of explaining or altering perception, emotion, cognition, or behavior. I expect that some of the treatments I currently administer may be considered malpractice in a few years. By using humor, I encourage humility. There is much we don't understand, and while we must take our work seriously, we do not need to take ourselves quite a seriously.

Humor conveys a sense of understanding. In order to find something humorous, a situation must be comprehended, as well as the incongruity or the psychological shift of the joke. Students that can comprehend levity included in didactic material have a solid understanding of what is being taught.

Humor conveys a humanistic approach to teaching, in effect saying, *"Relax, I'm your guide – you can trust me"* and *"This isn't such a terrible subject."* Adding humor lets readers know that the author was once a student who struggled to gain an understanding of the material, and now endeavors to make the process easier.

Humor is innovation, requiring a fresh perspective and an element of surprise. Getting readers to smile or laugh means that you've reached them. It takes a good deal of thinking, planning, and editing to include humor that it appropriate to the topic, and which enhances the material.

Because humor is subjective, I cannot include material that is mirthful for every reader on every occasion. Indeed, the same reader may have a different response to the material at different times.

My first disclaimer is that I have in no way set out to "make fun of patients" or trivialize mental illness. People who suffer from psychiatric difficulties have always been scorned and ridiculed. To be a clinician, yet alone an educator, and use mental illness as a source of humor is to me improper and unethical. I have never portrayed a patient in a humorous manner in my work. I have also never taken an experience of one of my patients and used it in a humorous way in my work. If there is a focus for my humor, it is the constructs we develop to explain, classify, and alter human behavior. For example, consider the assuredness with which clinicians engaged in such practices as physiognomy. As you may know, *Lavater's Essays on Physiognomy* was highly regarded – its author an internationally acclaimed expert whose opinion was given the utmost respect. Perusing old psychiatry texts from early in the 20th century reveals a complexity and forthrightness to some material, which has been thoroughly discredited (such as racial explanations for mental illness). Would these clinicians and writers not have been better off keeping a sense of perspective, and even humor, about their theories and explanations?

My next disclaimer is that I am not demeaning or trivializing the efforts of contemporary clinicians or theorists. We have a solid basis for continued research and understanding in many areas, but we do not have all-encompassing explanations. The DSM-IV, with its atheoretical approach and numerous artificial constructs, is not the final word in classifying mental illness. Is it not important to encourage in today's students a sense of humility? Can we not view today's constructs as being an improvement on physiognomy, but still a system that needs to be refined. Is there a better way of conveying this than with humor?

My books are thoroughly researched, accurate, and I hope, well written. Even without the humor, they are innovative and effective teaching resources. With the humor, they are enjoyable to read, and again I hope, achieve the goals I have listed here.

# Selected References

C.T. Beck
**Humor in Nursing Practice: A Phenomenological Study**
*International Journal of Nursing Studies* 34(5): 346 – 352, 1997

S. Freud
**Jokes and Their Relation to the Unconscious**
(J. Strachey, translator)
W.W. Norton, New York, 1960

M. Kuhrik, N. Kuhrik, & P.A. Berry
**Facilitating Learning With Humor**
*Journal of Nursing Education* 36(7): 332 – 334, 1997

K. Leidy
**Enjoyable Learning Experiences – An Aid to Retention?**
*The Journal of Continuing Education in Nursing* 23(5): 206 – 208, 1992

E.A. Lorenzi
**Humor in the Testing Situation**
*Nurse Educator* 21(1): 12 – 22, 1996

N.W. Moses & M.M. Friedman
**Using Humor in Evaluating Student Performance**
*Journal of Nursing Education* 25(8): 328 – 333, 1986

V. L. Nahas
**Humor: A Phenomenological Study Within the Context of Clinical Education**
*Nurse Education Today* 18: 663 – 672, 1998

E. Oring
**Jokes and Their Relations**
University of Kentucky Press, Lexington, Kentucky, 1992

J.M. Parfitt
**Humorous Preoperative Teaching: Effect on Recall of Postoperative Exercise Routines**
*AORN Journal* 52(1): 114 – 120, 1990

T.E. Parrott
**Humor As a Teaching Strategy**
*Nurse Educator* 19(3): 36 – 38, 1994

J. Robbins
**Using Humor to Enhance Learning in the Skills Laboratory**
*Nurse Educator* 19(3): 39 – 41, 1994

M.J. Watson & S. Emerson
**Facilitate Learning With Humor**
*Journal of Nursing Education* 27(2): 89 – 90, 1988

# Changes to the 2nd Edition

The first edition of **Brain Calipers** took around 1200 hours to write over the span of 15 months. This revision took another 300 hours, yet the changes are modest.

• The book was completely re-edited and re-typeset. The font (typeface) was changed to improve readability.

• Some of the humor pages between chapters were removed, as well as the blank pages for personal notes.

• Chapter 11 – *Insight & Judgment* was completely re-written, with sections on rating scales and proverb interpretation being added.

• Three new chapters were added:
    Chapter 15 – *Bedside Screening Tests*
    Chapter 16 – *The MSE and the Elderly*
    Chapter 17 – *The Child Mental Status Exam*

• New sections were added to several chapters:
    *Chapter 1* – Necessity of Conducting the MSE
    *Chapter 1* – Medicolegal Need for the MSE
    *Chapter 4* – Factitious Disorder
    *Chapter 8* – Protecting Yourself in Interviews
    *Chapter 9* – Congruence of Psychotic Symptoms in Mood
            Disorders
    *Chapter 14* – Other versions of the Mini-Mental State
            Exam

• The index was more than doubled in size.

• All of the references I used are now included at the end of the each chapter.

• Overall, there is approximately 12% more material in this edition.

# Acknowledgments

I am indebted to the following individuals for their unfailing support and enthusiasm in assisting me with this text.

- **Brian & Fanny Chapman**
- **Monty & Lilly Robinson**
- **Brad Groshok**
- **Dean Avola**
- **Dr. Donna Robinson & Dr. Robert Bauer**

I am fortunate to have a colleague –

- **Tom Norry, B.Sc.N.**

who devotes a considerable amount time and energy to correcting both the academic content, as well as the spelling and grammar, in my drafts. If there are mistakes that have crept into the final version, the fault is mine alone. Thank you, Tom.

I would also like to thank the following individuals for their numerous helpful suggestions which improved the content and presentation of this book:

- **Dr. Nina Desjardins**
- **Thomas Gantert, B.Sc.N.**
- **Dr. Michelle Kelly**
- **Dr. Sandra Northcott**
- **Dr. Lisa Bogue**
- **Dr. Janine Robertson**

# Publication Notes

## Terminology

Throughout this book, the term "patient" is used to refer to people who are suffering, and who seek help while bearing pain without complaint or anger. The terms "consumer" or "consumer-survivor" reflect an unfortunate trend that is pejorative towards mental health care, labeling it as if it were a trade or business instead of a profession. These terms are also ambiguous, as it is not clear what is being "consumed" or "survived." Where possible, I used the genderless "they" to refer to patients. When gender needed to be specified, I chose randomly between male and female.

## Graphics

All of the illustrations in this book are original works of art commissioned by Rapid Psychler Press and are a signature feature of our publications. Rapid Psychler Press makes available an entire library of color illustrations (including those from this book) as 35mm slides, overhead transparencies, and in digital formats (for use in programs such as PowerPoint®). These images are available for viewing and can be purchased from our website — **www.psychler.com**

These images from our color library may be used for presentations. We request that you respect our copyright and do not reproduce these images in any form, for any purpose, at any time.

## Bolded Terms

Throughout this book, various terms appear in bolded text to allow for ease of identification. Many of these terms are defined in this text. Others are only mentioned because a detailed description is beyond the scope of this book. Fuller explanations of all of the bolded terms can be found in standard reference texts.

# Brain Calipers 2nd Ed.
## Descriptive Psychopathology and the
## Psychiatric Mental Status Examination

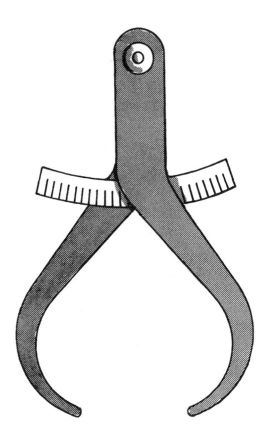

*A psychiatrist has to be a person who commits himself to making a person better. Nothing should be too menial for a psychiatrist to do.*

Willibald Nagler

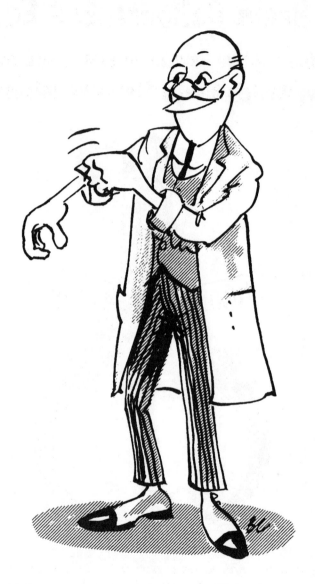

*A smart mother often makes a better diagnosis than a poor doctor.*

August Bier

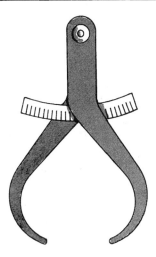

# Chapter 1

# Principles of the Mental Status Examination

## Psychiatry as a Branch of Medicine

Psychiatry is a fascinating area of medicine. Psychiatry and primary care take into account not only patients' illnesses, but their thoughts, emotions, and behaviors as well. Treating mental illness provides practitioners with perpetual variety because it involves a most complicated entity (the human brain, not managed care). Whereas most cases of congestive heart failure or glaucoma have set treatment protocols, psychiatric illnesses require creative interventions. In psychiatry, the pathognomonic findings or objective signs found in physical medicine are no longer present. No single sign or symptom is unique to a particular psychiatric diagnosis. We cannot rely on a blood test, MRI, or laparoscopy to clear up diagnostic uncertainty. Furthermore, substance use and general medical conditions can perfectly imitate almost any mental illness. For these reasons, among many others, psychiatrists must complete a full medical curriculum before embarking on specialist training.

Psychiatry is an all-encompassing field. Every patient on every service experiences emotional reactions to his illness. Convincing a patient to take medications, minimize risk factors, and to comply with discharge arrangements involves a multi-faceted understanding of human nature.

The exploration of the cause and effect of illness along the "mind-body continuum" is an area still in its infancy. For example, the interplay between emotions and changes in immune and endocrine function is now an established psychiatric subspecialty.

Psychological factors clearly have an effect on medical conditions, and an understanding of this association helps to make us better clinicians (in any field), as well as better students, teachers, spouses, parents, and indeed, human beings. Despite its current drawbacks and limitations, psychiatry offers a rich and varied approach to understanding and treating mental illness.

# A Method for Understanding Mental Illness

The illustration shown on the next page is helpful in conceptualizing mental illness. Any condition that affects one area will have an effect on all the others. Almost all the of the criteria used to diagnose mental illness in the DSM-IV can be categorized as being changes in perception, cognition, emotion, or behavior.

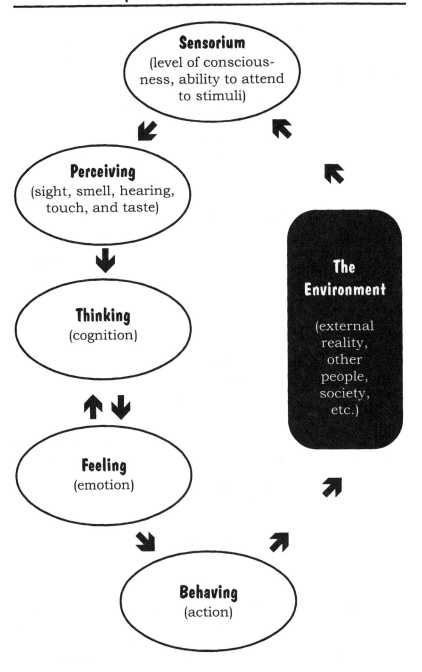

For example, consider depression, which is primarily a dis-order of mood that causes people to feel sad, blue, or empty. The effects that a depressed mood causes can be illustrated as follows:

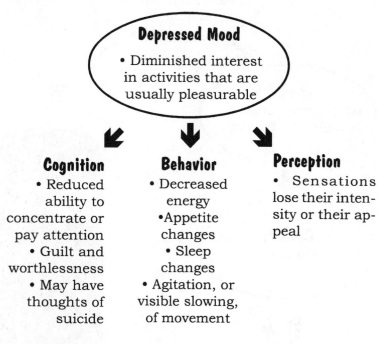

**Depressed Mood**
• Diminished interest in activities that are usually pleasurable

**Cognition**
• Reduced ability to concentrate or pay attention
• Guilt and worthlessness
• May have thoughts of suicide

**Behavior**
• Decreased energy
• Appetite changes
• Sleep changes
• Agitation, or visible slowing, of movement

**Perception**
• Sensations lose their intensity or their appeal

The assessment process in psychiatry relies primarily on the interviewing and observational skills of practitioners.

There are four components to making an accurate diagnosis:
• The psychiatric interview
• The mental status exam (**MSE**)
• Collateral sources of information
• Laboratory testing

An outline of the psychiatric interview appears on page 8, followed by a detailed introduction to the MSE. More information about the interview, collateral information, and laboratory testing is available in the *References* section at the end of this chapter.

# The Evaluation Process in Psychiatry

**STANDARD INTERVIEW PROCESS**

**MENTAL STATUS EXAM**

**PHYSICAL EXAM & ROUTINE INVESTIGATIONS**

**SPECIALIZED INVESTIGATIONS**

- Biochemical
- Neuro-imaging
- Other

# Anatomy of the Psychiatric Interview

The **American Psychiatric Association (APA)** published a set of practice guidelines for general psychiatric evaluation of adults. The following "domains of evaluation" comprise a complete psychiatric interview:

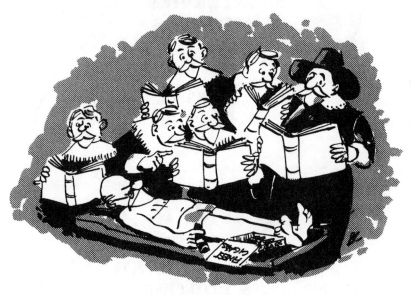

A. Reason for the Evaluation
B. History of the Present Illness
C. Past Psychiatric History
D. General Medical History
E. History of Substance Use
F. Psychosocial/Developmental History (Personal History)
G. Social History
H. Occupational History
 I. Family History
J. Review of Symptoms
K. Physical Examination
**L. Mental Status Examination (MSE)**
M. Functional Assessment
N. Diagnostic Tests
O. Information Derived From The Interview Process

# What Is the MSE?

The MSE is the component of an interview where cognitive functions are tested and inquiries are made about the symptoms of psychiatric conditions. It is a set of standardized observations and questions designed to evaluate:

- Sensorium and Level of Consciousness
- Perception
- Thinking
- Feeling
- Behavior

The MSE is an integral part of *any* clinical interview, not just one that takes place in a psychiatric context. An assessment of cognitive functioning must be made before information from patients can be considered accurate. *The MSE records only observed behavior, cognitive abilities, and inner experiences expressed during the interview.* The MSE is conducted to assess as completely as possible the factors necessary to arrive at a provisional diagnosis, formulate a treatment plan, and follow a patient's clinical course.

The MSE is a portable assessment tool that helps to identify the presence of psychiatric disorders and gauge their severity. With experience, it is a specific, sensitive, and inexpensive diagnostic instrument. The MSE takes only a few minutes to administer yet yields information that is crucial to making a diagnostic assessment and starting a course of treatment.

# What Are the Components of the MSE?

The MSE can be thought of as a psychiatric "review of symptoms." As outlined on page 5, the assessment of five main areas yields information necessary for a differential diagnosis and treatment plan.

Expanding on these five areas gives us the psychological functions that are assessed and recorded in the MSE.

## Sensorium & Cognitive Functioning
- Level of consciousness and attentiveness
- Orientation to person, place, and time
- Attention
- Concentration
- Memory
- Knowledge
- Intelligence
- Capacity for abstract thinking

## Perception
- Disorders of sensory input where there is no stimulus (hallucinations) or where a stimulus is misperceived (illusions), or of disorders of bodily experience (depersonalization or derealization)

## Thinking
- Speech
- Thought Content (*what* is said)
- Thought Form (*how* it is said or *the way* it is said)
- Suicidal or Homicidal Ideation
- Insight & Judgment

## Feeling
- Affect (objective, visible emotional state)
- Mood (subjective emotional experience)

## Behavior
- Appearance
- Psychomotor agitation or retardation
- Degree of cooperation with the interview

# How Do I Remember All That?

A mnemonic can help. The following memory aid not only lists the main areas, but does so in the order that they are usually asked about and presented.

## "ABC STAMP LICKER"

**A**ppearance
**B**ehavior
**C**ooperation

**S**peech
**T**hought – **form** and **content**
**A**ffect – moment-to-moment variation in emotion
**M**ood – subjective emotional tone throughout the interview
**P**erception – in all sensory modalities

**L**evel of Consciousness
**I**nsight & Judgment
**C**ognitive Functioning & Sensorium
      **O**rientation
      **M**emory
      **A**ttention & Concentration
      **R**eading & Writing
**K**nowledge base
**E**ndings – Suicidal and/or Homicidal Thoughts
**R**eliability of the Information

# Must I Conduct the MSE?

Yes. It is as essential to a complete psychiatric assessment as the physical examination is in other areas of medicine. The MSE has been adroitly called the "brain stethoscope." Remember, all psychiatric diagnoses are made clinically in interview situations. There is no blood test, X-ray, or single identifying feature for any psychiatric condition. This emphasizes the need for a thorough assessment, of which the MSE is an essential component.

# How Do I Start the MSE?

The MSE begins as soon as the patient is in view. A moment of observation before the interview reveals important information such as: grooming, hygiene, behavior, gait, level of interest in the surroundings, etc.

Other elements of the MSE are obtained as the interview proceeds. Most interviewers begin an interview with open-ended questions and allow patients at least five minutes of relatively unstructured time to say what is on their minds.

Invariably, there are items that will have to be asked about with specific questions. Such inquiries can be made in one of three ways:

**1.** Take the opportunity when it arises in the interview. This is the most natural approach, allowing the MSE to be woven into the fabric of the interview. For example, many patients will complain of poor memory and a decreased attention span, which presents an ideal opportunity to test cognitive functions. The disadvantage to this method is that it can disrupt the structure of an interview. For those new to interviewing and the MSE, this approach may be better left until more facility has been gained in coping with such tangents.

**2.** Take note of key points in the history that allow for a smooth transition for further investigation [called a **referred gate** – Shea (1998)]. If a patient mentions she has had difficulty getting along with co-workers, you can raise this again to ask about the presence of delusions – *"You mentioned some problems at work. Do you find that you have some ideas that no one else agrees with?"* This lets patients know that they have been listened to, while adhering to a more structured interview. If patients say something that opens this opportunity, but at an inopportune time, you can say something like, *"It's important for me to know about that, and we'll get back to it in a few minutes\*, but right now could you tell me more about. . ."* (\* Remember to ask about it later!).

**3.** Pose questions about the MSE at the end of the interview. This has the advantage of helping to preserve the structure of the interview. Additionally, opportunities for the two previous approaches don't always present themselves.

Specific parts of the MSE can be introduced as follows:

*"At this point, I'd like to ask you some questions that are separate from what we've been discussing so far, but will give me some important information about you."*

or

*"Right now, I'd like to ask you some questions to give me an idea about some aspects of your psychological functioning."*

or

*"I'd like to switch now and ask you a set of questions that will help me evaluate your. . . (thinking, memory, etc.)."*

or

*"There are some other areas that I need to test to get an idea about your. . . (concentration, attention, etc.). "*

or

*"In order to be as thorough as possible, I need to ask you some questions about your mental functions and inner experiences."*

These questions are only suggestions. Ask instructors or colleagues for their own patented phrases. While conducting the MSE is essential, it can be done in a variety of ways, and in any order. You can draw on the experiences of others initially, and then develop your own approach. Specific questions regarding certain sections of the MSE (e.g. hallucinations and delusions, suicidal or homicidal thoughts) are included in their respective chapters.

# How Does the MSE Differ From the Psychiatric History?

Many parts of the MSE are indeed covered in the body of the interview. However, it is rare for *all* aspects of the MSE to be covered without being specifically asked about.

On one hand, an interview can consist solely of the MSE. Patients who are delirious, severely demented, or grossly psychotic cannot provide reliable information. Interviews under these circumstances are principally a record of appearance, behavior, speech, thought form, etc.

On the other hand, someone can answer questions in a straightforward, logical manner and demonstrate no obvious abnormalities of behavior, but still have a serious mental illness. Most clinicians can recall a situation where they were fooled by not conducting a thorough MSE. The best example of this situation is a patient who suffers from a **delusional disorder**. Other than the theme of the delusion (paranoia, jealousy, etc.), the history can be largely unremarkable. Unless specific inquiries are made about the presence of these fixed, false ideas, these will be missed.

Other components of the psychiatric history and the MSE interact dynamically so interviewers learn where most profitably to direct their inquiries. Consider a patient who is disheveled, wearing a foil-wrapped jacket to ward off gamma radiation, and conversing with a light bulb using unusual language. Areas of immediate interest are:
• Recent ingestion of substances
• The presence of medical illnesses, head injuries, etc.
• A history of psychotic disorders and similar past episodes
• Compliance with recommended treatment
• The number and duration of hospital stays

The integration of the MSE and the psychiatric history is outlined on the next page.

# Integration of the MSE and History

| Psychiatric History | MSE Component |
| --- | --- |
| • Identifying Data<br>• Chief Complaint | • **Appearance**<br>• **Behavior**<br>• **Orientation**<br>(ask patients for their full name, if they had difficulty finding the room/clinic/hospital)<br>• **Level of Consciousness**<br>(this is usually obvious) |
| • **History of Present Illness (HPI)** 5 – 10 minutes of relatively unstructured questions using open-ended inquiries and other facilitating techniques | • **Cooperation**<br>• **Speech**<br>• **Thought Form**<br>• **Thought Content**<br>(this open format allows patients to talk about what concerns them, a valuable indicator of thought content) |
| • **Exploration of Symptoms from the HPI**<br>More focused assessment with elaboration of material from the HPI using closed-ended questions to get more specific information | • **Affect**<br>• **Mood**<br>• **Suicidal/Homicidal Ideation**<br>• **Elements of Cognitive Testing**<br>(it may be convenient to include these components at this point to help gauge the severity of reported symptoms) |
| **Direct Testing of Other MSE Components**<br>If certain areas aren't amenable to questions earlier in the interview, specific inquiries must be made at some point to assess these functions | • **Knowledge Base**<br>• **Perception**<br>• **Insight & Judgment**<br>• **Formal Cognitive Testing**<br>    **Memory**<br>    **Attention**<br>    **Concentration**<br>    **Reading & Writing**<br>    **Abstract Thinking** |

# The Unpopular MSE

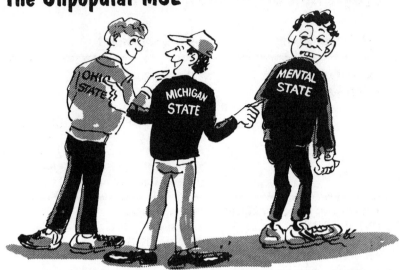

Despite the paramount importance of the MSE, it remains an unpopular exercise, and in many cases is simply not completed by physicians.

Kiernan (1976) reported on the completeness of 100 case records written by trainees. Three main sections of the record were scored for completeness: history, MSE, and formulation. While Kiernan found significant inadequacies in the history and formulation sections, he had this to say about the MSE: *Items in the MSE were even less satisfactorily recorded. An adequate assessment of the MSE is the acid test of the competent psychiatrist. It is also the area most strange to the recent entrant to psychiatry.*

Riba (1990) documented the steps taken in the evaluation of patients with psychiatric complaints who were "medically cleared" prior to being referred from the emergency room. In total, 137 patient referrals were studied. The least popular evaluations were: complete neurological exam (20%); laboratory testing (8%); dermatologic assessment (4%); musculoskeletel assessment (1%); pelvic/rectal exam (0%); and the MSE (0%).

The MSE is usually unpopular for two reasons:
• The questions are difficult to formulate because they are not asked in other types of interviews or in other areas of medicine, psychology, nursing, etc.
• The questions appear to be of dubious relevance

Once these two difficulties are surmounted, the MSE becomes an enjoyable and interesting aspect of interviewing. To achieve this level of comfort, it helps to realize that almost half of the MSE is obtained "free" through observation and discussion from the initial parts of the interview.

| "Free" Parameters | Parameters to Ask About |
|---|---|
| Level of Consciousness | Orientation |
| Appearance | Cognitive Functioning |
| Behavior | Suicidal/Homicidal Thoughts |
| Cooperation | Knowledge Base |
| Reliability | Perception |
| Affect | Mood |
| Thought Form | Thought Content |

# How Else Can I Conceptualize the MSE?

The MSE can be considered the "physical examination" of psychiatry. Eliciting somatic symptoms in physical medicine warrants examination of the affected area via **I.P.P.A.**

• **I**nspection
• **P**alpation
• **P**ercussion
• **A**uscultation

Further "looking into," "touching on," "sounding out," and "listening to" is required to fully evaluate psychiatric symptoms. Unlike the physical exam, the MSE is at least partly integrated with the history. Both the physical exam and MSE are recorded separately from the body of the history.

The MSE can also be considered part of the objective portion of the **S.O.A.P.** approach to recording information:

- **Subjective** — Consists of sections from the interview:
  Chief Complaint
  History of Present Illness
  Medical and Psychiatric History
  Family and Personal History

- **Objective** — Recording of observations
  Mental Status Exam
  Physical Examination
  Laboratory Testing

- **Assessment** — Provisional (or Preferred) Diagnosis
  & Differential Diagnoses

- **Plan** — Further Investigations, Short-Term, & Long-Term
  Treatment

# Diagnostic Decision Making and the MSE

Seasoned clinicians generate hypotheses early in interviews with limited data. In a group of psychiatrists studied by Gauron (1966), the most efficient diagnosticians generated hypotheses after two pieces of information were given (e.g. age, and reason for referral), and needed only 8 to 14 infobits to arrive at a diagnosis (the least efficient interviewers needed up to 36). Maguire (1976) observed a group of senior medical students conducting a standardized 15-minute interview. In this time period, students elicited an average of 14 useful pieces of information, which was estimated to be about one-third of the data available under the imposed time constraints.

In other studies, it was found that physicians generated their initial hypotheses in less than one minute, containing an average of six possible diagnoses (Feightner, 1975 & Barrows, 1979). At just five minutes into the interview, they had finalized their hypotheses about which illnesses they thought the patient might have. Over half of the relevant information was obtained in the first quarter of the interview. By necessity, diagnostic decision-making must begin early. In many situations, interviewers do not have the chance to spend extended periods of time with patients. In situations where a specific task is required (e.g. triaging patients in an emergency room; consultation interviews focusing on a question from the consultee), **hypothesis generation** begins immediately upon speaking with the patient.

Gauron (1966) determined that the following pieces of information were the most helpful in arriving at a diagnosis (presented in order of importance):

1. Reason for Referral
2. Previous Personality/Level of Functioning
3. Thought Disorder (Content and Process) on the MSE
4. Previous Psychiatric Illnesses
5. Testing for Organic Conditions
6. Personality Testing
7. Insight and Judgment on the MSE
8. Appearance and Behavior on the MSE
9. Affect and Mood on the MSE
10. Physical Examination

Note that of the 10 most important pieces of information, four are from the MSE.

# Are There Some Practical Examples?

**Scenario A**

An elderly male patient had hip surgery two days ago. Since that time, he has been persistently disoriented, disruptive, and agitated. At the outset of the interview, he is grasping at invisible objects and mumbling to himself.

**Evaluation**

This man is delirious, and the information obtained from him at this point is of questionable reliability. His mental status needs to be assessed first, with questions involving the following areas:
• Orientation
• What he's experiencing at the moment (What is he picking

at? Are there sounds, sights, smells, or sensations that are diverting his attention?)
• Have him speak up or repeat what he's been saying

### Scenario B
A woman in her late twenties is seen in the emergency department due to intermittent attacks of shortness of breath and wheezing. After answering some preliminary questions, she reveals that these episodes occur only when her neighbors fill her apartment with poison gas.

### Evaluation
This woman more likely has a paranoid disorder than a respiratory ailment. At this point, the MSE becomes the principal component of the interview. The next step might involve exploring her thoughts of being persecuted (onset of the attacks, identity of conspirators, etc.).

In these two brief examples, a full MSE becomes paramount because an understanding of thinking, feeling, behavior, perception, sensorium, and cognitive functioning is integral to making a correct diagnosis and instituting treatment. Positive findings on the MSE help target areas for further questioning, investigations, the need for collaborative history, etc., and are a guide to clinical course and prognosis.

# Is the MSE the Only Examination Needed?

Not at all. The MSE is a component of an interview like the *Medical History* or *Personal History*. The MSE consists of a range of questions inquiring about the features of certain mental illnesses and assessing a number of psychological functions. It is by no means the end of the investigative or diagnostic process. The MSE assists with **hypothesis generation**, and helps determine which further investigations might be necessary.

Beyond the interview and MSE, collateral history, a physical exam and appropriate laboratory testing are warranted.

# Medicolegal Need for the MSE

Performing and recording a complete MSE is one of the most important steps a clinician can take to avoid malpractice actions (or limiting one's liability).

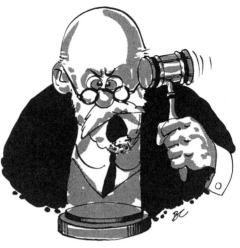

Many medical communications (i.e. *Psychiatric News, Psychiatric Times*) have reported that lawsuits were dropped, or damages minimized, because the MSE supported a psychiatrist's actions in certain situations.

The MSE is an integral component of competence/capacity assessments:

**Competence** refers to having the ability to understand and act reasonably; competence is a legal term, and the decision about someone's competence is made by a judge.

**Capacity** is having the mental ability to make a rational decision (based on understanding and appreciating all relevant information); capacity is determined by a clinician.

## Areas of Competence/Capacity

- Execution
- Be sentenced
- Live independently
- Enter into a contract
- Stand trial
- Manage financial affairs
- Make medical decisions
- Get married
- Be a witness (**Testimonial Capacity**)
- Vote
- Make a will (**Testamentary Capacity**)

# Interviewing Skills

Because psychiatric symptoms and diagnoses are made in interview situations, developing skills in the art of obtaining information is crucial. Particularly relevant to the MSE are the following:

• A psychiatric interview is not a conversation, but an active period of questioning and observation. All aspects of the person being interviewed are subject to scrutiny: body odors, unusual movements, grooming habits, etc. Areas that might tactfully be avoided in social situations are pursued in assessments to further the understanding of that person.

• Be interested! Pursue hints, suggestions, and insinuations. Psychiatric interviews allow the privilege of asking about personal matters and making repeated inquiries for further information.

• Exude a neutral, calm manner. All aspects of patients' lives (sexual, religious, fantasy) are relevant. Information involving sensitive areas is best obtained using a straightforward, non-judgmental demeanor. Your task is to understand patients and empathize with them. An attitude of curiosity and acceptance helps to facilitate this exchange.

• Be flexible. Adjust your tone. Avoid the use of psychiatric jargon – pose questions that your patients will understand.

• At regular intervals, take a break to check your understanding of patients' problems with them. This clearly conveys your interest, and helps clarify which areas need further exploration.

• Attend to the comfort of your patients. Provide tissues, ashtrays, water, etc. to see that their needs are met. Taking care of these preliminary considerations expresses empathy and avoids interruptions. A list of references for interviewing skills is provided at the end of this chapter.

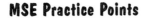

## MSE Practice Points

• The Mini-Mental State Examination (**MMSE**) **IS NOT** the same as a complete MSE. See the *Chapter 14 – The MMSE* for a fuller presentation.

• The MSE was originally a component of the neurological examination.

• The MSE is an evaluation of the patient at the time of the interview. The findings on an MSE can and do change (invariably in front of a senior colleague). It is a record of observations made at the time of a particular evaluation.

• The MSE provides an assessment to help monitor course and prognosis. It has a high "test-retest" value and reveals important information about clinical course.

• The MSE consists of a relatively standardized approach and list of inquiries. However, every instructor will have his or her own rationale for doing things a certain way. It is important to have exposure to as many styles as possible. Then, assimilate this knowledge into an approach that suits you best. Different approaches can be used at different times in different ways; there is no single "correct" approach.

• The aim of the MSE is to have completed a thorough evaluation by the end of the interview. You are free to develop your own style – as long as you have covered the main areas, your approach is not "wrong," and you have latitude in how this is accomplished. You can always benefit from the ideas of others, but critically review their suggestions before automatically incorporating them into your interview style.

# Summary

It is not prudent to remove vital organs from a woman who has the delusion of being infested with extraterrestrial microbes, even if she demands the procedure. Similarly, a man who wanted a blood transfusion with type A blood so it could combine with his own type B blood – to make type AB – would also be denied. In both these examples, the psychotic thought processes elicited in the MSE have a direct bearing on diagnostic and therapeutic interventions.

An evaluation of a patient's mental status is an integral part of any clinical interview, regardless of whether symptoms are obvious or subtle. From the first moment of contact with patients, clinicians begin the process of **hypothesis generation**, which is refined by further observation, questioning, and investigations. The psychiatric interview, like the scalpel in surgery, is the instrument that reveals what lies beneath the surface. A well-conducted interview is no less revealing than an operation, and is a skill that takes an equal amount of time and effort to master. The MSE is no less an instrument of psychological functioning than the stethoscope is an instrument for cardiac or respiratory assessments. Along with the history, physical exam, and specialized testing, the MSE is a cornerstone of psychiatric assessment and descriptive psychopathology.

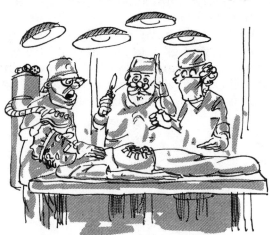

"Not again – another case of delusional appendicitis!"

# Dr. Meador's Rules*

7. There is no blood or urine test to measure mental function. There probably never will be.

9. If in doubt about dementia, do a Mental Status Exam.

31. The interview is the beginning of treatment.

133. Let patients ramble for at least 5 minutes when you first see them. You will learn a lot.

135. Listen for what the patient is *not* telling you.

314. The last statement a patient makes as you leave the room is very important.

323. The error of missing a diagnosis of dementia in hospitalized patients is common. This occurs because cognitive mental status evaluations are too often omitted.

326. A test of orientation to time must include the day, date, month, and *year*. Orientation to time can remain intact to everything except *the year*.

398. Do not make the error of accepting the first abnormality found as the cause for the patient's symptoms.

421. You cannot diagnose what is not in your differential diagnosis.

* Clifton K. Meador, M.D.
**A Little Book of Doctors' Rules**
Hanley & Belfus Inc., Philadelphia, 1992
Reprinted with permission.

# References

## Reference Books for the MSE

American Psychiatric Association
**Practice Guidelines for the Treatment of Psychiatric Disorders – Compendium 2000**
American Psychiatric Association, Washington D.C., 2000

N.C. Andreason & D.W. Black
**Introductory Textbook of Psychiatry, 2nd Ed.**
American Psychiatric Press, Inc., Washington D.C., 1995

R. Hales, S. Yudofsky, & J. Talbott, Editors
**Textbook of Psychiatry, 2nd Ed.**
American Psychiatric Press, Inc., Washington D.C., 1994

H.I. Kaplan & B.J. Sadock, Editors
**Synopsis of Psychiatry, 8th Ed.**
Williams & Wilkins, Baltimore, 1998

B.J. Sadock & V.A. Sadock, Editors
**Comprehensive Textbook of Psychiatry, 7th Ed.**
Lippincott, Williams & Wilkins, Philadelphia, 2000

R. Waldinger
**Psychiatry for Medical Students, 3rd Ed.**
American Psychiatric Press, Inc., Washington DC, 1997

## Articles on the MSE

W.E.S. Kiernan, R.G. McCreadie & W.L. Flanagan
**Trainees' Competence in Psychiatric Case Writing**
*British Journal of Psychiatry* 129: 167 – 172, 1976

D. O'Neill
**Brain Stethoscopes: The Use and Abuse of Brief Mental Status Schedules**
*Postgrad. Medical Journal* 69: 599 – 601, 1993

M. Riba & M. Hale
**Medical Clearance: Fact or Fiction in the Hospital Emergency Room**
*Psychosomatics* 31(4): 400 – 404, 1990

## Reference Books for Interviewing Skills

E. Othmer & S.C. Othmer
**The Clinical Interview Using DSM-IV**
American Psychiatric Press, Inc., Washington D.C., 1994

J. Morrison
**The First Interview: Revised for DSM-IV**
Guilford Press, New York, 1994

J. Morrison & R. Muñoz
**Boarding Time, 2nd Ed.**
American Psychiatric Press, Inc., Washington, D.C., 1996

S.C. Shea
**Psychiatric Interviewing: The Art of Understanding, 2nd Ed.**
W.B. Saunders Co., Philadelphia, 1998

D.J. Robinson
**Three Spheres: A Psychiatric Interviewing Primer**
Rapid Psychler Press, Port Huron, Michigan, 2000

# Articles on Interviewing Skills

A. Cox, K. Hopkinson, & M. Rutter
**Psychiatric Interviewing Techniques II: Naturalistic Study: Eliciting Factual Information**
*British Journal of Psychiatry* 138: 283 – 291, 1981

A. Cox, M. Rutter, & D. Holbrook
**Psychiatric Interviewing Techniques V: Experimental Study: Eliciting Factual Information**
*British Journal of Psychiatry* 138: 29 – 37, 1981

A. Cox, D. Holbrook, & M. Rutter
**Psychiatric Interviewing Techniques VI: Experimental Study: Eliciting Feelings**
*British Journal of Psychiatry* 138: 144 – 152, 1981

K. Hopkinson, A. Cox, & M. Rutter
**Psychiatric Interviewing Techniques III: Naturalistic Study: Eliciting Feelings**
*British Journal of Psychiatry* 138: 406 – 415, 1981

L.M. Lovett, A. Cox, & M. Abou-Saleh
**Teaching Psychiatric Interview Skills to Medical Students**
*Medical Education* 24: 243 – 250, 1990

J.R. McCready & E.M. Waring
**Interviewing Skills in Relation to Psychiatric Residency**
*Canadian Journal of Psychiatry* 31: 317 – 322, 1986

D.C. Pollock, D.E. Shanley, & P.N. Byrne
**Psychiatric Interviewing and Clinical Skills**
*Canadian Journal of Psychiatry* 30: 64 — 68, 1985

M. Rutter & A. Cox
**Psychiatric Interviewing Techniques I: Methods and Measures**
*British Journal of Psychiatry* 138: 273 – 282, 1981

M. Rutter, A. Cox, S. Egert, D. Holbrook, & B. Everitt
**Psychiatric Interviewing Techniques IV: Experimental Study: Four Contrasting Styles**
*British Journal of Psychiatry* 138: 456 – 465, 1981

# Collateral History

E.S. Gershon & J.J. Guroff
**Information From Relatives**
*Archives of General Psychiatry* 41: 173 – 180, 1984

J. Mendlewicz, J.L. Fleiss, M. Cataldo, & J.D. Rainer
**Accuracy of the Family History Method in Affective Illness**
*Archives of General Psychiatry* 32: 309 – 314, 1975

W.D. Thompson, H. Orvaschel, B.A. Prusoff, & K.K. Kidd
**An Evaluation of the Family History Method for Ascertaining Psychiatric Disorders**
*Archives of General Psychiatry* 39: 53 – 58, 1982

# Diagnosis

American Psychiatric Association
**Diagnostic and Statistical Manual of Mental Disorders, 4th Ed.**
American Psychiatric Association, Washington D.C., 1994

J. Morrison
**DSM-IV Made Easy: The Clinician's Guide to Diagnosis**
Guilford Press, New York, 1995

R.L. Spitzer, M. Gibbon, A.E. Skodol & M.B. First
**DSM-IV Casebook: A Learning Companion to the Diagnostic and Statistical Manual of Mental Disorders**
American Psychiatric Press Inc., Washington D.C. 1994

M.B. First, H.A. Pincus, & A. Frances
**DSM-IV Handbook of Differential Diagnosis**
American Psychiatric Press, Inc., Washington D.C., 1995

M.R. Morrison & R.F. Stamps
**DSM-IV Internet Companion**
W.W. Norton & Co., New York, 1998

# Diagnostic Decision Making

H.S. Barrows
**An Overview of Medical Problem Solving**
University of Vermont Office of Continuing Medical Education, Burlington, Vermont, 1979

A.R. Feinstein
**An Analysis of Clinical Reasoning II: The Strategy of Intermediate Decisions**
*Yale Journal of Biology and Medicine* 46: 264 – 283, 1974

J.W. Feightner, G.R. Norman, H.S. Barrows, & V.R. Neufeld
**A Comparison of the Clinical Methods**
Association of American Medical Colleges, Washington D.C., 1975

E.F. Gauron & J.K. Dickinson
**Diagnostic Decision-Making in Psychiatry I: Information Usage &
II: Diagnostic Styles**
*Archives of General Psychiatry* 14: 225 – 232 & 233 – 237, 1966

G.P. Maguire & D.R. Rutter
**History Taking For Medical Students: Evaluation of a Training Program**
*Lancet* ii: 558 – 560, 1976

B. Nurcombe & I. Fitzhenry-Coor
**Clinical Reasoning in the Psychiatric Interview**
*Australian & New Zealand Journal of Psychiatry* 16: 13 – 24, 1982

## Medical Evaluation of Psychiatry Patients

T.J. Anfinson & R.G. Kathol
**Screening Laboratory Evaluation in Psychiatric Patients: A Review**
*General Hospital Psychiatry* 14: 248 – 257, 1992

J.G. Dolan & A.I. Mushlin
**Routine Laboratory Testing for Medical Disorders in Psychiatric Inpatients**
*Archives of Internal Medicine* 145: 2085 – 2088, 1985

H.C. Sox, L.M. Koran, C.H. Sox, K.I. Marton, F. Dugger, & T. Smith
**A Medical Algorithm for Detecting Physical Disease in Psychiatric Patients**
*Hospital and Community Psychiatry* 40: 1270 – 1276, 1989

W.K. Summers, R.A. Muñoz, & M.R. Read
**The Psychiatric Physical Examination – Part I: Methodology**
*Journal of Clinical Psychiatry* 42(3): 95 – 98, 1981

W.K. Summers, R.A. Muñoz, & M.R. Read
**The Psychiatric Physical Examination – Part II: Findings in 75 Unselected Psychiatry Patients**
*Journal of Clinical Psychiatry* 42(3): 99 – 102, 1981

A.J. White & B. Barraclough
**Benefits & Problems of Routine Laboratory Investigations in Adult Psychiatric Admissions**
*British Journal of Psychiatry* 155: 65 – 72, 1989

## Medicolegal Issues

D. J. Wear-Finkle
**Medicolegal Issues in Clinical Practice**
Rapid Psychler Press, Port Huron, Michigan, 2000

F. Flach, Editor
**Malpractice Risk Management in Psychiatry**
Hatherleigh Press, New York, 1998

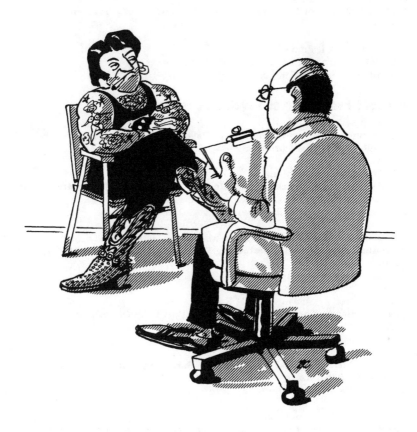

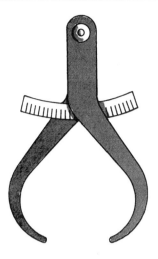

# Chapter 2

# Appearance

## Which Aspects of Appearance are Recorded in the MSE?

The purpose of recording information about appearance is to convey an accurate description of a patient's physical characteristics. This is done not only for the purposes of complete documentation, but also to convey to others as closely as possible what it was like to see the patient. Features of appearance that are recorded in the MSE are:

- **Gender & Cultural Background (Section I)**
- **Actual & Apparent Age (II)**
- **Attire (III)**

- **Grooming & Hygiene (IV)**
- **Body Habitus (V)**
- **Physical Abnormalities & Assistive Devices (VI)**
- **Jewelry & Cosmetics (VII)**
- **Other Notable Features (VIII)**

# What is the Diagnostic Significance of Observations Made Regarding Appearance?

(Note: Each DSM-IV disorder has a unique identifying number, which is included after the name of the condition. Additionally, each criterion has its own designation, which is the letter/number combination listed to the left of the description.)

• **Trichotillomania** 312.39
A.  Recurrent pulling out of one's hair resulting in noticeable hair loss.

• **Anorexia Nervosa** 307.1
A.  Refusal to maintain body weight at or above a minimally normal weight for age and height (e.g. weight loss leading to a maintenance of body weight less than 85% of that expected; or failure to make expected weight gain during a period of growth, leading to a body weight less than 85% of that expected).

• **Major Depressive Episode** 296.X
A. (3) Significant weight loss when not dieting, or weight gain (i.e. a change of more than 5% of body weight in a month).

• **Schizophrenia** 295.X
A. (5) Negative symptoms (see also the *Behavior* Chapter).
Negative symptoms are also diagnostic criteria for:
    **Schizophreniform Disorder** 295.40
    **Schizoaffective Disorder** 295.70

• **Gender Identity Disorder** 302.X
A. (2) In boys, preference for cross-dressing or simulating female attire; in girls, insistence of wearing only stereotypical masculine clothing (coded as a separate disorder depending on whether it occurs in children or adolescents/ adults).

• **Histrionic Personality Disorder** 301.50
(4) Consistently uses physical appearance to draw attention to self.
Diagnostic criteria are from the DSM-IV.
© American Psychiatric Association, Washington, D.C. 1994
Reprinted with permission.

# The Psychiatric Physical Exam
## Head and Neck

| | |
|---|---|
| • altered pupil size | drug intoxication/withdrawal |
| • Argyll Robertson pupil | neurosyphilis |
| • corneal pigmentation | Wilson's disease |
| • body piercing | borderline or antisocial personality |
| • dental caries | eating disorders (from vomiting) |
| • esophagitis | eating disorder (from vomiting) |
| • parotid enlargement | anorexia/bulimia nervosa |
| • nasal septal defect | cocaine use |
| • arcus senilis | alcohol use |

## Skin

| | |
|---|---|
| • tattoos | borderline or antisocial personality disorder |
| • callus/laceration on knuckles | eating disorder (due to self-induced vomiting) |
| • scars from slashing | borderline personality disorder |
| • scars from trauma | antisocial personality; alcohol use |
| • needle marks/tracks | IV drug use |
| • piloerection | opioid withdrawal |
| • palmar erythema | alcohol use |
| • bruising | alcohol use; seizure disorders |

| | |
|---|---|
| • cigarette burns | dementia; alcohol use; other neurologic conditions; self harm |
| • dermatitis or excoriated skin | OCD – compulsive hand washing; may occur on knees from cleaning in a kneeling position |
| • unusual pattern of hair loss | trichotillomania |
| • pretibial myxedema | Graves' disease |
| • Kaposi's sarcoma | AIDS; HIV encephalopathy |
| • lanugo hair | anorexia nervosa |
| • café-au-lait macules | neurofibromatosis |
| • red-purple striae | Cushing's syndrome/disease |
| • edema | MAOI drugs, anorexia nervosa |
| • spider angiomata | alcohol use disorder |

## Cardiovascular

| | |
|---|---|
| • mitral valve prolapse | anorexia nervosa |
| • hypotension | anorexia nervosa |

## Abdomen and Chest

| | |
|---|---|
| • enlarged liver | alcohol use disorder |
| • gynecomastia | alcohol use disorder |
| • dilated abdominal veins | alcohol use disorder |
| • decreased motility | pica (with a bezoar); anorexia nervosa |

## Genitals

| | |
|---|---|
| • chancre | syphilis (primary) |
| • mutilation | psychotic disorder; paraphilia, gender identity disorder |
| • testicular atrophy | alcohol use disorder; anabolic steroid use |

## Musculoskeletal & Nervous System

| | |
|---|---|
| • gait abnormalities | normal pressure hydrocephalus; dementia paralytica or high stepping gait (syphilis); festinating gait (Parkinson's |

| | disease); alcohol use (cerebellar degeneration); Wernicke-Korsakoff syndrome |
|---|---|
| • tremor | Parkinson's disease; lithium use; caffeine intoxication; alcohol withdrawal; anxiety disorders |
| • repeated movements | Tourette's disorder; tic disorders; autism; tardive dyskinesia; OCD; mental retardation |
| • muscle wasting | alcohol use disorder |

> \* The implications listed here are speculative. They are not meant to be pejorative or to indicate that diagnostic criteria have been met. Furthermore, other diagnoses need to be considered beyond the ones listed here (e.g. there may be many other reasons beyond trichotillomania for unusual patterns of hair loss).

# I — Gender & Cultural Background

Gender and cultural background are descriptive features.

# II — Actual & Apparent Age

Actual age is a factual identifying feature. Apparent age is a judgment made by the interviewer based on actual age and other factors (e.g. hair and skin condition, style of clothing, behavior, etc.). This is generally recorded as:
• *Appears his or her stated age*
• *Appears younger/older than the stated age*

Interviewers with experience in booths at county fairs or exhibitions may attempt a more precise estimate ("This is a 40-year-old man who doesn't look a day over 39.").

Many factors contribute to an older-looking appearance, the most common being:
- Serious and prolonged physical illnesses
- Protracted exposure to strong weather elements
- Alcohol and other substance abuse
- Chronic and severe psychiatric disorders
- Disadvantaged **socioeconomic status (SES)**
- Homelessness

# III – Attire

Attire describes how patients are dressed and how they have presented themselves for the interview. Attire is a reflection of many factors: SES, occupation, self-esteem, interest in attending to convention, etc. Descriptions often include a comment on the overall impression or "gestalt" of patients' attire, and then the details of how they are dressed, for example:

*The patient was meticulously dressed in a tuxedo with a top hat and white gloves. . .*

Medical records are legal documents. Your comments can surface again in a variety of settings (e.g. legal proceedings). Patients usually have the right to read their charts. For this reason, descriptions are best made with regard to the congruity of patients' attire to the context of the interview, followed by an objective description:

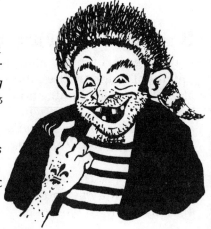

Wrong: *This rube had on a très gauche, fake raccoon fur hat, and a cheap-looking sweater worn over a Bert & Ernie style undershirt.*

Right: *This man is dressed as if prepared for the outdoors. He has on a fur hat, black jacket, and a striped shirt.*

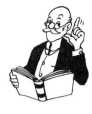

Attire, when taken in context with other signs and symptoms, provides useful information:
• Patients who are manic or hypomanic often dress flamboyantly, and seem to have a predilection for the color red
• Schizophrenia, depression, dementia, and substance use are common causes for a decline in self-care
• Patients with personality disorders can reflect their character traits in their style and choice of clothing
• Anorectic patients often dress in loose, baggy clothing to hide their state of emaciation
• Intravenous drug users may wear long-sleeved shirts and long pants to hide needle marks (called "tracks")

# IV – Hygiene & Grooming

Hair, attention to facial hair, skin condition, nails, body odor, oral hygiene, and condition of clothing are the major aspects surveyed. Common descriptions are:
• *Disheveled* (ruffled as if by a strong wind)
• *Unkempt* (not initially well groomed)
• *Immaculately/ neatly/ adequately/ poorly groomed*

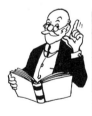

As with attire, the level of grooming and hygiene can help to make a diagnosis and gauge the severity of the condition.
• Patients with OCD may wash so frequently that they cause skin damage
• Delusional disorders can affect patients' level of grooming (e.g. not washing as a means of warding off some feared entity)
• Patients with an obsessive-compulsive or narcissistic personality disorder are fastidiously groomed and spend a considerable amount of time attending to their appearance
• Chronic, severe mental illness reduces the level to which patients maintain their self-care

# V – Body Habitus

Body habitus refers to the body type or build. To help convey an accurate mental image, descriptions can be made using the following terms:
- *Ectomorphic*: thin or slight body build
- *Mesomorphic*: muscular or sturdy build
- *Endomorphic*: heavy or portly body build

An overly muscular build can be relevant to a psychiatric assessment for the following reasons:
- Some patients with a history of abuse (of any variety) engage in intense physical training to decrease their vulnerability (or their sense of vulnerability)
- Paranoid patients may wish to increase their ability to physically ward off future attackers
- Anabolic steroid abuse should be considered

An excess of adipose tissue can be an indication of:
- Metabolic abnormalities (e.g. hypothyroidism)
- Past or current abuse; for example, in cases of sexual abuse, some patients reported that they made themselves less attractive to potential perpetrators by gaining weight
- Poor impulse-control with food or alcohol

Additionally, the following unusual body proportions should be noted:
- Truncal obesity and wasting of the arms and legs occurs in Cushing's disease/syndrome, and liver disease
- A barrel chest which is disproportionate to the rest of the body can be caused by emphysema or chronic bronchitis, raising the possibility of a neoplastic growth

# VI – Physical Abnormalities

Physical abnormalities should be noted, as well as the resulting handicap and need for assistive devices. In social situations it is often polite to avoid discussing handicaps, but exploring these areas during the interview is important to recording a complete MSE.

A sensitive line of questioning indicating your interest will be helpful in exploring these areas, with the following inquiries being a guide:
• Is the missing/disfigured part a congenital or an acquired abnormality?
• If congenital, what difficulties did this pose during development?
• If acquired, was it through an accident? An assault? An attempt at self-harm?
• What limitations does this currently impose?
• Has the patient experienced any losses related to the handicap? How has he or she adjusted to the loss?

Exploring these areas also conveys to patients that you are willing to discuss any aspect of their lives, and creates a greater degree of openness in the interview.

Physical handicaps can be significant for the following reasons:
**1.** The level of adjustment gives a good idea of someone's overall ability to cope with stress and losses; the ability to adapt gives a good indication of insight and judgment.
**2.** They can be of relevance to the etiology of psychiatric disorders. For example, a child who is continually ridiculed and ostracized may well develop a paranoid personality features. Other common outcomes are the development of depressive disorders, dysthymia, anxiety disorders, and substance abuse or dependence.

# VII – Jewelry & Cosmetic Use

Jewelry and cosmetic use are extensions of attire and grooming, respectively. They can convey a strong and personal sense of how patients see themselves and what they consider important. Examples of the usefulness of these observations are as follows:
• Make-up can be bizarrely applied by patients with psychotic conditions, and lavishly so by patients who are manic or have personality disorders (usually borderline or histrionic)

• Patients with schizophrenia or schizotypal personality disorder may wear amulets or trinkets to which they have attached some mystical significance

• The study of rings is a fascinating pastime. More than just marital status, they can indicate occupation (e.g. school rings, engineers wear a steel or iron ring on the fifth finger of their working hand), achievements (if you have never seen a Super Bowl or World Series ring, they are worth a look), organizations (e.g. Freemasons), etc.

• Chains, necklaces, ear and nose rings are often of significance for personal, cultural, and religious reasons

# VIII — Other Notable Features

## Are Tattoos Significant?

The word "tattoo" in Tahitian (or other Polynesian languages) means "to knock or strike." The word also has two military meanings: a signal (e.g. drumbeat) to return to quarters, or an outdoor display.

Tattooing has been in existence for thousands of years, extending back at least as far as the time of Ancient Egypt. Captain Cook visited Tahiti in the late 1700's and made the first recorded reference in Europe to the word tattoo. On subsequent voyages, sailors to these islands became interested in the ornate designs they saw.

Wearing a tattoo was initially associated with the lower classes and criminal elements. This association persists today, though in the intervening centuries the upper classes and royalty have been no strangers to the art (including King George V and Winston Churchill's mother!).

Tattoos are made by the injection of permanent or indelible ink into the dermal layer of the skin. Tattoos can be made professionally with the use of an electric needle, or in a more crude manner by hand (often referred to as "jail-house").

"Tats" as they are commonly known today, have an unprecedented level of popularity. Many celebrities sport them. They are frequently displayed in movies, and are often central to the plot. There are conventions, magazines, associations, and renowned artists that have created a tattoo subculture.

Tattoos reflect a myriad of meaning. For example, they can signify membership in criminal organizations (e.g. the Japanese Mafia or Yakuza) or convictions for certain crimes. Alternatively, they can be expressions of attachment to a person or lifestyle (e.g. sexual orientation or sexual practices).

People seek to express themselves through their appearance. Tattoo wearers have used their skin as a canvas with which to make a permanent and highly personal statement. It is important to ask about tattoos, even if they are not visible.

Questions that you might ask of patients are:
• *"What is the tattoo? What does it represent?"*
• *"What does the tattoo symbolize to you?"*
• *"What was going on in your life when you got the tattoo?"*
• *"What made this person/group/event so significant?"*
• *"How much time did you spend thinking about the tattoo, and what steps did you take before getting it?"*
• *"What gave you the. . . (confidence/hope/etc.) that you would always feel as strongly towards the. . . (person/organization/ etc.)?"*
• *"Have you regretted getting the tattoo? Have you taken any steps to have it removed?"*

From these questions, you can learn about:
• Significant relationships, level of commitment, etc.
• Affiliation with groups, subcultures, etc.
• Sexual practices, legal involvement, etc.
• Level of impulse-control, insight, judgment, etc.

Tattoos can serve a number of psychological functions. At the core, they help define an identity and boost esteem. Whether this serves as a compensation for perceived inadequacies needs to be determined with information from the rest of the interview. The psychiatric relevance of tattoos has spawned considerable debate. Raspa & Cusack (1990) associated tattoos with alcohol and drug abuse, and with antisocial or borderline personality disorders. Studies investigating the strength of this association are lacking. Gittleson (1969) looked at the usefulness of tattoo content, but was unable to correlate a psychiatric diagnosis with the theme of the tattoo.

It may be that patients with the above-mentioned diagnoses have a greater likelihood of having a tattoo, but the presence of a tattoo should not imply that patients have these disorders. Larger tattoos in visible areas, or that have a menacing or sinister appearance, have a higher probability of being associated with psychiatric conditions.

Tattoo removal can be accomplished in several ways:
• A "cover up" tattoo, which is by necessity larger and usually has a more benign theme
• Abrading the skin with salt, which has a sanding action
• Surgical excision, which can include prior tissue expansion
• Laser removal

## Media Examples of Tattoos

Interesting movie examples of tattoos can be seen in:
• *Tattoo* (a case of "tattoo rape")
• *Blues Brothers* (their names are tattooed on their fingers)
• *Cape Fear* (1962 original, 1991 remake)
• *Raising Arizona* (Woody Woodpecker tattoo)
• *Irezumi* (Japanese film)
• *The Illustrated Man* (movie and story by Ray Bradbury)
• *The Night of the Hunter* (1955 original, 1991 remake)
• *Heat* (1996 film with DeNiro and Pacino!)

## Bead Insertion

The implantation (under the skin) of various sized beads is becoming a popular practice.

## Body Piercing

Body piercing has become common in recent years. Typical sites for this include the nose, eyebrows, cheeks, lips, tongue, nipples, belly-button, and genitals. Like tattoo wearers, there are devotees who have developed subcultures based on this practice. At the time of writing, there are other alternative "body art" forms gaining popularity. These include cuttings, scarring/scarification, and branding. The medical literature on these practices is scant. Whereas tattoos can be quite beautiful and ornate, the potential for significant disfigurement and the historical precedents for some of these practices may well indicate a higher level of psychopathology.

# Isn't It Judgmental to Make Inferences About a Patient's Appearance?

Appearance is too important a feature to not include when gathering information for the MSE. While inferences can be drawn and hypotheses made regarding certain features, further information is required for confirmation. Diagnosis requires more than appearance alone. People wear particular clothing, jewelry and cosmetics, and adapt their grooming styles to express themselves. In clinical situations, we strive to interpret more than fashion statements. A wealth of information is available to an experienced observer.

To illustrate this, we turn to the famous Victorian detective Sherlock Holmes. In the short story called *The Yellow Face,* he examines a pipe and informs Watson:

*"The owner is obviously a muscular man, left-handed, with an excellent set of teeth, careless in his habits, and with no need to practice economy."*

How Holmes arrives at these conclusions makes perfect sense once he reveals both his observations and their significance. It is widely believed that Sir Arthur Conan Doyle used as a role model for Holmes a lecturer at the University of Edinburgh named Dr. Joseph Bell.

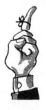

### Practice Points

• Examiners are impressed by succinct and detailed summaries of appearance. This indicates that you were observant and looked for other sources of information during the interview. Avoid the overused phrase, *"The patient was appropriately dressed."*

• Race and cultural background are important factors to consider, especially if these are different than your own. Signs and symptoms have different meanings in other cultures. For example, there are several **culture-bound syndromes** which seem as unusual to us as aspects of our society appear to them. Some of these are described in the chapter on *Thought Content.*

# Summary

With over one-third of our brains involved in the direct or indirect interpretation of visual images, humans can be said to be visual creatures. For many, the ultimate truth is observing, hence the saying "seeing is believing."

Appearance in our culture is often a highly significant statement about who we are, and what we consider to be important. Though we do not live in an era where as much can be gleaned from someone's attire as in Holmes' Victorian England, a good deal of useful information is still conveyed through appearance. No psychiatric diagnosis is made, nor is any treatment recommended, purely on the basis of appearance. It is one of the first modes of assessment during an interview, and as such provides important clues for further exploration.

Have the curiosity and initiative to ask about attire. This aids in the process of **hypothesis generation**. To paraphrase Holmes, *"We cannot theorize without data."* Our job is to try and understand patients; every effort should be made to keep our opinions and biases from influencing interviews.

# Physiognomy

In the late 1700's and early 1800's great attention was given to facial appearance (called countenance) and the significance of certain features. This study, called **physiognomy**, proposed that *"the correspondence of external figure with internal qualities is not the consequence of circumstances... but related like cause and effect...the form and arrangement of the muscles determine the mode of thought and sensibility."* John Caspar Lavater (1741 – 1801) was a Swiss scholar who wrote essays on physiognomy that were so well received they were considered "standard" works of literature. What makes his essays so entertaining is the fervor with which he asserts his opinions. For example, here are his interpretations of the following two countenances:

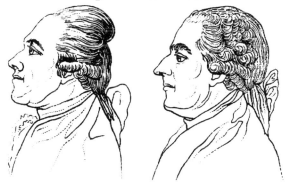

*Two profiles, German and English. Which is which? Hesitation is unnecessary. How fine, how desirable is the head on the right side. The head on the left, if not stupid, is at least common; if not rude, clumsy. The left side is a caricature I grant, yet there is something sharp and fine in the eye and mouth which a connoisseur will discover, but very different from the fineness and delicacy of the other.*

Lavater goes on to list 100 rules of physiognomy. His advice on seeking a partner is as follows: *If thou hast a long, high forehead, contract no friendship with an almost spherical head; if thou hast an almost spherical head, contract no friendship with a long, high, bony forehead. Such dissimilarity is especially unsuitable to matrimonial union.*

# References

## Books

American Psychiatric Association
**Diagnostic and Statistical Manual of Mental Disorders, 4th Ed.**
American Psychiatric Association, Washington D.C., 1994

N.C. Andreason & D.W. Black
**Introductory Textbook of Psychiatry, 2nd Ed.**
American Psychiatric Press, Inc., Washington D.C., 1995

A. Conan Doyle
**The Complete Sherlock Holmes**, Vol.1, p. 352
Doubleday & Co. Inc., New York, 1971

R. Hales, S. Yudofsky, & J. Talbott, Editors
**Textbook of Psychiatry, 2nd Ed.**
American Psychiatric Press Inc., Washington D.C., 1994

H.I. Kaplan & B.J. Sadock, Editors
**Synopsis of Psychiatry, 8th Ed.**
Williams & Wilkins, Baltimore, 1998

J.C. Lavater
**Lavater's Essays on Physiognomy, 9th Ed.**
William Tegg & Co., London, England, 1855

B.J. Sadock & V.A. Sadock, Editors
**Comprehensive Textbook of Psychiatry, 7th Ed.**
Lippincott, Williams & Wilkins, Philadelphia, 2000

A. Sims
**Symptoms in the Mind, 2nd Ed.**
Saunders, London, England, 1995

R. Waldinger
**Psychiatry for Medical Students, 3rd Ed.**
American Psychiatric Press, Inc., Washington DC, 1997

E.L. Zuckerman
**The Clinician's Thesaurus, 5th Ed.**
Clinician's Toolbox, The Guilford Press, New York, 2000

## Articles

K.A. Phillips
**Body Dysmorphic Disorder: The Distress of Imagined Ugliness**
*American Journal of Psychiatry* 148(9): 1138 – 1149, 1991

# References for Information on Tattoos

J. Appleby
**Letter to the Editor re: Psychiatric Implications of Tattoos**
*American Family Physician* 43(4): 1162/1171, 1991

M.L. Armstrong, K.P. Murphy, A. Sallee, & M.G. Watson
**Tattooed Army Soldiers: Examining the Incidence, Behavior, and Risk**
*Military Medicine* 165(2): 135 – 141, 2000

J. Farrow, R. Schwartz, & J. Vanderleeuw
**Tattooing Behavior in Adolescence**
*Am. J. of Diseases of Children* 145(2): 184 – 7, 1991

N. Gittleson, G.D. Wallen, & K. Dawson-Butterworth
**The Tattooed Psychiatric Patient**
*British Journal of Psychiatry* 115: 1249 – 53, 1969

A. Martin
**On Teenagers and Tattoos**
*J. Am. Acad. Child Adolesc. Psychiatry* 36(6): 860 – 1, 1997

R. Raspa & J. Cusack
**Psychiatric Implications of Tattoos**
*American Family Physician* 41: 1481 – 6, 1990

K. Sperry
**Tattoos and Tattooing: Part I**
*Am. J. of Forensic Med. & Path.* 12(4): 313 – 9, 1991
**Tattoos and Tattooing: Part II**
*Am. J. of Forensic Med. & Path.* 13(1): 7 – 17, 1992

The Internet is an excellent source of current information on all forms of body art. Check out the following sites:
• http://www.bme.freeq.com
• http://www.bodytattoos.com
• http://www.tattoos.com
• http://www.tattoo-art.com
• http://www.tattoospa.com
• http://www.tattoos4you.com
• http://www.tattoostudios.com
• http://www.safetattoos.com
• http://www.zelacom.com/~nyctattoo

The **rec.arts.bodyart** newsgroup contains postings and FAQ's (frequently asked questions) about tattoos, piercing, scarification, bead insertion, etc.

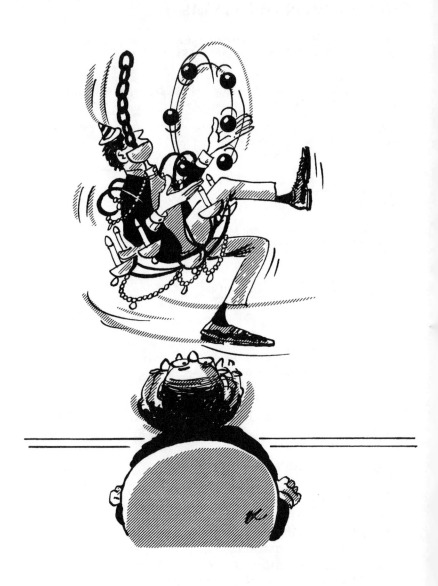

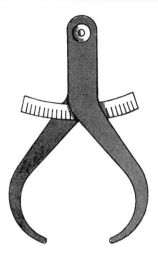

# Chapter 3

# Behavior

## Which Aspects of Behavior are Important?

Behavior refers to activity during the interview, and is one of the cardinal means of describing mental illness. It provides the only outwardly observable manifestation of psychiatric conditions. Patients may be delusional, suicidal, or plagued by hallucinations, but these are all internal experiences to which a clinician has no direct access. Behavior also reveals information about other parameters of the MSE, such as mood, cooperation & reliability, thought content, etc. As with appearance, the assessment of behavior begins as soon as patients are in visual contact, which may be the only opportunity to observe certain actions (e.g. tics, compulsions, etc.). The major aspects of behavior are:

# General Observations

## Activity Level
### Habits & Mannerisms
### Psychomotor Agitation & Retardation

# Specific Movement Abnormalities

- **Akathisia (Section I)**
- **Automatisms (II)**
- **Catatonia (III)**
- **Choreoathetoid Movements (IV)**
- **Compulsions (V)**
- **Dystonias (VIa) & Extrapyramidal Symptoms (VIb)**
- **Tardive Dyskinesia (VII)**
- **Tics (VIII)**
- **Tremors (IX)**
- **Negative Symptoms (X)**

# What is the Diagnostic Significance of Observations Made Regarding Behavior?

- **Schizophrenia** 295.X
A. (4) Grossly disorganized or catatonic behavior

- **Major Depressive Episode** 296.X
A. (5) Psychomotor agitation or retardation nearly every day (observable by others, not merely subjective feelings of restlessness or being slowed down)

- **Manic/Hypomanic Episode** 296.X
B. (6) Increase in goal-directed activity (either socially, at work or school, or sexually) or psychomotor agitation

• **Generalized Anxiety Disorder** 300.02
C. (1) Restlessness or feeling keyed up or on edge
C. (5) Muscle tension

• **Obsessive-Compulsive Disorder** 300.3
A. Compulsions – repetitive behaviors (e.g. hand washing, ordering, checking) or mental acts (praying, counting, repeating words silently) that the person feels driven to perform in response to an obsession

• **Posttraumatic Stress Disorder** 302.X
D. (4) Hypervigilance
D. (5) Exaggerated startle response

• **Exhibitionism** 302.4
A. . . . behaviors involving the exposure of one's genitals to an unsuspecting stranger

• **Frotteurism** 302.89
A. . . . behaviors involving touching and rubbing against a non-consenting person

• **Narcolepsy** 347
B. (1) Cataplexy (i.e. brief episodes of sudden bilateral loss of muscle tone, often in association with intense emotion)

• **Kleptomania** 312.32
A. Recurrent failure to resist impulses to steal objects that are not needed for personal use or for their monetary value

• **Schizotypal Personality Disorder** 301.22
A. (7) Behavior or appearance that is odd, eccentric or peculiar
A. (9) Excessive social anxiety . . .

• **Borderline Personality Disorder** 301.83
A. (5) Recurrent suicidal behavior, gestures or threats, or self-mutilating behavior

• **Narcissistic Personality Disorder** 301.81

A. (9) Shows arrogant, haughty behaviors or attitudes

• **Tourette's Disorder** 307.23

A. Both multiple motor and one or more vocal tics have been present at some time during the illness, although not necessarily concurrently (a tic is a sudden, rapid, recurrent, non-rhythmic, stereotyped movement or vocalization)

• **Neuroleptic-Induced Acute Dystonia** 333.7

A. (1) Abnormal positioning of the head and neck. . .
(2) Spasms of the jaw muscles
(3) Impaired swallowing, speaking, or breathing. . .
(5) Tongue protrusion or tongue dysfunction
(6) Eyes deviated up, down, or sideways
(7) Abnormal positioning of the distal limbs or trunk

• **Neuroleptic-Induced Parkinsonism** 332.1

A. (1) Parkinsonian tremor
(2) Parkinsonian muscular rigidity
(3) Akinesia

• **Neuroleptic-Induced Postural Tremor** 333.1

A. A fine postural tremor that has developed in association with the use of a medication

B. The tremor has a frequency between 8–12 Hz

• **Neuroleptic-Induced Tardive Dyskinesia** 333.82

B. The involuntary movements occur in a variety of patterns:
(1) Choreiform movements
(2) Athetoid movements
(3) Rhythmic movements

• **Neuroleptic-Induced Acute Akathisia** 333.99

B. At least one of the following is observed:
(1) Fidgety movements or swinging of the legs
(2) Rocking from foot to foot while standing
(3) Pacing to relieve restlessness
(4) Inability to sit or stand still for several minutes

Diagnostic Criteria are from the DSM-IV.
© American Psychiatric Association, Washington, D.C. 1994
Reprinted with permission.

The behaviors listed above are among the most likely to be observed in interview situations. However, the contribution of behavior to diagnosing mental illness goes beyond specific criteria. Behaviors that are reported but not seen are presented in the body of the history, since the MSE is a record of what happens only during the interview.

Observation of behavior is the critical element in descriptive psychopathology. **Phenomenology** is the study of observed events without inferring a cause, which was the original basis for classifying mental disorders. The other major division is **explanatory psychopathology**.

N.B. *Behavior, movement,* and *activity* are used synonymously in this chapter.

# How Do I Describe the General Aspects of Activity?

**Activity level** is a global description of patients' physical movements. Individual factors assessed are:
• Posture
• Range and frequency of spontaneous movements
• Cooperation, and the ability to carry out requested tasks

Activity level is generally recorded as:
• *Increased* (also referred to as speeded up or agitated)
• *Decreased* or *Slowed* (also called **hypokinesis** or bradykinesia)
• *Within Normal Limits* (WNL)

Even in cases where there are no obvious behavioral abnormalities, a brief description provides a visual image of what it was like to be in the interview. For example:

*"Mr. Y.K.K. sat comfortably in the room with his arms folded across his chest and absent-mindedly fidgeted with the zipper on his jacket. . ."*

It can be helpful to classify movements in three ways:
• **Conscious voluntary movements** – such as getting up to clean the dirt from a light switch
• **Unconscious voluntary movements** – such as adjusting eyeglasses or clearing one's throat; habits and mannerisms are included in this category
• **Involuntary movements** – such as tremors or dystonias; these are usually considered to be neuropsychiatric abnormalities

The MSE records only observed behavior, not the patients' internal experiences motivating the behavior. For example, patients who clean light switches may have a **compulsion** to do so; patients who frequently adjust their eyeglasses may have a **motor tic**, however, only the action itself is recorded.

**Agitation** is used to describe physical restlessness, which is usually accompanied by a heightened sense of tension or level of arousal. Common signs of agitation are:
• Hand-wringing, finger tapping, or fidgeting
• Frequent shifts in posture or position
• Foot-tapping or rhythmic leg movements
• Frequent shifts in the focus of attention
• Decreased ability to concentrate due to the distracting influence of feeling restless (as opposed to other causes such as a decreased level of consciousness, etc.)

Agitation can also be used to describe an emotional state, in that patients can both feel and appear agitated.

**Psychomotor** refers to movements that are psychically determined, as opposed to those caused by external sources. For example, a high intake of caffeine can cause people to feel restless or agitated. This distinction is important because there are many causes of agitation (see the list below). In recognition of this distinction, the DSM-IV specifies **psychomotor agitation** in the diagnostic criteria for mania, hypomania, and depression.

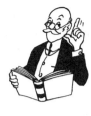

Agitation is seen in the following conditions:
• Substance ingestion or withdrawal – commonly with ethanol, benzodiazepines, or stimulants
• General medical conditions such as hyperthyroidism, hypoparathyroidism, or delirium
• Psychiatric conditions such as schizophrenia, depression, mania/hypomania, any of the anxiety disorders, and Cluster A & C personality disorders*
• Agitated depression; patients may be experiencing a **mixed state** of manic and depressive symptoms; this is very unpleasant to endure and more highly correlated with completed suicide than other bipolar states

**\* Cluster A** — Paranoid, Schizoid, Schizotypal Personality Disorders
**Cluster B** — Histrionic, Borderline, Antisocial, Narcissistic Personality Disorders
**Cluster C** — Obsessive-Compulsive, Dependent, Avoidant Personality Disorders

**Hyperactivity** refers to an increased level of physical energy. It is distinguished from agitation by the absence of inner tension, and by the fact that energy is used in a goal-directed manner. Patients often speak quickly and at length, and may become unusually assertive or even aggressive.

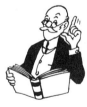

Hyperactivity is most often seen with:
• Mania or hypomania
• Attention-Deficit/Hyperactivity Disorder
• Obsessive-compulsive personality disorder
• **Catatonic excitement** (covered in the section on *Catatonia* later in this chapter)
• Seizure disorders, particularly in the **interictal periods** (after one seizure and before the onset of another)
• Head injuries, delirium, or other causes of acute confusion
• Dissociative states or **culture-bound syndromes**

**Akathisia** is an inner drivenness to keep moving. It occurs as a side effect of medication (usually antipsychotics, but other categories can cause this as well – e.g. SSRIs). Patients often seem ill at ease, move their legs rhythmically, or have to get up and walk around the room. Akathisia cannot be differentiated from other states of agitation by observation alone. It is a subjective experience, and must be inquired about when patients are on neuroleptics. More information on akathisia is included later in this chapter and in the chapter on *Suicidal & Homicidal Ideation.*

**Restless Leg(s) Syndrome** is characterized by uncomfortable sensations in the legs compelling the sufferer to keep moving. This usually occurs at the onset of sleep, and is classified as a sleep disorder (**dyssomnia**). Prolonged inactivity, uremia, and anemia (often seen in pregnancy) are known causes. An autosomal dominant inheritance has been found. Benzodiazepines, among other medications, provide effective treatment.

**Psychomotor retardation** refers to a slowness of voluntary and involuntary movements. Other terms used to describe this observation are **hypokinesia** or **bradykinesia**, and in extreme cases the virtual absence of movement is called **akinesia**. This description applies to the initiation, execution, and completion of movement. It excludes those who may have trouble initiating tasks, but can complete them readily (such as obsessive-compulsive or dependent personalities), or those who start tasks readily but can't complete them (such as patients with dementia or mania).

Often accompanying the slowed movements are changes in voice and **prosody of speech** (the natural emotional tone or inflection of speech). Most people move spontaneously when speaking, often gesturing with their hands to facilitate speech or to accentuate what they are saying. Other typical movements include adjusting eyeglasses, scratching, shifting posture, crossing and uncrossing legs, folding and unfolding arms, etc. Keeping track of a patient's repertoire of spontaneous movements is valuable in assessments. Make a point of asking about unusual or repetitive actions, or the absence of typical movements. Descriptions of behavior must also be prefaced by an indication of the **level of consciousness (LOC)**. You would not be surprised that obtunded or comatose patients demonstrated severely diminished body movements (akinesia in these cases), but you'd probably like to hear about their level of consciousness first.

**Facial expression** is another important aspect to observe. Check to see if patients convey a sense of what they are discussing with appropriate facial expressions. **Mask-like** or **masked facies** refers to the absence of facial expression, leading to an appearance reminiscent of a mask.

**Abulia** is the reduced will to take action or initiate thought, often with an indifference to the consequences. Spontaneity of speech and response to stimuli are also slowed in patients with abulia.

In general, mental processes are slowed along with movements, with patients reporting that they are unable to think as fast as usual. This needs to be distinguished from **mental retardation (MR)**, which is an intellectual deficit or mental subnormality. The distinction is that patients who are mentally retarded have permanent learning disabilities, not ones that will clear with time. Mental retardation is defined as subaverage mental functioning prior to 18 years of age. It differs from dementia in that patients with dementia have achieved a normal level of intelligence, and then acquired an illness or injury causing them to lose their mental faculties.

Depression can affect cognitive functioning so strongly that the person appears to be demented. This is called **pseudodementia**, or more recently, the **dementia syndrome of depression**. While this latter term more accurately reflects the pathology of this process, pseudodementia is seen in other conditions and is still widely used as a descriptive term.

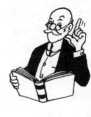

Paucity of movement is seen in:
• Depression, which is the most common psychiatric cause; in past diagnostic nomenclature, there was a subtype of depression called *retarded depression*
• Schizophrenia, and in particular, the presence of **negative symptoms**
• Medication side effects, especially in response to antipsychotics
• Catatonia (explained in detail later in this chapter)
• Dementia, of any cause
• General medical conditions, in particular illnesses which have fatigue as a prominent symptom, such as hypothyroidism, Addison's disease, mononucleosis, arthritis, Parkinson's disease, multiple sclerosis, etc.

Occasionally, only certain parts of a patient's body may have diminished or absent movements. Common causes are:
• Pain syndromes, e.g. affecting the use of extremities
• Paralysis of one or more limbs
• **Conversion disorders**, which are psychogenic impairments of motor or sensory function

# I – Akathisia

Akathisia has been mentioned previously. It is called **neuroleptic-induced** when it is caused by antipsychotic medication. The usual manifestations are rocking, fidgeting, pacing, or generally feeling compelled to keep moving. Akathisia can be quite uncomfortable – suicides and violence have been reported because it was not detected or adequately treated. Trying to voluntarily suppress akathisia-driven movements only increases the level of discomfort.

# II – Automatisms

Automatisms are "automatic" involuntary movements that can range from relatively minor to complex behaviors. They occur most commonly in epileptic seizures of the **partial complex** or **absence** type. Automatisms may be the only outward manifestations of a seizure disorder. They are also seen in head injuries, substance ingestion, catatonia, and dissociative and fugue states. By definition, automatisms occur during an altered state of consciousness. During automatisms, actions can range from purposeful to disorganized, and may or may not be appropriate for the situation or the person displaying them. Patients may be partially aware of their surroundings. They may continue with their actions, but do not seem "quite right" at the time, and are amnestic for the episode. Common automatisms are:
• Lip-smacking or uttering words (which are still understandable)
• Fumbling with clothing (e.g. doing/undoing a button)
• Eye blinking or staring with an unwavering stare
• Continuing with activities such as driving a car, or repetitive actions such as sorting or cleaning

Automatisms are occasionally complex actions that result in violence towards self or others, and for this reason also have a legal significance and definition.

# III – Catatonia

Catatonia is a term applied to a diverse number of postural and movement disturbances. The motor disorders can include both increased and decreased levels of activity. The term catatonia was developed by Kahlbaum and was initially a diagnostic entity on its own. If Kahlbaum had been a dog person, he would have called it *dogatonia*. In the DSM-IV, catatonia is diagnosed as:
• A subtype of schizophrenia
• A specifier for a mood episode
• As part of a general medical condition

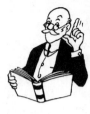

Catatonia is also found in:
• **Periodic catatonia**, a rare variant involving an alteration of thyroid function and nitrogen balance
• Neurologic illnesses that involve the basal ganglia, frontal lobes, limbic system, and extrapyramidal pathways
• Syphilis and viral encephalopathies
• Head trauma, arteriovenous malformations
• Toxic states (e.g. alcoholism, fluoride toxicity)
• Metabolic conditions (e.g. hypoglycemia, hyperparathyroidism)

The features of catatonia listed in the DSM-IV are contained in the following mnemonic:

# "WRENCHES"

**W**eird (peculiar) movements
**R**igidity
**E**chopraxia – copying the body movements of others
**N**egativism – automatic opposition to all requests
**C**atalepsy (waxy flexibility)
**H**igh level of motor activity
**E**cholalia – repeating the words of others
**S**tupor – immobility

**Weird** (peculiar) voluntary movements given as examples in the DSM-IV consist of:
• Inappropriate or bizarre **postures** that are often uncomfortable and maintained for extended periods of time (e.g. kneeling or squatting when a chair is available). Most people would find this uncomfortable, but patients experiencing catatonia appear to be

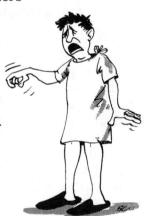

able to endure this without apparent discomfort. Another example is the **psychological pillow**, where muscle contractions elevate patients' heads when they are laying down.

• **Stereotyped movements** are repetitive, driven, non-purposeful actions. These movements are thought to have something of personal, autistic significance. Examples include body rocking, head banging, self-biting, picking at one's skin or orifices, hitting one's self, etc. They are usually "socially unacceptable" behaviors and have no adaptive function (except in mosh pits at rock concerts).

• Prominent **mannerisms** are exaggerated, crude, or unusual behaviors. They are more socially appropriate than stereotyped movements, but often occur out of context or have some other odd component. For example, some patients make a very grand show of seeking out new people and giving a prolonged, firm handshake accompanied by repeated nodding, a stern expression, and a loud greeting.

• Prominent **grimacing** refers to a particularly hollow smile. This humorless baring of the teeth with deadened, unblinking eyes is seen most frequently among patients with catatonia.

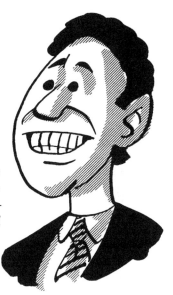

**Rigidity** is central to the definition of catatonia (Sims, 1995 p. 336), as "*a state of increased tone in muscles at rest, abolished by voluntary activities, and thereby distinguished from extra-pyramidal rigidity.*" In the latter condition, muscle tone would not be reduced with movement.

Extreme rigidity can lead to muscle breakdown, acute renal failure, and even death. This is referred to as **lethal catatonia**, which can result from any form of catatonia. This is a medical emergency and after supportive measures, is effectively treated with **electroconvulsive therapy (ECT)**.

Various types of rigidity are seen:
• **Lead pipe**: resistance to movement in all directions
• **Cogwheel**: a stop-and-go pattern, seen in parkinsonism
• **Clasp Knife**: resistance to a certain point, then giving way

**Echopraxia** is the involuntary repetition of the movements of others (mimicry would be voluntary). For example, a patient who is instructed to touch her left ear when you cross your arms will not be able to comply, and will instead copy your actions as if she were a mirror image. This phenomenon has been called **echokinesis**, **echomimia**, and **copying mania**, and is seen with seizure disorders, tic disorders, and dementias. Echopraxia is also one of the automatic behaviors (covered in this chapter).

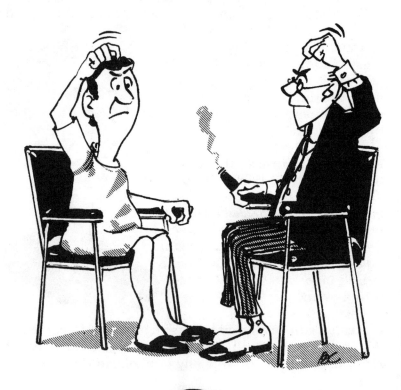

**Negativism** refers to the automatic refusal to cooperate. Even simple requests are strongly opposed for no obvious reason, even in cases where patients would benefit by participating. Patients typically either refuse, or do the exact opposite of what is asked of them. If patients are given gentle physical encouragement, they will passively resist. A large but as yet unpublished group of parents have proposed that this is a developmental stage that most teenagers seem to pass through.

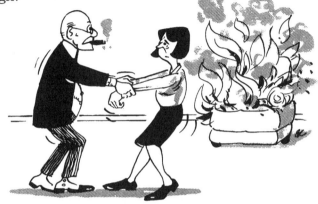

**Catalepsy (waxy flexibility, flexibilitas cerea)** is a phenomenon whereby patients can be moved and stay in position for periods of thirty seconds or more. This condition was so named because early phenomenologists likened patients' malleability to that of candle wax. Patients with waxy flexibility give some resistance to being moved (in contrast to catatonic rigidity, where patients cannot be moved).

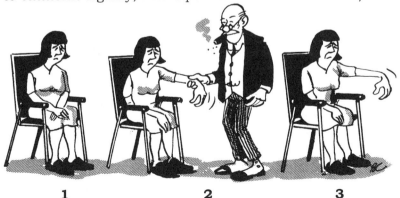

1    2    3

**High level of motor activity**, called **catatonic excitement**, is an episode of hyperactive behavior consisting of a high-pitched "running amok" that ends when the patient collapses in exhaustion or when treatment is started. This can progress to the point of becoming a medical emergency due to fever, dehydration, electrolyte abnormalities, autonomic instability, and an altered level of consciousness. During this episode, patients may display any of the other movement abnormalities that are part of catatonia: bizarre postures, grimacing, echopraxia, rigidity, waxy flexibility, etc.

**Echolalia** is the involuntary repetition of words, such as greetings, statements and questions, without patients being able to express their own thoughts. Again, this differs from mimicry in that patients don't do this of their own volition.

**Stupor** is probably the most commonly known catatonic behavior. Patients can become mute and akinetic. They may also have a reduced awareness of their environment. A stupor can last for a prolonged time, and lead to the point where an intervention is necessary for nutritional or hygienic reasons. An episode can end abruptly with a sudden outburst or impulsive act that is not in response to external stimuli. A similar condition is **akinetic mutism** (also called a **coma vigil**) – a state of unconsciousness where patients are mute and unresponsive but may follow objects with their eyes. A number of vascular, traumatic, or neoplastic conditions produce this syndrome.

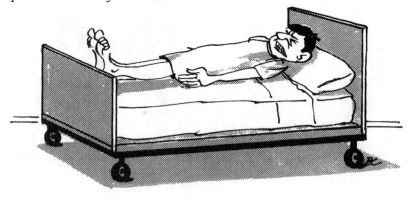

There are other catatonic behaviors beyond those listed in the DSM-IV. Another group, the **automatic behaviors**, involves instantaneous obedience:
• **Echopraxia** and **echolalia** have been discussed
• **Mitgehen** (a German term meaning "going with") can be demonstrated by directing patients with a very light touch; a typical example is to have a patient extend an arm, which can be lowered or elevated with a very light touch even when she is instructed to resist
• **Mitmachen** (German, meaning "making with") is the patient's slow, spontaneous return to the original position
• **Automaton-like behavior** involves patients carrying out requests immediately in stilted, concrete fashion
• **Advertence** is the heedful facing towards the interviewer when being addressed, as if required by strict discipline

These conditions should be suspected in situations involving an excessive and mechanistic level of cooperation, and can be tested by instructing patients not to perform them.

**Negativism** has been mentioned. However, it should be emphasized that patients actively resist all attempts to reach them. This is differentiated from uncooperative patients who display a passive-aggressive behaviors and sabotage efforts in an interview. Other features of negativism are:
• **Gegenhalten** (German, meaning "to hold against") describes the situation where patients resist being moved with a force equal to that being applied
• **Aversion**, which is the opposite of **advertence** in that patients automatically shun examiners upon hearing them speak

Patients can shift from automatic obedience to negativism without obvious precipitants, which is known as **ambitendency**.

A final feature of catatonia is a facial expression called **schnauzkramp** (German, meaning "snout cramp"), which is a puckering or protruding of the lips and jaw.

# IV – Choreoathetoid Movements

The term choreoathetoid is an amalgamation of two different movement disorders:

• **Choreiform** movements are involuntary and appear as irregular, jerky, spasmodic, and quasi-purposeful; they are irregularly timed and generally not repeated; these movements most often affect the face and arms; an example would be a man whose hand shot up towards his face and who incorporates this movement into an adjustment of his hair

• **Athetoid** movements are slow, writhing (snake-like), and twisting, and have the appearance of following a pattern; any muscle group can be affected; an episode might look like someone practicing *tai chi*, or using a hand to imitate an airplane climbing and diving

• **Ballismus** is a larger-amplitude, faster, and more violent motion (it has the same word root as ballistics); it usually occurs on one side of the body (**hemiballismus**) and resembles speeded-up athetoid movements (like punching into the air)

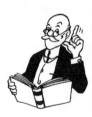

The most common causes for choreoathetoid movements are:
• Huntington's chorea
• Sydenham's chorea (rheumatic fever)
• Wilson's disease (hepatolenticular degeneration)
• Multiple sclerosis
• Tourette's disorder
• Liver or kidney failure
• Aging/hereditary causes
• Cerebral infarcts, trauma, or tumors

Causes of particular interest in psychiatry are:
• Use of antiparkinsonian (dopaminergic) agents
• Use of stimulants (e.g. to treat ADHD)
• Use of anticonvulsants (e.g. phenytoin)
• Lithium toxicity
• Tardive dyskinesia (covered in this chapter)

# V – Compulsions

**Compulsions** are defined in the DSM-IV as:
(1) Repetitive behaviors or mental acts that the person feels driven to perform in response to an obsession, or according to rules that must be applied rigidly
(2) Behaviors or mental acts aimed at preventing or reducing distress or preventing some dreaded event or situation; however, these behaviors or mental acts are either not connected in a realistic way with what they are designed to neutralize or prevent, or are clearly excessive

Two points bear emphasis with this definition:
• Compulsions can be entirely mental experiences (prayers, sayings), though the majority are actions
• The "rules that must be applied rigidly" are self-imposed, and not due to involvement with an organization with a strict code of conduct (e.g. mom, the military, boarding schools)

Compulsions are also:
• Unwanted and ego-dystonic (insight is preserved)
• Purposeful or semi-purposeful actions performed to lessen anxiety (anxiety is increased if they are not carried out)
• Performed consciously (though compulsions are often resisted to at least some degree, at least initially)
• Stereotyped (repeated over and over)
• Ritualistic (performed the same way each time)
• Usually linked to obsessions – those with obsessional doubt, check things; those obsessed with dirt, clean things

Compulsions can occur individually, but are usually preceded by obsessions, (which are also described in the chapter on *Thought Content*). Briefly, obsessions are recurrent thoughts, images, or impulses that are:
• Recurrent and recognized as excessive or unreasonable
• Not simply excessive concerns about realistic problems
• Recognized as a product of the person's mind, as opposed to thoughts being inserted from elsewhere

A patient's current compulsions may or may not be evident

in interview situations. Some patients can endure the anxiety that stems from suppressing compulsions for the duration of the time spent being observed. If compulsions are reported but not seen, they should be listed in the case presentation as part of the present illness or psychiatric history, but not in the MSE.

The most common compulsions are:
• Excessive or ritualized grooming (hand-washing, showering, brushing teeth, etc.)
• Excessive cleaning of objects (e.g. decontamination)
• Rituals of repetition (circling a room in a certain manner, putting clothes on in a certain order, etc.)
• Checking (e.g. doors to see if they are locked, the stove to see if it is turned off, containers to see if they're closed, etc.)
• Counting, touching, or measuring
• Ordering or arranging (usually in a logical sequence, e.g. size, alphabetical order, for symmetry and precision)
• Hoarding and collecting
• Asking or confessing

The following questions can help screen for compulsions:
• *"Are there actions that you perform repetitively?"*
• *"Do you feel you must perform acts against your will?"*
• *"Do you spend time doing something over and over?"*
• *"Do you have a sense of doom if you do not carry through with a certain action?"*
• *"Do you, for example, clean, check, count, or arrange things on a repetitive basis?"*

The DSM-IV stipulates that obsessions or compulsions involve at least one hour per day. Some patients have multiple compulsions, and a quick "laundry list" of common ones may help screen for their presence. Compulsions can change over time. In some cases, patients will defend their compulsions as being proper (e.g. cleaning or washing) despite the psychosocial cost to them (e.g. marital discord, losing their jobs, etc.).

# VIa – Dystonias

A dystonia is an (involuntary) increase in muscle tone, and is a specific type of **extrapyramidal symptom**. Dystonias are manifested as sustained torsion or contraction of muscles (usually muscle groups) that give patients a contorted appearance. They generally occur:
• As a reaction to antipsychotic medications
• As a consequence of chronic schizophrenia
• As the consequence of a neurologic condition

Acute dystonias usually occur within the first five days of neuroleptic administration. Young males and patients who receive high-potency neuroleptics (e.g. haloperidol) are at greater risk for dystonic reactions. Some clinicians advocate that antiparkinsonian agents be used prophylactically to prevent such reactions in higher-risk groups.

Common dystonias are:
• **Oculogyric crisis** or **spasm** – a fixed upward gaze, or the eye muscles being forced into a dysconjugate gaze

• **Torticollis** or **wry neck** – spasmodic contraction of neck muscles that causes the head to rotate and the chin to point to the side opposite the spasm

• **Opisthotonos**, also known as **arc de cercle** – a spasm in the neck and back that causes an arching forward; in severe cases, recumbent patients have only their heels and the backs of their heads touching the floor

• **Laryngospasm** – a dystonia of the muscles controlling the tongue and throat; it can lead to difficulty speaking and swallowing, and in severe cases, even breathing

These reactions are very uncomfortable and frightening for patients. The presence of a dystonic reaction requires immediate intervention. Prolonged reactions are a major reason that patients do not comply with their medications. Untreated, these reactions can last at least an hour. Fortunately, dystonias can usually be treated effectively and quickly with antiparkinsonian/anticholinergic medications.

The groups of medications that are commonly used to treat dystonias are:
• Antiparkinsonian agents/**anticholinergic agents (ACAs)**
• Antihistamines
• Benzodiazepines
• Beta-blockers
• Dopamine agonists

Most acute dystonias seen in practice are caused by **conventional** (as opposed to **novel** or **atypical**) **antipsychotic medications**. However, dystonias have been well documented in patients with schizophrenia who have never been exposed to neuroleptic medication. Not only have extrapyramidal reactions been recorded, but a whole range of motor disorders have been seen, including:
• Posture, tone, and gait abnormalities
• Abnormal eye movements and blinking rates
• Abnormal facial, head, trunk, and limb movements
• Difficulties with speech production
• Problems with purposeful movements relating to completing tasks

Next to **torticollis**, the most common dystonia is **blepharospasm** (the involuntary closure of both eyes), though muscles controlling head movements and chewing are often affected. Dystonias can be **tardive** as opposed to acute and have a delayed onset (months to years). Dystonia itself is a neurologic condition. It is classified on the basis of its etiology, age of onset, and distribution. Dystonia is differentiated from other motor disorders (such as choreoathetoid) by the presence of repetitive, patterned, and sustained movements.

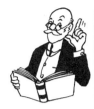 Additional causes of dystonia of interest to psychiatrists are:
• Lesch-Nyhan syndrome, Rett's disorder, and Reye's syndrome
• Huntington's disease, Wilson's disease, Parkinson's disease, multiple sclerosis
• Head trauma or peripheral nerve trauma
• Methane or carbon monoxide poisoning
• Medications – particularly anticonvulsants, bromocriptine, and fenfluramine
• Psychogenic

# VIb – Extrapyramidal Symptoms (EPS)

The pyramidal tracts are made up of axons that originate in the posterior frontal and anterior parietal lobes. Ninety percent of the fibers pass through the pyramid of the medulla, and form a tract found laterally in the spinal cord. The group of nuclei known as the **basal ganglia** make up the major component of the extrapyramidal system.

The following is a list of extrapyramidal symptoms (in their usual order of occurrence after neuroleptic administration):
• Dystonic reactions (occur in hours to days)
• Akathisia (hours to weeks)
• Akinesia or bradykinesia (days to weeks)
• Rigidity (days to weeks)
• Tremors (weeks to months)
• **Pisa** and **Rabbit syndrome** – see p. 75 (months to years)

**Parkinsonism** refers to the symptoms but not the presence of Parkinson's disease, which is an idiopathic depletion of dopaminergic neurons in the basal ganglia. Parkinson's disease occurs in sporadic and familial forms.

The causes of parkinsonism most relevant to psychiatry are:
• Medication-induced dopamine blockade – neuroleptics, (which are dopamine-receptor blockers) and others with this action such as the antidepressant **amoxapine** and several

**antiemetics** – prochlorperazine, metoclopramide, promethazine, trimethobenzamide, thiethylperazine, trifluopromazine

• Medication-induced dopamine depletion, which occurs with reserpine and tetrabenazine

• Lithium, disulfiram, methyldopa, and some of the calcium channel blockers

• Toxins such as carbon monoxide, cyanide, methanol, MPTP

• Head trauma

## Parkinsonism Practice Points

• The features of parkinsonism are listed in the mnemonic "TRAP" – **T**remor, **R**igidity, **A**kinesia, **P**ostural changes

• **T**remor at rest is one of the most common signs of parkinsonism; it has been called a **pill-rolling tremor** due to the action of the fingers; the tremor occurs at 3 – 5 Hz (see p. 82) and can also be seen in the facial muscles and legs; in medication-induced parkinsonism, a coarser tremor is usually seen

• **R**igidity in EPS is of the **lead pipe** or **cogwheel** type; these are descriptions of what it feels like for an examiner to passively move the limb

• **A**kinesia (or more often, **bradykinesia**) is present because the basal ganglia fails to activate cortical areas that are involved in the initiation of movement

• **P**ostural changes occur both because of muscle rigidity and the impairment of postural reflexes; because of this, falls are common in patients with parkinsonism

• Other common signs are stiffness, shuffling or festinating gait, mask-like facies, drooling, stooped posture, and **at-araxia** (an indifference towards the environment)

• Drug-induced parkinsonism is clinically indistinguishable from Parkinson's disease, and stopping the medication is the only way of making a distinction between the two; in some cases, patients continue to have parkinsonism as long as three months after the neuroleptic was stopped, and require antiparkinsonian medication. In some of these in-

stances, patients have subclinical Parkinson's disease.
• Fluoxetine (Prozac®) has been reported to cause parkinson-like side effects
• About 15% of patients taking neuroleptics experience parkinsonism; women are twice as likely to be affected as men; those over age forty also have a higher risk
• The features of parkinsonism can be confused with the **negative symptoms of schizophrenia** (covered in this chapter), and the anergia of depression
• The DSM-IV lists **neuroleptic-induced parkinsonism** 332.1 as a research diagnosis to be coded on Axis I

Parkinsonism can be understood by looking at the two major neurotransmitters in the basal ganglia, **acetylcholine** and **dopamine**. The basal ganglia contain the highest concentration of $D_2$ receptors in the brain, which are thought to be the site of action of **conventional neuroleptics** (**novel** or **atypical antipsychotics** such as: olanzapine, clozapine, risperidone, and quetiapine have other sites of action).

• When the neurotransmitters are in balance, no movement disorder is present (Figure 1).

 **Fig. 1**

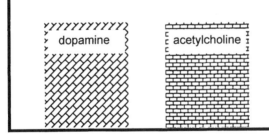

• With the decreased availability of dopamine (Figure 2), an imbalance is created causing the group of disordered movements known as **parkinsonism**. This happens regardless of the cause of the lowered amount of dopamine. Dopamine may be decreased by the receptor-blocking action of neuroleptics, or by idiopathic cell loss in the substantia nigra leading to degeneration of dopaminergic tracts, (which is what happens in Parkinson's disease).

**Fig. 2**

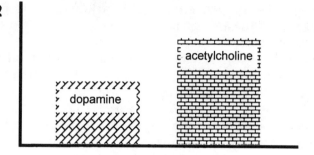

To correct this mismatch, two strategies can be used (Figure 3):

**Fig. 3**

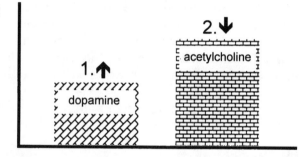

**1.** Pharmacologically increasing the amount of dopamine. This doesn't work in psychiatry because dopamine agonists generally worsen the symptoms of psychosis. However, this is one of the main strategies in treating Parkinson's disease.

**2.** Pharmacologically decreasing acetylcholine. This is the approach taken to treat parkinsonism caused by psychiatric medications. There are several **anticholinergic agents** available – benztropine, biperiden, procyclidine, ethopropazine, and trihexyphenidyl. Complications can arise because neuroleptics themselves have anticholinergic side effects. The additive effects can result in adverse peripheral reactions (dry mouth, blurred vision, constipation, flushed skin) or central reactions (confusion, restlessness, impaired memory, hallucinations, incoherence, etc.).

Other extrapyramidal symptoms (EPS) are:
• **Pisa syndrome**, so named because patients' posture bears a resemblance to the Leaning Tower of Pisa. It is a **tardive dystonia** that causes a torsion spasm of the torso muscles with the result that patients bend to one side (also called **pleurothotonus**).

**Rabbit Syndrome**, a quick, perioral movement that resembles the chewing action of a rabbit's mouth (like Bugs Bunny eating a carrot), often with a smacking of the lips. This syndrome is more rapid and regular than the oral-facial-bucco-lingual movements seen in tardive dyskinesia.

# VII — Tardive Dyskinesia (TD)

TD is an involuntary movement disorder associated with chronic neuroleptic use. **Tardive** refers to the delayed onset, which is from months to years after starting medication. **Dyskinesia** is a distortion of voluntary movement. This condition is composed of **choreoathetoid** movements, but is considered separately due to its importance in psychiatry. Dyskinesias of other etiologies can occur in patients taking neuroleptics, and in order to standardize the findings, the DSM-IV lists research criteria for **Neuroleptic-Induced Tardive Dyskinesia** 333.82:

A. Involuntary movements of the tongue, jaw, trunk, or extremities have developed in association with the use of neuroleptic medication.

B. The involuntary movements are present over a period of at least 4 weeks and occur in any of the following patterns:
(1) Choreiform movements (i.e. rapid, jerky, nonrepetitive)
(2) Athetoid movements (i.e. slow, sinuous, continual)
(3) Rhythmic movements (i.e. stereotypies)

C. The signs or symptoms in Criteria A and B develop during exposure to neuroleptic medication or within 4 weeks of withdrawal from an oral neuroleptic or 8 weeks from a depot neuroleptic.

D. There has been exposure to neuroleptic medication for at least 3 months (1 month if age 60 or older).

E. The symptoms are not due to a neurological or general medical condition.

F. The symptoms are not better accounted for by a neuro-leptic-induced movement disorder.

Diagnostic Criteria are from the DSM-IV.
© American Psychiatric Association, Washington, D.C. 1994
Reprinted with permission.

TD occurs in three areas:
**1. Facial and oral movements** (present in 75% of those affected)
• Facial expressions – frowning, blinking, grimacing
• Lips and mouth – pouting, puckering, lip smacking
• Jaw – opening and closing, chewing, teeth grinding
• Tongue – tremor, protrusion, rolling

**2. Extremities** (present in 50% of those affected)
• Choreoathetoid movements in the upper or lower limbs
• Tremors or rhythmic movements may be present
• Range from rapid, purposeless, and spontaneous, to slow and complex motions

**3. Trunk** (present in 25% of those affected)
• Twisting, rocking or gyrating of the back, neck, shoulders or pelvis

In the early stages of development, TD can easily be missed, and only an observant interviewer who is looking for the initial manifestations will notice them. TD is not usually reported by patients, but by those around them who are aware of the repetitive movements (often smacking or chewing). It can easily be passed off as being due to gum or tobacco chewing, or even ill-fitting dentures.

The movements of TD are more pronounced during stressful periods (such as interviews), and with use of non-affected body parts. Lessening of the signs and symptoms is seen during periods of relaxation, use of affected parts, and voluntary suppression. TD is typically absent during sleep. An increase in neuroleptic dosage temporarily improves the symptoms, whereas the use of an ACA worsens some forms of TD. In severe cases, TD can also cause irregularities in speaking, breathing, and swallowing. Swallowing air (**aerophagia**) can lead to chronic belching or grunting. Limb involvement can leave patients incapacitated.

The risk factors that increase the likelihood of TD are:
• Advancing age; being female
• Longer duration of neuroleptic administration
• Increasing neuroleptic dosage
• Presence of a nonpsychotic disorder
• **Drug holidays** – these are not "summer trips," but planned discontinuations of prescription medication
• Brain damage, and other neurologic conditions
• Severe EPS early after neuroleptic administration

A research instrument was designed by the National Institute of Mental Health to assess TD, called the **Abnormal Involuntary Movement Scale (AIMS).** The AIMS involves both observation, and performing actions that will assist in the detection of TD. These activated movements are scored on a 5-point scale (from 0 to 4), allowing quantification and a means by which to assess future changes. A summary of the protocol for activated movements is as follows:

**Facial and Oral Movements**
• Have the patient remove extraneous material from mouth
• Open mouth, and protrude tongue

**Extremities**
• Ask the patient to sit with hands hanging unsupported over or between knees
• Tap each finger on the thumb of the same hand
• Flex and extend the arms

**Trunk**
• Ask the patient to stand up and walk, then turn around
• While standing, extend both arms, palms down

N.B. Recall that distraction makes movements in affected areas worse. Observe body parts not currently being evaluated for the presence of abnormal movements.

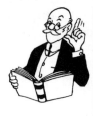

Dyskinesias occur in a wide variety of conditions:
• Disorders of the basal ganglia – Huntington's disease, Wilson's disease, Sydenham's chorea, etc.
• Metabolic conditions – hyperthyroidism, hypoparathyroidism
• Medications – levodopa, amphetamines, bromocriptine, amantadine
• Spontaneous dyskinesias (senile chorea)

TD is not rare, and is worth taking the time to detect. Up to 5% of younger patients who take neuroleptics for one year develop at least one sign. This increases to 30% in elderly patients. TD has been reported in schizophrenic patients who have never taken neuroleptic medication. It has been proposed as a late complication of schizophrenia that has been spuriously associated with neuroleptic administration. Nevertheless, there have been successful lawsuits brought about because of a lack of **informed consent**. Until the connection is either more formally proved or disproved, it is prudent to examine patients as carefully as possible prior to giving neuroleptics and at regular intervals (three to six months) throughout the period of administration.

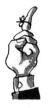

## TD Practice Points
• There are other types of tardive phenomena – dystonia, akathisia, and Tourette's
• The management of TD involves early detection, use of as little neuroleptic medication as possible, and switching to an atypical antipsychotic

• Several medication schemes have been reported as helping to diminish TD once it is present; this list is extensive and keeps growing; consult recent journal articles for current recommendations
• **Withdrawal dyskinesias** can occur as neuroleptic dosages are decreased
• The proposed mechanism for TD is dopamine receptor super-sensitivity (from prolonged blockade) in the basal ganglia

# VIII – Tics

Tics are defined in the DSM-IV as involuntary, sudden, rapid, recurrent, non-rhythmic, stereotyped, irresistible movements or vocalizations. Tics generally mimic all or part of a normal movement, and may be seen as "purposeful" in this regard. They can range from simple to complex, though their duration is about 1 second. Most patients with tics have a unique "repertoire" that varies in type, location, degree, and frequency. Tics often occur in paroxysmal bouts.

Patients can voluntarily suppress tics during interviews. However, this becomes increasingly difficult and is associated with escalating discomfort. Prior to a tic occurring, patients may experience premonitory urges or sensations. As with compulsions, a feeling of relief comes with expressing the tic. Stress, fatigue, new situations, or even boredom can exacerbate tics. Other illnesses, concentration on other matters, relaxation, alcohol, and orgasm can diminish tics. Like other movement disorders, tics are virtually absent during sleep.

Examples of simple motor tics are:
• Blinking or **blepharospasm**
• Facial twitches, grimaces, head jerking
• Abdominal tensing
• Shrugging or rotation of the shoulders
• Jerking movements in the extremities
• Grinding teeth (**bruxism**)
• Oculogyric movements

Examples of complex motor tics are:
- Grooming behaviors
- Head shaking
- Jumping or kicking
- Hitting or biting oneself
- Touching or smelling objects
- **Copropraxia** (making obscene gestures)
- **Echopraxia** (copying the movements of another)

Examples of simple vocal tics are:
- Coughing, humming
- Grunting, gurgling
- Throat clearing, clicking, or clacking
- Sneezing, sniffing, snorting, or snuffling
- Screeching, barking, squealing
- Whistling, hissing

Examples of complex vocal tics are:
- Sudden utterances of inappropriate syllables or words
- **Copralalia** (saying or shouting obscenities)
- **Palilalia** (repeating one's own phrases)
- **Echolalia** (repeating others' phrases – this is also one of the behaviors in **catatonia**)

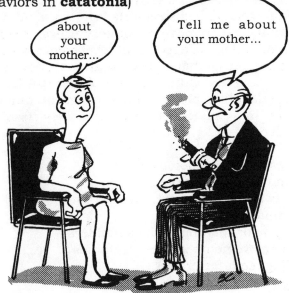

Tics can be present in up to one-sixth of boys and about one-twelfth of girls. The highest prevalence is in children aged seven to eleven. Tics are considered pathological when they are present nearly every day for at least one month. As with other movement disorders, the pathology is thought to occur at the level of the basal ganglia. Tics often disappear without consequence.

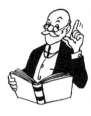

Tics occur in a wide variety of conditions:
• Physiologic tics – mannerism or gestures
• Primary tic disorders (see below)
• Chromosomal abnormalities – e.g. Down's syndrome, Fragile X syndrome)
• Medications – anticonvulsants, neuroleptics, levodopa; stimulants used for the treatment of ADHD – pemoline, methylphenidate, and amphetamine; caffeine
• Head trauma
• Mental retardation – including pervasive developmental disorders
• Neurologic conditions – e.g. Huntington's disease, Sydenham's chorea, Wilson's disease
• Infections – e.g. encephalitis, Creutzfeldt-Jakob disease
• Schizophrenia
• Gasoline or carbon monoxide poisoning

The DSM-IV lists four tic disorders (the diagnostic criteria are abbreviated):

**Tourette's Disorder** 307.23
• Both multiple motor and one or more vocal tics have been present, although not necessarily concurrently
• The tics occur many times a day (usually in bouts), nearly every day or intermittently throughout a period of more than one year, and during this time there is no tic-free period of more than three consecutive months
• Causes marked distress or significant impairment in social, occupational, or other important areas of functioning

**Transient Tic Disorder**  307.21
- Single or multiple motor and/or vocal tics
- Tics occur many times per day
- Duration is between four weeks and one year

**Chronic Motor or Vocal Tic Disorder**  307.22
- Duration is longer than one year

**Tic Disorder Not Otherwise Specified**  307.20
- The catch-all diagnosis for other tic conditions

Motor tics can be subdivided into **clonic** and **tonic** forms. Clonic tics are abrupt and simple movements, such as head twitching or nose wrinkling. Tonic tics are more sustained movements and may be painful, such as **torticollis**, **blepharospasm**, or prolonged mouth opening.

Diagnosing tic disorders may take years. Tics usually start with eye-blinks, head-jerks, or grimaces, which are common twitches in children. The tics in Tourette's disorder are often accompanied by irritability, attentional deficits, or a low frustration tolerance, which can lead to a misdiagnosis of a behavioral disorder (e.g. conduct disorder). Also, there are comorbid conditions that complicate diagnostic issues (e.g. obsessive-compulsive disorder)

# IX — Tremors

Tremors are involuntary movements consisting of regular, rhythmic oscillations of some part of the body. They are usually seen in the hands, arms, head, neck, lips, mouth or tongue, but can also occur in the legs, voice, or trunk. Classification of tremors is made using the following criteria:
- Speed, which is measured in cycles per second, called Hertz (abbreviated Hz)
- Presence of **resting tremors,** tremors that appear with movement (**action** or **intention tremors**), and tremors seen when the affected part is held in a sustained manner (**postural tremors**)
- Small (fine) or large (coarse) degrees of movement

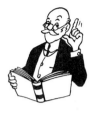

The causes of tremors which are most relevant to psychiatry are:
• Stress-induced – situational anxiety, anxiety disorders (e.g. panic disorder), strong emotion, fatigue, hypothermia
• Psychotropic medication-induced – lithium, valproic acid, neuroleptics, **tricyclic antidepressants (TCAs)**, **selective serotonin re-uptake inhibitors (SSRIs)**
• Other medication – dopaminergic medications (levodopa, bromocriptine), beta-adrenergic agonists (isoproterenol, theophylline), stimulants (caffeine, amphetamines, cocaine)
• Endocrine – hyperthyroidism, pheochromocytoma
• Substance withdrawal – alcohol, benzodiazepines
• Familial – essential tremor
• Neurologic conditions – Parkinson's disease or parkinsonism, Wilson's disease, brain tumors, conditions affecting the cerebellum
• Physiologic tremor
• Hysterical tremor

The most likely tremors to be encountered are:
• **Pill-rolling tremor**: a passive or resting tremor where the thumb is rolled across the other fingers; this is the classic tremor of parkinsonism
• **Postural tremor**: a physiologic tremor that occurs when maintaining a position or posture
• **Essential tremor**: an action tremor of the hands (but can include head or voice tremors); this is inherited as an autosomal dominant trait in most cases
• **Wing-beating tremor**: an abduction of the shoulder with flexion of the elbow; often seen in Wilson's disease
• **Liver flap (asterixis)**: can be seen in patients with liver failure; the wrist exhibits rapid flexion-extension

The DSM-IV includes research criteria for **medication-in-**

**duced postural tremor**. This condition has been most frequently reported with the use of lithium. Its features include the following:
• It is dose-related and can affect up to 50% of patients
• Pre-existing tremors or a family history increase the risk
• It is most often confined to the fingers, is irregular in amplitude and rhythm, variable throughout the day, interferes with hand-writing, and worsens with anxiety
• It occurs at 8 – 12 Hz
• It can be managed with propranolol 10 mg qid

The tremor of **parkinsonism** has the following features:
• It is present in the hands and wrists
• It occurs at 4 – 7 Hz and is more rhythmic
• It occurs in about 15% of patients receiving antipsychotics
• **Micrographia** is present, as opposed to jagged handwriting (this can also refer to handwriting that gets smaller across the line on the page)
• It is managed by reducing the neuroleptic dose, using anticholinergic agents (ACAs), and if necessary, amantadine or diphenhydramine

# X – Negative Symptoms

Part of developing skills as an interviewer is to not only pay attention to what *is* being said or done, but to what *is not* being said or done. For example, patients who talk about their families but omit certain members (like a parent) often betray the presence of a conflict with that person. Similarly, there are certain behavioral aspects that are remarkable for their absence.

Many clinicians divide the signs and symptoms of schizophrenia into **positive** and **negative symptoms**, also referred to as Type I and Type II schizophrenia, respectively. One way to conceptualize this distinction is that positive symptoms are *added* to the picture, negative ones are *deficits* in the clinical presentation. **Positive symptoms** are: **hallucinations, delusions, a formal thought disorder** and **bizarre** or **disorganized behavior**. Positive symptoms are findings added to the clinical picture that are not present in unaffected people. Negative symptoms are features that are present in unaffected patients (a range of emotion, volition, intact attention span, enjoyment of activities), but are missing from the clinical picture of affected patients. A mnemonic for remembering negative symptoms is:

## "NEGATIVE TRACK"

**N**egligible response to conventional antipsychotics
**E**ye contact is decreased
**G**rooming & hygiene decline
**A**ffective responses become flat
**T**hought blocking
**I**nattentiveness
**V**olition diminished
**E**xpressive gestures decrease

**T**ime – increases the number of negative symptoms
**R**ecreational interests diminish; **R**elationships decrease
**A**'s – the 5 'A' or principal symptoms from the DSM-IV
**C**ontent of speech diminishes (poverty of thought)
**K**nowledge – cognitive deficits increase

• Since Kraepelin and Bleuler described schizophrenia, they made distinctions between *fundamental* (positive) and *accessory* (negative) symptoms
• Negative symptoms are not usually treated effectively by traditional antipsychotic medication, whereas positive symptoms generally do respond. Newer antipsychotics appear to treat negative symptoms much more effectively
• Of the five 'A' or principal criteria for schizophrenia from the DSM-IV, only one includes negative symptoms; the DSM-IV requires six months of **prodromal** or **residual symptoms**, which may consist largely or entirely of negative symptoms
• Negative symptoms tend to become more prominent with time and are significantly disabling to patients
• Statistically, those with primarily negative symptoms are unmarried males who have an earlier onset, poorer course, and higher incidence of other behavioral abnormalities

Dr. Nancy Andreason developed standardized scales to more fully assess the presence of positive and negative symptoms. The scale for positive symptoms is called the **SAPS (Scale for the Assessment of Positive Symptoms)**. The other is the **SANS (Scale for the Assessment of Negative Symptoms**; for those who appreciate puns, *sans* in French means "without"). The major headings in this scale are in the following mnemonic:

| | |
|---|---|
| a**P**athy/Avolition<br>a**L**ogia<br>**A**ffective Flattening<br>a**N**hedonia<br>a**T**tenional deficits | PLANT mnemonic for the five A's from the Scale for the Assessment of Negative Symptoms provided by:<br>**Dr. David Wagner**<br>**Indiana University** |

N.B. While these symptoms start with the letter 'a' these are not the 'A' criteria from the DSM-IV referred to earlier.

## Behavior Practice Points

• **Regressed behavior** refers to age-inappropriate behaviors exhibited by patients; the overall decline may be present as neediness, poor motivation, emotional lability, diminished self-care, etc.

• **Yawning** can be an indication of opioid withdrawal

• **Cigarette smoking** is common among patients with schizophrenia – it is estimated that up to 90% smoke; smoking may alter the metabolism of antipsychotic medications and diminish side-effects

• **Perseveration** is both a verbal and behavioral phenomenon, and is defined as an inability to switch tasks (e.g. patients asked to stand up will do this when asked to perform a different task)

• Patients with **dystonia** may not be able to let go of your hand after shaking it

• Frequent water drinking may be seen in schizophrenia; this can lead to **water intoxication**, seizures from hyponatremia, and even death

• **Cataplexy** is the sudden involuntary loss of postural muscle tone, and is a feature of narcolepsy (don't confuse it with **catalepsy**)

# Comparison of Repetitive Behaviors

Tics

Compulsions

Repetitive
Behaviors

Stereotyped
Behaviors

Habits &
Mannersims

| FEATURE | Compulsions | Stereotypies | Habits | Tics |
|---|---|---|---|---|
| conscious | + | + | – | + |
| voluntary | + | + | + | – |
| "purposeful" | + | – | – | + |
| complex movements | + | + | – | –/+ |
| rhythmic | – | + | – | – |
| paroxysmal | – | – | – | + |
| ritualistic | + | – | – | –/+ |
| decrease anxiety | + | – | – | – |
| premonitory urge | – | – | – | + |

## Summary

According to the esteemed philosopher Forrest Gump, *"Stupid is as stupid does."* While there are numerous and far-reaching interpretations of his wisdom, in this context he tells us that behavior is the principal means of classification.

No less an authority on psychiatry than Hannibal "The Cannibal" Lecter behooves us to read Marcus Aurelius, *"Of each particular thing, ask: What is it in itself, in its own constitution? What is its causal nature?"*

What others look like is one of the first things we notice – another is what they are doing. The human brain is exquisitely attuned to appearance and action, and for this reason one of the major means of recording psychiatric illness is through the classification of abnormal behavior.

Psychopathology can be categorized from an **explanatory** viewpoint (i.e. psychodynamic theory) or a **descriptive** one involving the *observation of behavior* and *recording of the inner experiences of patients*. **Phenomenology** is the study of events as they occur, rather than by attempting an explanation. In psychiatry, this involves the translation of aberrant perception, cognition, emotion, and behavior into the signs and symptoms of mental illness.

The key to phenomenological classification is precision. While patients may "look depressed," "act schizophrenic," or "seem anxious," more accurate descriptions help classify these observations.

The immense range of behaviors that might be seen in interview situations could fill an entire book. This chapter provides a basis for not only recognizing certain key behaviors, but also understanding their significance to hypothesis generation, and the rationale for diagnosing psychiatric illnesses.

# References

## Books

American Psychiatric Association
**Diagnostic and Statistical Manual of Mental Disorders, 4th Ed.**
American Psychiatric Association, Washington D.C., 1994

N.C. Andreason & D.W. Black
**Introductory Textbook of Psychiatry, 2nd Ed.**
American Psychiatric Press, Inc., Washington D.C., 1995

R. Campbell
**Psychiatric Dictionary, 7th Ed.**
Oxford University Press, New York, 1996

W. Groom
**Forrest Gump**
Doubleday, New York City, 1994

T. Harris
**The Silence of The Lambs**
St. Martin's Press, New York City, 1988
(Lecter said something slightly different in the movie version)

H.I. Kaplan & B.J. Sadock, Editors
**Synopsis of Psychiatry, 8th Ed.**
Williams & Wilkins, Baltimore, 1998

J. Maxmen & N. Ward
**Psychotropic Drugs Fast Facts, 2nd Ed.**
W. W. Norton & Co., New York, 1995

G.W. Rockville, Editor
**Abnormal Involuntary Movement Scale**, in ECDEU Assessment Manual
National Institute of Mental Health, 1976

L. Rolak
**Neurology Secrets**
Hanley & Belfus, Philadelphia, 1993

B.J. Sadock & V.A. Sadock, Editors
**Comprehensive Textbook of Psychiatry, 7th Ed.**
Lippincott, Williams & Wilkins, Philadelphia, 2000

A. Sims
**Symptoms in the Mind, 2nd Ed.**
Saunders, London, England, 1995

R. Waldinger
**Psychiatry for Medical Students, 3rd Ed.**
American Psychiatric Press, Inc., Washington DC, 1997

# Articles
## Akathisia

G.D. Blaisdell
**Akathisia: A Comprehensive Review and Treatment Summary**
*Pharmacopsychiatry* 27(4): 139 – 146, 1994

A. Rappoport, D. Stein, A. Grinshpoon, & A. Elizur
**Akathisia and Pseudoakathisia: Clinical Observations and Accelometric Recordings**
*J. Clin. Psychiatry* 55(11): 473 – 477, 1994

P. Sachdev
**Research Diagnostic Criteria for Drug-Induced Akathisia: Conceptualization, Rationale, and Proposal**
*Psychopharmacology* 114(1): 181 – 186, 1994

P. Sachdev & J. Kruk
**Clinical Characteristics and Predisposing Factors in Acute Drug-Induced Akathisia**
*Archives of General Psychiaty* 51(12): 963 – 974, 1994

P. Sachdev
**The Development of the Concept of Akathisia**
*Schizophrenia Res.* 16(1): 33 – 45, 1995

## Automatisms

R.G. Beran
**Automatisms – The Current Legal Position Related to Clinical Practice and Medicolegal Interpretation**
*Clin. Exp. Neurology* 29: 81 – 91, 1992

E.A. Serafinides
**Automatisms (letter)**
*Neurology* 46(4): 61 – 64, 1995

## Catatonia

G. Bush, M. Fink, G. Petrides, F. Dowling, & A. Francis
**Catatonia I: Rating Scale and Standardized Examination**
*Acta Psychiatr Scand.* 93(2): 129 – 136, 1996

G. Bush, G. Petrides, & A. Francis
**Catatonia and Other Motor Syndromes in a Chronically Hospitalized Psychiatric Population**
*Schizophrenia Res.* 27(1): 83 – 92, 1997

T. Clark & H. Richards
**Catatonia I: History and Clinical Features**
*Hospital Medicine* 60(10): 740 – 742, 1999

T. Clark & H. Richards
**Catatonia II: Diagnosis, Management, and Prognosis**
*Hospital Medicine* 60(11): 812 – 814, 1999

C.P Tang, C.M. Leung, G.S. Ungvari, & W.K. Leung
**The Syndrome of Lethal Catatonia**
*Singapore Med. J.* 36(4): 400 – 402, 1995

## Compulsions

A. Heinz
**Neurobiological & Anthropological Aspects of Compulsions and Rituals**
*Pharmacopsychiatry* 32(6): 223 – 229, 1999

R. Joseph
**Frontal Lobe Psychopathology: Mania, Depression, Confabulation, Catatonia, Perseveration, Obsessive-Compulsions, and Schizophrenia**
*Psychiatry* 62(2): 138 – 172, 1999

F. Klemperer
**Compulsions Developing Into Command Hallucinations**
*Psychopathology* 29(4): 249 – 251, 1996

P. Muris, H. Merckelbach, & M. Clavan
**Abnormal and Normal Compulsions**
*Behav. Res. Ther.* 35(3): 249 – 252, 1997

## Extrapyramidal Symptoms

T.R. Barnes & M.A. McPhillips
**Novel Antipsychotics, Extrapyramidal Side Effects, and Tardive Dyskinesia**
*Int. Clin. Psychopharmacology* 13 (Suppl. 3): S49 – 57, 1998

S. Dollfus, J.M. Ribeyre, & M. Petit
**Objective and Subjective Extrapyramidal Side Effects in Schizophrenia: Their Relationships with Negative and Depressive Symptoms**
*Psychopathology* 33(3): 125 – 130, 2000

W.M. Glazer
**Extrapyramidal Side Effects, Tardive Dyskinesia, and the Concept of Atypicality**
*J. Clin. Psychiaty* 61(Suppl. 3): 16 – 21, 2000

G. Muscettola, G. Barbato, S. Pampallona, M. Casiello, & P. Bollini
**Extrapyramidal Syndromes in Neuroleptic-Treated Patients: Prevalence, Risk Factors, and Association With Tardive Dyskinesia**
*J. Clin. Psychopharmacology* 19(3): 203 – 208, 1999

## Positive & Negative Symptoms

I. Berman, B. Veigner, A. Merson, E. Allan, D. Pappas, & A.I. Green
**Differential Relationships Between Positive and Negative Symptoms and Neuropsychological Deficits in Schizophrenia**
*Schizophrenia Res.* 25(1): 1 – 10, 1997

M.E. Kelley, D.P. van Kammen, & D.N. Allen
**Empirial Validation of Primary Negative Symptoms: Independence From Effects of Medication and Psychosis**
*American Journal of Psychiaty* 156(3): 406 – 411, 1999

S.E. Roitman, R.S. Keefe, P.D. Harvey, L.J. Siever, & R.C. Mohs
**Attentional and Eye Tracking Deficits Correlate With Negative Symptoms in Schizophrenia**
*Schizophrenia Res.* 26(2–3): 139 – 146, 1997

D. Schuldberg, D.M. Quinlan, & W. Glazer
**Positive and Negative Symptoms and Adjustment in Severely Mentally Ill Outpatients**
*Psychiatry Res.* 85(2): 177 – 188, 1999

T. Tsutsumi & H. Uchimura
**Algorithm for the Treatment of Negative Symptoms in Chronic Schizophrenia**
*Psychiatry Clin. Neurosci.* 53(Suppl): 15 – 17, 1999

## Neuroleptic Malignant Syndrome

R.C. Christensen
**Recognizing Early Signs of Neuroleptic Malignant Syndrome (letter)**
*Am. J. Emergency Medicine* 16(1): 95 – 96, 1998

A.L. Peloner, J.L. Levenson, & A.K. Pandurangi
**Neuroleptic Malignant Syndrome: A Review**
*Psychiatric Services* 49(9): 1163 – 1172, 1998

K.G. Rasmussen
**Risk Factors for Neuroleptic Malignant Syndrome (letter)**
*American Journal of Psychiatry* 155(11): 1639 – 1640

V.R. Velamoor
**Neuroleptic Malignant Syndrome: Recognition, Prevention, and Management**
*Drug Safety* 19(1): 73 – 82, 1998

## Tardive Dyskinesia

W.M. Glazer
**Review of Incidence of Tardive Dyskinesia Associated With Typical Antipsychotics**
*J. Clin. Psychiatry* 61(Suppl. 4): 15 – 20, 2000

D.V. Jeste
**Tardive Dyskinesia in Older Patients**
*J. Clin. Psychiatry* 61(Suppl. 4): 27 – 32, 2000

N.S. Kaye & T.J. Reed
**Tardive Dyskinesa: Tremors in Law and Medicine**
*J. Am. Acad. Psychiatry Law* 27(2): 315 – 333, 1999

R. Slovenko
**Upadate on Legal Issues Associated With Tardive Dyskinesia**
*J. Clin. Psychiatry* 61(Suppl. 4): 45 – 57, 2000

J.R. Swartz, K. Burgoyne, M. Smith, R. Gadasally, J. Ananth, & K. Ananth
**Tardive Dyskinesia and Ethnicity: A Review of the Literature**
*Ann. Clin. Psychiatry* 9(1): 53 – 59, 1997

## Tics

V. Eapen & M.M. Robertson
**All That Tics May Not Be Tourette's (letter)**
*British Journal of Psychiatry* 164(5): 708, 1994

J. Jankovic
**Tourette Syndrome: Phenomenology and Classification of Tics**
*Neurol. Clin.* 15(2): 267 – 275, 1997

K. Kompoliti & C.G. Goetz
**Tourette Syndrome: Clinical Rating and Quantitative Assessment of Tics**
*Neurol. Clin.* 15(2): 239 – 254

C.C. Santos & E.W. Massey
**Tourette's Syndrome: Tics, Jerks, and Quirks**
*Postgraduate Medicine* 87(2): 71 – 78, 1990

E. Stern, D.A. Silbersweig, K.Y. Chee, A. Holmes, & M.M. Robertson
**A Functional Neuroanatomy of Tics in Tourette's Syndome**
*Archives of General Psychiatry* 57(8): 741 – 748, 2000

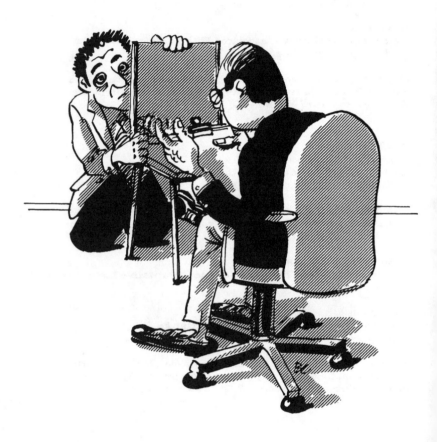

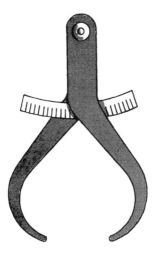

# Chapter 4

# Cooperation & Reliability

## Which Factors Determine Cooperation and Reliability?

Cooperation from patients is required so that the information they provide is useful in forming a diagnostic impression. Some patients *can't* or *won't* share information. This needs to be included in the presentation of the MSE at an early stage, as it colors the rest of the information obtained. In a sense, cooperation refers to the *quantity* of information given. This doesn't imply that taciturn patients are uncooperative if questions can be answered succinctly. Cooperation is best gauged by the responses to open-ended questions, which have no clear end-point. Most patients share information freely and participate readily in interviews.

Of course, a cornucopia of information is not useful unless it is accurate. In a similar vein, reliability refers to the *quality* of data obtained in the interview. The following parameters provide an assessment of cooperation and reliability:

- **Eye Contact (Section I)**
- **Attitude/Demeanor (II)**
- **Attentiveness to the Interview(III)**
- **Level of Consciousness (IV)**
- **Affect (V)**
- **Secondary Gain (VI)**
- **Malingering (VII)**
- **Factitious Disorder (VIII)**

# What is the Diagnostic Significance of Cooperation and Reliability?

• **Malingering** V65.2
The essential feature of malingering is the intentional production of false or grossly exaggerated physical or psychological symptoms motivated by external incentives

• **Factitious Disorder** 300.1X
A. Intentional production or feigning of physical or psychological signs or symptoms
B. The motivation for the behavior is to assume the sick role
C. External incentives for the behavior are absent

• **Antisocial Personality Disorder** 301.7
A. (2) Deceitfulness, as indicated by repeated lying, use of aliases, or conning others for personal profit or pleasure

• **Paranoid Personality Disorder** 301.0
A. (1) Suspects, without sufficient basis, that others are exploiting, harming or deceiving him or her
• **Manic/Hypomanic Episode** 296.X
A. A distinct period of abnormally and persistently elevated, expansive or irritable mood
B. (5) Distractibility

• **Major Depressive Episode** 296.X
A. (8) Diminished ability to concentrate, or indecisiveness, nearly every day. . .

• **Dementias (of various etiologies)** 290.X
A. (1) Memory impairment. . .

Diagnostic Criteria are from the DSM-IV.
© American Psychiatric Association, Washington, D.C. 1994
Reprinted with permission.

# I — Eye Contact

Eye contact is a universal indicator of interest. Generally speaking, continuous eye contact indicates cooperation. Patients may avert their gaze momentarily to think about details that are not readily available. A sustained aversion of gaze can be an indication that some area of difficulty for the patient has been encountered.

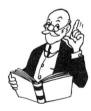

Poor eye contact may have several causes:
• Paranoid patients (due to schizophrenia, a delusional disorder, or personality disorder) are often vigilant about their surroundings
• Hallucinations (usually auditory or visual)
• Patients with a social phobia may show fleeting eye contact at the outset of an interview, which improves as rapport develops
• In some cultures, direct eye contact can mean disrespect
• An unwavering gaze can be an act of intimidation, a veiled threat, or a challenge to your position as an interviewer

Eye contact is described as *continuous/good/intermittent/ fleeting/absent*. If aberrations are present, describe them in detail:

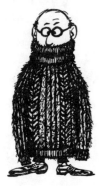

*"Mr. Gunn avoided direct eye contact for the majority of the interview but remained wary of his surroundings. After a cursory inspection of the room, he cast furtive glances at the heating vent, light switch, and overhead speaker. Then he spent a great deal of time staring out the window at a parked vehicle outside the clinic."*

## Eye Contact Practice Points

• Patients with schizophrenia have a high rate of blinking, which is thought to be due to a hyperdopaminergic state

• **Smooth-pursuit eye movement (SPEM)** abnormalities occur in schizophrenia, mood disorders, and organic brain disorders; they also occur at a higher rate in the first-degree relatives of schizophrenic patients than the general population and may be a marker for this illness; **saccades** are fast eye movements under voluntary control – for example, eyes make several discrete movements across a line when reading; saccades are abnormal when tracking an object moving smoothly across the visual field (e.g. watching a moving car or train)

• **Wilson's disease** causes an abnormal deposit of copper in the cornea called a Kayser-Fleischer ring; sunflower cataracts are another ocular finding

• A common observation regarding sociopaths is their cold, unfeeling, "reptilian" gaze; several authors have commented on this both in fiction and in the medical literature

• An **oculogyric crisis** is one form of dystonia consisting of a forced upward gaze; in psychiatric patients this is almost always due to a reaction to antipsychotic medications, though it also occurs in other neurologic disorders

• **Wernicke's triad** consists of ataxia, mental changes (confusion), and **ophthalmoplegia**; the eye muscle most commonly affected is the lateral rectus muscle resulting in a conjugate gaze palsy, though a diverse number of other ocular abnormalities can occur
• Pin-point pupils are a sign of opioid use
• Injected conjunctiva are a sign of marijuana use
• Glassy eyes may be a sign of substance ingestion, usually with alcohol (or it may in fact be a glass eye)
• **Nystagmus** is an involuntary oscillating movement of the eyes consisting of alternating slow and quick movements; it occurs normally at the extremes of gaze (called **end-point** or **physiologic nystagmus**); movement can occur laterally, vertically or in a rotatory fashion and is almost always a sign of pathology

# II – Attitude and Demeanor

Attitude and demeanor towards the interview and interviewer are other important factors. Patients may have biases from previous contact with mental health professionals. Usually, this becomes obvious early in the interview and can pose a significant obstacle to obtaining information.

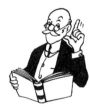

Cooperation may be compromised with patients who:
• Have personality disorders, usually from Cluster B (typically borderline or antisocial)
• Are under duress to attend the interview (e.g. from a spouse, business partner, etc.)
• Suffer from chronic conditions that have resulted in numerous contacts with different caregivers
• Have an agenda (e.g. **secondary gain**) to carry out in the interview and seek to gain the upper hand at the outset
• Are cognitively impaired due to organic processes or substance ingestion/withdrawal
• Are in emotional or physical pain
• Are involuntarily committed

Demeanor can be described globally as being cooperative or uncooperative. Cooperative patients can be further described as:
- *Obsequious/solicitous/effusive*
- *Seductive/flattering/charming*
- *Over-inclusive/eager to please*
- *Entitled/controlling*

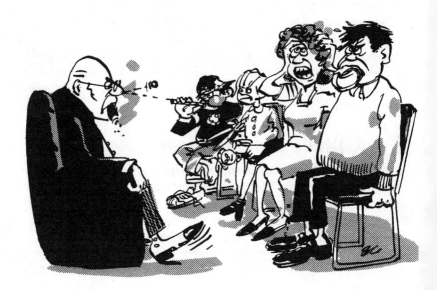

The manner in which patients are uncooperative requires elaboration, for example:
- *Hostile/defensive*
- *Suspicious/guarded*
- *Antagonistic/critical*
- *Childish/regressed*
- *Sullen/withdrawn*

To illustrate your choice of adjectives, include a quote or observation from the interview.

# III — Attentiveness to the Interview

Attentiveness impacts on cooperation and reliability. Patients can be distracted by external (noise) or internal stimuli (hallucinations) while speaking, and may preferentially pay attention to these other events.

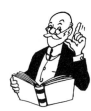

Patients can lose interest in an interview for any of a number of reasons:
• Borderline or antisocial personalities often become bored in interview situations
• Narcissistic or histrionic personalities can develop an abrupt need for affirmation of their specialness or attractiveness
• Patients experiencing a manic or hypomanic episode may be highly distractible
• Delirious patients drift in and out of lucidity; they may lapse into a clouded state of consciousness during an interview
• Obsessive-compulsive disorder can cause patients to succumb to the intrusive thoughts; they may engage in a number of ritualized behaviors
• Anxiety disorders can cause a sudden, overwhelming distraction for patients
• Patients who are psychotic may experience hallucinations or incorporate interview material into delusions, which then reduces their ability to attend to questions

These findings are recorded in the MSE as patients being *attentive* or *inattentive*. A further description is given for diminished attention span, which may be due to:
• Being preoccupied
• A reduced or fluctuating level of consciousness
• Being distracted by activity in and around the interview
• Sudden shifts in affect or mood state

A formal test of attention for the MSE is covered in the chapter on *Sensorium & Cognitive Functions*.

# IV – Level of Consciousness (LOC)

LOC refers to the degree of alertness. In typical interview situations, patients are attentive and responsive to questions. This can be recorded in the MSE as, "*The patient was fully alert and attentive to the interview.*" Changes in the level of arousal are important to include early in recording or reporting the MSE. The reader or listener needs to be aware of this at the outset, because an altered level of consciousness affects the quality of the information that follows. A diminished LOC immediately calls into question the possibility of an organic condition, and warrants an urgent investigation. While the LOC can't be increased, an increased level of attentiveness can be observed, and is referred to as:

• *Hyperarousal* if patients are agitated or anxious
• *Hypervigilant* if they unduly focus on minor stimuli

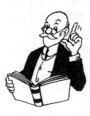

Hyperarousal occurs most commonly in the following:

• Mania – patients are highly distractible, and will shift their attention to any new or competing stimulus (e.g. overhead announcements, the color of your name tag, strains of conversations they can overhear, etc.)

• Anxiety disorders – if patients have a panic attack or a flashback (posttraumatic stress disorder) during the interview, their level of arousal will increase

• Paranoia – patients are typically hypervigilant for evidence that they are being conspired against (e.g. hidden cameras, tape recorders, microphones, etc.)

• Substance abuse – this most frequently occurs with stimulants such as cocaine or amphetamines; it can also occur with caffeine or phencylidine (PCP) ingestion

• General medical conditions, such as hyperthyroidism or pheochromocytoma

Decreased LOC is recorded using the following terms (listed in order of increasing severity):
• **Drowsy** or **lethargic** – the patient responds with a minimal effort (raised voice or gentle nudging); thought is slowed and lacks goal-directedness; patients may drift off to sleep

• **Obtunded** – greater efforts are needed to bring arousal to the point where questions can be answered; persistent efforts (i.e. direct, closed-ended, or even "yes or no" questions) are required to maintain focus

• **Stupor** – refers to a state where patients make occasional returns to a wakeful state; vigorous or even painful stimulation is needed to accomplish this; mild stimuli may produce groaning or movement away from an annoying sound or touch

• **Coma** – a persistent state of unconsciousness

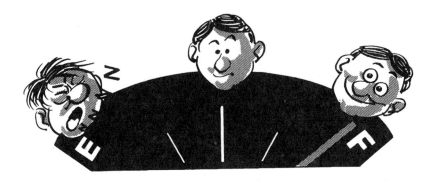

Following the time course of a change in LOC can help delineate the cause. For example:
• **Deteriorating LOC**: may mean intracranial bleeding, edema, or infection; structural lesions; overdoses, etc.
• **Fluctuating LOC**: this is the hallmark of delirium
• **Improving LOC**: possibilities include alcohol or drug intoxication that lessens with time; a post-ictal state; concussion; hypoglycemia; period of anoxia; ischemic neurologic event; sleep deprivation; etc.

# V – Affect

Affect is introduced here, and is fully covered in the chapter on *Affect & Mood*. Affect is defined as:
• The observable or objective quality of an emotional state
• The moment-to-moment variability of visible emotions based on what is occurring in the interview (external events) or feelings (internal events)
• The range of reactions to questions/events that would usually be considered of emotional significance

A financial analogy is as follows: **affect** is the minute-to-minute variation in the worth of a company stock, **mood** is the general trend over a longer time period. Another analogy is that affect is like weather, while mood is like climate.

In the DSM-IV, the conditions previously referred to as "Affective Disorders" were renamed "Mood Disorders." This was done to more accurately reflect the nature of the pathology. The conditions being described (depression, mania, etc.) are of a sustained nature and are more aptly described as disorders of mood. While "affective disorders" are no longer diagnosed, there are situations where the emotional component of other disorders interferes with interviews.

Some patients experience rapid shifts in their emotional state in interviews, which interferes with the quality and quantity of the information obtained. Of particular relevance is that patients with Cluster B Personality Disorders (antisocial, borderline, histrionic, and narcissistic) frequently experience dramatic changes in emotional state as a reaction to the interviewer. More often than not, these affective changes involve hostility, irritability, or anger. However, affective changes that accompany flirtation or idealization can be just as detrimental to the interview.

Affect is reported in a separate section along with mood. In situations where intense affect interferes with obtaining information, describing this in the *Cooperation & Reliability* section helps put subsequent information in perspective.

# VI – Secondary Gain

Secondary gain (also called **morbid** or **epinosic** gain) refers to an actual or external advantage that patients gain from being ill. Common examples include:
- Being relieved of occupational responsibilities
- Prescription medication (e.g. opioids, benzodiazepines)
- Avoiding military service
- Gaining leverage in personal relationships
- Postponing exams
- Deferring legal proceedings; transfer out of prison or jail
- Shelter and/or food; financial reward

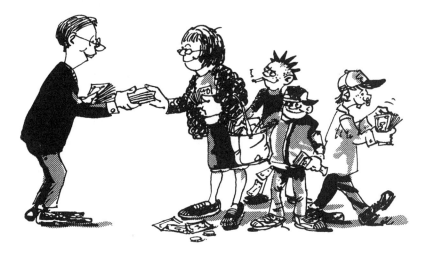

In psychoanalytic theory, a symptom functions to decrease intrapsychic conflict and distress, which is called the **primary gain**. The best example of this can be demonstrated with a conversion disorder. Here, a psychological conflict is "converted" into a physical one that is often symbolically linked to the conflict. For example, a wife catching her husband in the act of infidelity develops blindness; a son who wishes to strike his father "converts" this conflict into a paralyzed arm.

**Tertiary gain** is the advantage that others receive from the patient's illness (e.g. disability income).

# VII – Malingering

Any mental disorder can be mimicked by medical conditions, or by someone skilled in the production of psychiatric symptoms. There is no way of objectively assessing auditory hallucinations, paranoia, flashbacks, or any other internal experience. For this reason, mental illnesses are favored by malingerers, who consciously produce symptoms for secondary gain. The history of malingering is the history of civilization itself. As soon as there were unpleasant tasks or situations, people found ways out of them by faking illness. An account of malingered psychosis appears in the Bible. The antics of Corporal Klinger on M*A*S*H provide another example.

Malingering can occur in a variety of contexts:
• *"Faking bad"* – this can range from the exaggeration of actual symptoms to their complete fabrication
• *"Faking good"* – minimizes or denies current symptoms
• *Staged events* provide a witnessed or otherwise verifiable record of an injury or traumatic event, which can be used later to feign illness
• *Alteration of documentation*, e.g. altered photocopies, forged referral notes, stolen letter- head, etc.
• *Tampering with diagnostic procedures*, e.g. scars that are self-in- flicted to look like surgical incisions, blood added to urine, feces injected to cause septice- mia

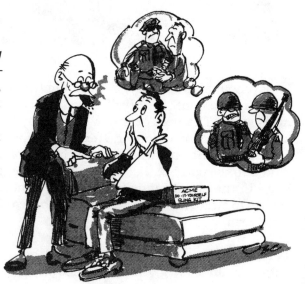

## How Can Malingering Be Detected?

Reliable clues to unveil malingering have been sought for centuries. There are some reports that even experienced interviewers do little better than mere chance in making the distinction. It should not be your primary goal in an interview to detect the malingering. You will cause yourself less grief in being fooled by a stream of malingerers than you will by incorrectly confronting one legitimate patient. Additionally, not all false information provided by patients is due to malingering.

Nevertheless, an attitude of "benevolent skepticism" where there is obvious secondary gain helps keep the possibility of manufactured symptoms in mind. It is usually not difficult to determine that secondary gain is present. This is perhaps most prevalent with incarcerated individuals. Mental illness can mean a transfer out of the general population into medical segregation, called "soft time," which is more lenient. Of even greater significance is the issue of a mental illness being a contributing factor in criminal behavior. Such a finding in court means that the perpetrator is sent to a forensic psychiatry unit instead of prison. In less obvious situations, patients often guide the interview to address their agenda, or even voice their requests, and hope to exploit the compassion of the interviewer.

Signs that patients may be malingering are as follows (adapted from Sadock & Sadock, 2000):
• Anxiety expressed as a high-pitched voice, grammatical mistakes, or **parapraxes** ("slips of the tongue")
• Anxiety expressed as agitation, hand wringing, etc.
• Delays in answering questions, evasive answers
• Discrepancies between facial expression and physical movement (especially anxious fidgeting)
• Statements that obliquely address the truth e.g. "Would I lie to you?"

N.B. Eye contact and facial expression may not be reliable clues to the detection of feigning information.

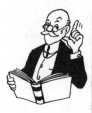

Certain psychological symptoms, or mental illnesses, are among the most likely to be malingered:
- Mental retardation or deficiency
- Cognitive disorders (e.g. dementias)
- Amnesia
- Psychosis
- Delusions
- Hallucinations
- Posttraumatic stress disorder

Sadock & Sadock (2000) include a summary of factors to help distinguish between real and malingered symptoms for each of these disorders. They also note that malingering is difficult to maintain in a lengthy interview and suggest that the evaluative process should be extended for as long as possible. In such situations, patients can be asked to repeat segments of their histories to verify what they said earlier.

While interviewing skills are important in the detection of malingering, other methods to investigate the veracity of interview material are (Rogers, 1997):
- Interview patients on separate occasions to corroborate earlier information
- Obtain medical records and/or speak with prior contacts of patients
- The **Minnesota Multiphasic Personality Inventory, Second Version (MMPI-2)**; this test includes the F and K Scales that can be used individually or in combination to detect malingering; test patients with other **objective personality inventories**
- **Projective testing** with such tests as the **Rorschach** or **Thematic Apperception Tests (TAT)**
- Sodium amytal and other drug-assisted interviews
- Hypnosis
- Polygraph (lie-detector) testing (this is not used in typical clinical situations)

# VIII – Factitious Disorder

The hallmark of factitious disorder (FD) is the conscious production of symptoms in order to "assume the sick role." The goal appears to gaining admission to hospital, and to be the focus of clinical investigation and treatment. It is both a fascinating and disturbing disorder. FD is of particular interest in psychiatry, both because of the interest in human motivation, and because the symptoms that make up the diagnostic criteria can be faked (sometimes with incredible accuracy). FD does not appear to be explainable on the basis of an obvious gain. For example, opioid (narcotic) medications can be relatively easily obtained – one needn't be admitted to a hospital solely to obtain them.

Patients often have some familiarity with health-care terminology and procedures, and know which symptoms to emphasize. They are often eager to have invasive procedures performed – possibly in the hope that a complication develops or a coincidental finding is made. The etiology of this disorder remains obscure, but clearly involves profound disturbances in identity and personality formation. This disorder has also been called **Münchausen's syndrome**, which is a misnomer because he was more of a raconteur than someone fabricating a serious illness. Other terms describing this disorder are **hospital addiction** and **pseudologia fantastica**.

Management involves early detection, limiting investigations, and avoiding unnecessary medication.

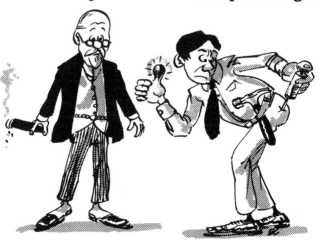

# In What Other Situations is False Information Provided?

• **Confabulation** is the "invention of stories" to fill in memory gaps. Patients are not consciously trying to be deceptive; they do so to avoid calling attention to their cognitive deficits; this is most commonly seen in **Korsakoff's psychosis** and is due to **anterograde amnesia** caused by thiamine (vitamin B$_1$) deficiency (usually as a result of chronic alcohol ingestion.)

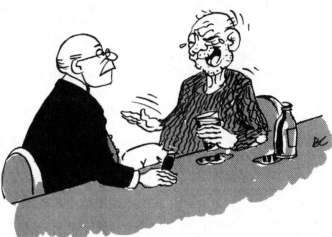

• **Ganser's syndrome** originally referred to episodes of transient psychosis and clouding of consciousness. Currently, the syndrome refers to the situation where approximate answers are given. Answers like "there are *six* fingers on a normal hand" or "*five* quarters in a dollar" are typical. Controversy surrounds this disorder. In some studies, Ganser-like answers were given by subjects trying to imitate mental disorders. Others have shown that it occurs in response to stress, head injuries, or mental illness, and that it is not under voluntary control. There is an overlap of malingering, dissociative, and psychotic symptoms in this syndrome.

• Ego defense mechanisms such as **denial** or **repression** operate to keep certain information beyond conscious retrieval; patients may quite legitimately not be aware of events that are documented in their medical records

# Summary

Cooperation from patients is required for psychiatric diagnoses to be made. A number of factors can interfere with patients' volition, and a distinction needs to be made as to whether someone *can't* or *won't* share information. Patients who *can't* cooperate are often severely ill with medical and/or psychiatric conditions. Those who *won't* share information are usually angry at events that take place in or around interviews. Factors such as involuntary committal, appearing under duress, or the presence of a personality disorder are common reasons for a willful lack of cooperation. This is referred to as **resistance**. It is a maxim that resistance must be dealt with before other aspects of an assessment can begin. To paraphrase the *Borg* from *Star Trek*, not addressing resistance can be futile!

Whereas **cooperation** makes reference to the *quantity* of information shared, **reliability** reflects the *quality* of the data obtained. Patients can create the illusion of cooperation while providing little useful information. For an excellent example of this, see Kevin Spacey's role in the movie, *The Usual Suspects*.

An understanding of what **secondary gain** is available to patients is important. Psychiatric diagnoses, being determined largely through interviews, are more easily malingered than physical conditions. Collateral information is always important to obtain, and may be the only way of detecting malingering or factitious disorder. These are important conditions to keep in mind during any assessment, but are "diagnoses of exclusion." Their presence does not rule out the possibility of concurrent or future legitimate medical or psychiatric conditions.

There are many other conditions in which information is distorted for reasons other than deception (e.g. denial in alcohol abuse or confabulation in cortical blindness, also known as **Anton's syndrome**).

# Dr. Meador's Rules* — Part II

29. Patients with factitious disease do not remain with the physician who makes the diagnosis.

60. All patients will lie about something. Some will lie about everything.

177. Illness behavior attracts attention. All illness has some secondary gain.

215. Factitious skin lesions do not appear between the scapulae.

299. Patients who are receiving money for disability rarely get well. After the first year they never get well even if the money is less than they could earn working.

333. Think of factitious disorder when there are unusual findings, especially when caring for a physician's spouse or any health-care worker.

418. If a patient is clearly lying to you, remember:
• The lie is usually directed to "the doctor," not you as a person.
• The facts, like the lies, are important medical symptoms
• No patient's lie should be held against the patient or make you angry.

* Clifton K. Meador, M.D.
**A Little Book of Doctor's Rules**
Hanley & Belfus, Philadelphia, 1992
Reprinted with permission.

# References
## Books

American Psychiatric Association
**Diagnostic and Statistical Manual of Mental Disorders, 4th Ed.**
American Psychiatric Association, Washington D.C., 1994

K. Artingstall
**Practical Aspects of Münchausen by Proxy and Münchausen Syndrome Investigation (Practical Aspects of Criminal and Forensic Investigations)**
CRC Press, Boca Raton, Florida, 1998

R. Campbell
**Psychiatric Dictionary, 7th Ed.**
Oxford University Press, New York, 1996

M.D. Feldman & C.V. Ford
**Patient or Pretender: Inside the Strange World of Factitious Disorders**
John Wiley & Sons, New York, 1995

M.D. Feldman & S.J. Eisendrath, Editors
**The Spectrum of Factitious Disorders (Clinical Practice, 40)**
American Psychiatric Press, Inc., Washington, D.C., 1996

C.V. Ford
**Lies! Lies!! Lies!!!: The Psychology of Deceit**
American Psychiatric Press, Inc., Washington, D.C., 1999

J.T. McCann
**Malingering and Deception in Adolescents: Assessing Credibility in Clinical and Forensic Settings**
American Psychological Association Press, Washington, D.C., 1997

R. Rogers
**Clinical Assessment of Malingering and Deception, 2nd Ed.**
The Guilford Press, New York, 1997

R. Rogers & D.W. Shuman
**Conducting Insanity Evaluations**
The Guilford Press, New York, 2000

B.J. Sadock & V.A. Sadock, Editors
**Comprehensive Textbook of Psychiatry, 7th Ed.**
Lippincott, Williams & Wilkins, Philadelphia, 2000

# Articles

S. Albert, H.M. Fox, & M.W. Kahn
**Faking Psychosis on the Rorschach: Can Expert Judges Detect Malingering?**
*J. Pers. Assess.* 44(2): 115 – 119, 1980

C. Brems & K. Harris
**Faking the MMPI-2: Utility of the Subtle-Obvious Scales**
*J. Clin. Psychol.* 52(5): 525 – 533, 1996

D.G. Brunetti, R.S. Schlottmann, A.B. Scott, & J.L. Mihura
**Instructed Faking and MMPI-2 Response Latencies: The Potential for Assessing Response Validity**
*J. Clin. Psychol.* 54(2): 143 – 153, 1998

M.W. Carney, T.K. Chary, P. Robotis, & A. Childs
**Ganser Syndrome and its Management**
*British Journal of Psychiatry* 151: 697 – 700, 1987

G. Dalla Barba
**Different Patterns of Confabulation**
*Cortex* 29(4): 567 – 581, 1993

J.R. Hanley, G.A.Baker, & S. Ledson
**Detecting the Faking of Amnesia: A Comparison of the Effectiveness of Three Different Techniques for Distinguishing Simulators From Patients With Amnesia**
*J. Clin. Exp. Neuropsychol.* 21(1): 59 – 69, 1999

M.W. Kahn, H. Fox, & R. Rhode
**Detecting Faking on the Rorschach: Computer Versus Expert Clinical Judgment**
*J. Pers. Assess.* 52(3): 516 – 523, 1998

J. Kalivas
**Malingering versus Factitious Disorder (letter)**
*American Journal of Psychiatry* 153(8): 1108, 1996

J. Kerbeshian & L. Burd
**More on Ganser's Syndrome and DSM-III**
*American Journal of Psychiatry* 144: 119–120, 1987

P.D. Kiester & A.D. Duke
**Is It Malingering, or Is It "Real?" Eight Signs That Point to Non-Organic Back Pain**
*Postgraduate Medicine* 106(7): 77 – 80, 1999

L.E. Krahn
**Paranoid Schizophrenia – Malingering or Factitious Disorder (letter)**
*American Journal of Psychiatry* 156(3): 498 – 499, 1999

A.E. Kuisak
**Validity of Malingering Signs Questioned (letter)**
*Postgraduate Medicine* 107(2): 31, 2000

C.J. LoPiccolo, K. Goodkin, & T.T. Baldewicz
**Current Issues in the Diagnosis and Management of Malingering**
*Ann. Med.* 31(3): 166 – 174, 1999

N. Newmark & K.J. Adityanjee
**Pseudologia Fantastica and Factitious Disorder: A Review of the Litera-
ture and a Case Report**
*Compr. Psychiatry* 40(2): 89 – 95, 1999

T.A. Stern
**How to Spot the Patient Who's Faking It**
*Med. Econ.* 76(10): 105 – 106, 1999

M. Turner
**Malingering (editorial)**
*Br. J. Psychiatry* 171: 409 – 411, 1997

W.G. Van Gorp & R.G. Meyer
**The Detection of Faking on the Millon Clinical Multiaxial Inventory
(MCMI)**
*J. Clin. Psychol.* 42(5): 742 – 747, 1986

S. Wetzler & D. Marlowe
**"Faking Bad" on the MMPI, MMPI-2, and Millon-II**
*Psychol. Rep.* 67(3 Pt. 2): 1117 – 1118, 1990

R.W. Wildman
**The Detection of Malingering**
*Psychol. Rep.* 84(2): 386 – 388, 1999

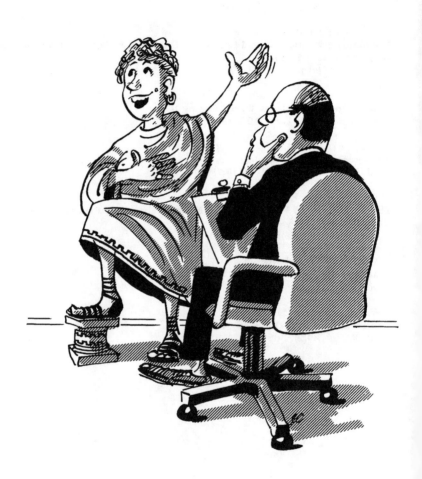

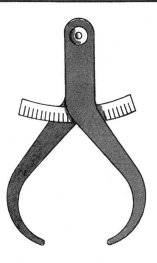

# Chapter 5

# Speech

## Which Aspects of Speech Are Important in the MSE?

- **Speech** refers to verbal expression, which consists of utterances, words, phrases, and sentences.

• **Language** refers to the communication of comprehensible ideas. Not all speech is language (e.g. vocal tics, campaign promises). Language can be conveyed by means other than speech, e.g. posture, gestures, expressions, actions, and sign language (signing) all transmit clear meanings without requiring verbal expression. Language consists of ideas (usually expressed as words) that convey meaning (**semantics**) and are properly produced or pronounced (**articulation**).

• **Thought process** is the way in which thought is organized. Thought cannot be accessed directly, and is inferred from speech and language (including writing or signing).

Many clinicians view the above distinction as arbitrary and coalesce speech and thought process together in the MSE. This chapter outlines the mechanical (motor) aspects, and various qualities of, speech production that are not generally included in the presentation of thought process. Thought and language have a large interplay, but describe different processes. Language is the principal means by which thought process is assessed. Animals and preverbal humans demonstrate that thought occurs without the ability to express syntactical language. While humans are anatomically capable of speech, language is an acquired ability. Understandable sounds are uttered by eighteen months, with phrases being spoken between two and three years of age. A decision tree for speech abnormalities is as follows:

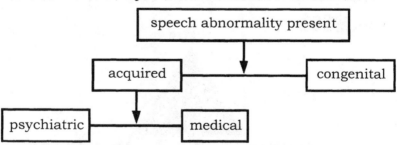

The aspects of speech presented in this chapter are:

• **Primary Language Disorders (Section I)**

• **Quality of Speech (II)**

• **Prosody (III)**

# What is the Diagnostic Significance of Abnormal Speech?

## Congenital/Onset in Childhood

• **Mental Retardation** 31X.X
B. Concurrent deficits or impairments in present adaptive functioning in. . . use of communication

• **Expressive Language Disorder** 315.31
A. The scores obtained from standardized individually administered measures of expressive language are substantially below those of nonverbal intelligence . . .

• **Stuttering** 307.0 (explained in detail on p.138)

• **Autism** 299.00
A. (2) (a) Delay in, or total lack of, the development of spoken language (not accompanied by an attempt to compensate through alternative modes of communication such as gesture or mime)
(b) In individuals with adequate speech, marked impairment in the ability to initiate or sustain a conversation with others
(c) Stereotyped and repetitive use of language or idiosyncratic language

## Medical

• **Delirium** 293.0
B. A change in cognition (such as memory deficit, disorientation, language disturbance) . . .

• **Dementia** 290.X
A. (2) (a) Aphasia (language disturbance)

## Psychiatric

• **Schizophrenia**  295.X
A. (3) Disorganized speech (e.g. frequent derailment or incoherence)

• **Brief Psychotic Disorder**  298.8
A. (3) Disorganized speech (e.g. frequent derailment or incoherence)

• **Manic Episode & Hypomanic Episode**  296.X
B. (3) More talkative than usual or pressure to keep talking

• **Schizotypal Personality Disorder**  301.22
(4) Odd thinking and speech (e.g. vague, circumstantial, metaphorical, overelaborate or stereotyped)

• **Histrionic Personality Disorder**  301.50
(5) Has a style of speech that is excessively impressionistic and lacking in detail

Diagnostic Criteria are from the DSM-IV.
© American Psychiatric Association, Washington, D.C. 1994
Reprinted with permission.

# I – What Are the Primary Language Disorders?

In order to understand the primary language disorders it is necessary to review the neuroanatomy of speech production. The brain is lateralized, with the areas responsible for speech being found in the dominant cerebral hemisphere. Hand dominance is related to lateralization:
• Right-handers make up 90% of the population and almost all have the speech center on the left side of their brains
• Among left-handers, about two-thirds have a dominant left cerebral hemisphere; the remainder have right-sided or bilateral dominance
• Gauging handedness by using the writing hand is about 85% accurate in determining dominance, while footedness

is about 98% accurate; in addition to asking about writing, find out which hand the patient would peel a potato or throw a ball with; the dominant foot is the one used for kicking
• Handedness is a hereditary trait, but the hand used for writing can be changed (e.g. by hand/arm accidents or teachers opposed to the use of the left hand for writing)

The cerebrum has four lobes: frontal, temporal, parietal, and occipital. The areas involved in speech are found around the **sylvian fissure** (also called the **peri-sylvian area**) which separates the temporal from the frontal lobe. The Sylvian fissure is also called the **lateral cerebral sulcus**. **Broca's area** is in the frontal lobe and controls the motor expression of speech. **Wernicke's area** is in the superior part of the temporal lobe and controls the center for the receptive or sensory aspects of speech. These areas are connected by a group of neurons called the **arcuate fasciculus**. There are many classification systems for specifying locations in the brain. One of the most practical ones for psychiatric considerations was developed by Korbinian **Brodmann**, which divides the brain into 47 areas based on differences in cortical regions.

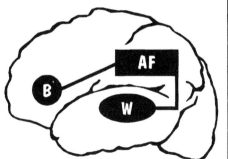

### B – Broca's Area
Frontal lobe – Brodmann Area 44

### W – Wernicke's Area
Superior Temporal Gyrus, Brodmann Area 22

### AF – Arcuate Fasciculus

While the dominant hemisphere (usually left) controls most of the functions of speech; the right hemisphere provides an integrative function. In order to "get the whole picture" or see "the forest and the trees" or understand a *Far Side* cartoon, the non-dominant hemisphere must be functioning. Other non-dominant functions include the inflection, rhythm, and emotional components of language. Interest-

ingly, second and later languages and obscenities are not controlled by the dominant hemisphere. Damage to the **corpus callosum** (the neurons connecting the two halves of the brain) can result in a number of language abnormalities. The following cranial nerves (**CN**) are required for the comprehension and production of speech:
• CN 5 – control of articulation via jaw muscles
• CN 7 – control of articulation via facial muscles
• CN 8 – (cochlear part) carries auditory information
• CN 9, 10, 11, & 12 – control the soft palate, pharynx, larynx, and tongue to facilitate speech

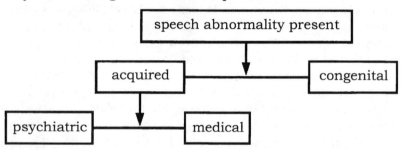

Based on the above decision tree, obtaining information to answer the following questions starts the formal assessment of speech abnormalities:
1. Is the patient's speech abnormal?
2. In what way is it abnormal?
    Abnormal speech patterns form the basis of the rest of this chapter and the *Thought Process* Chapter

3. Was the patient's speech ever normal?
    A list of conditions affecting speech development and the speech patterns of certain illnesses follows later.

4. Is anything else abnormal in addition to speech?
        • reading
        • writing/drawing
        • comprehension
        • repetition
        • copying
        • naming
        • response to directions

} these tasks can be carried out during the MSE to further deliniate a patient's deficits

Given that speech is encoded thought, the chance to hear patients speak gives us valuable clues about their mental functioning. It is not unusual to have a patient present for an interview who is shabbily dressed and acting in an eccentric manner. While you are busy (prematurely) considering some heavy-duty diagnosis, you are taken aback by the person's intelligence and eloquent speech. Conversely, patients can be demented, delirious, or mentally retarded and appear neatly groomed with no obvious behavioral abnormalities.

## Which Conditions Affect the Acquisition of Normal Language Skills?

• **Mental Retardation** is a combination of significantly sub-average intellectual functioning and limitations in adaptation occurring before age 18 years. The IQ falls below 70 – 75, which takes into account an error of 5 points on testing. Mild-to-moderate retardation affects learning to the point that mental abilities are arrested at about the level of grade six. Vocabulary is accordingly limited. Clinical findings include repeated verbalizations and the use of behavior to express feelings (e.g. throwing things).

• **Autism** is characterized by delayed social relationships and language, and resistance to environmental changes. Common findings are **echolalia**, and the reversal of pronouns. For example, "You want" is verbalized instead of "I want." **Neologisms** (made up words with idiosyncratic meanings) are also common. Words and sentences may be used once and then dropped from the vocabulary for days to weeks. Odd voice quality and rhythm patterns have also been noted.

## Pervasive Developmental Disorders

• **Rett's disorder** – encephalopathy beginning between 6 to 24 months in otherwise normal infant girls

• **Asperger's disorder** – currently defined in the DSM-IV as impaired social interaction and stereotyped behaviors, but language deficits have been included previously.

• **Heller's syndrome (Childhood Disintegrative Disorder)** – has a typical onset between ages 3 to 4 years and involves a loss of previously acquired language skills

• **Tourette's disorder** involves vocal and motor tics, which are apparent on average by age seven and must be present by age eighteen. Vocal tics can take several forms, such as repeated words or phrases (out of context to the situation) and **coprolalia** (the involuntary utterance of obscene words). Coprolalia can occur alone or as an interruption during a sentence.

## Primary Language Disorders

• **Aphasias** (also called **dysphasias**) are disturbances in the ability to express and comprehend language. The pathology is in the brain itself and not in the nerves or muscles involved in speech production. Aphasias are manifested as errors in word choice and grammar. The main types of aphasias are outlined later in this chapter.

• **Dysarthria** is poorly articulated speech due to a dysfunction in the physical ability to produce sounds (e.g. mouth, tongue, lips, cranial nerves, larynx, throat). The speech of dysarthric patients is distorted and indistinct. In particular, consonant sounds are difficult to distinguish. Other abnormalities include added, deleted or substituted sounds.

• **Alexia** is the inability to read (for neurological reason, as opposed to illiteracy). **Dyslexia** is defined as an impairment in learning to read that leads to difficulties with spelling and the perception of the shapes of words and letters. Dyslexia is usually a developmental disorder, whereas alexia is usually acquired and involves a lesion in the occipital lobe.

• **Agraphia** (or **dysgraphia**) is an inability to write in someone who had acquired this skill. The ability to copy can persist. The deficits with written language usually parallel those with verbalization.

• **Agnosia** is an inability to recognize objects despite intact sensory and intellectual abilities and language function. For example, patients can physically describe an object but not its function.

• **Apraxia** is the inability to perform learned movements as a result of disruption of areas controlling motor and language function. The ability to comprehend the movement remains intact. Apraxia often occurs with aphasia.

• **Anomia** is a specific inability to name or label things even though they are familiar. This occurs whether the object to be named is shown or recalled from memory.

## How Do I Distinguish Medical From Psychiatric Causes of Speech Disturbance?

The distinction between aphasias and disorders of thought process can be difficult because they both affect verbal expression. In the case of severe psychiatric disturbances, it may not be possible in one interview to make the distinction (a classic example is the confusion between schizophrenic and aphasic speech). Additionally, some patients can have both simultaneously; for example, **Broca's aphasia** (defined later) can be complicated by hypomania or paranoia, and **Wernicke's aphasia** can cause depression. The following is a list of potential distinguishing features:

| Parameter | Medical | Psychiatric |
|---|---|---|
| • greater severity | + | − |
| • continuous duration | + | − |
| • abrupt onset | + | − |
| • older age of onset | + | − |
| • related language symptoms | + | − |
| • word finding difficulties | + | − |
| • awareness of difficulty (partial) | + | − |
| • loss of repetition, naming, and comprehension abilities | + | − |

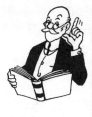

Speech abnormalities are caused by:
- Cerebrovascular accidents (CVAs) involving the left middle cerebral artery (in right handers and most left handers) is the most common cause
- Tumors, head trauma, seizures, sleep deprivation
- Infections – meningitis, encephalitis
- Degenerative disorders – Parkinson's disease, Huntington's disease, Pick's disease

The major psychiatric conditions that involve speech abnormalities were listed at the beginning of the chapter along with their specific diagnostic criteria. Other conditions, such as anxiety and lithium toxicity, also affect language abilities by causing stuttering and dysarthria, respectively.

## What are the Specific Aphasias?

Because of the potential difficulties in distinguishing primary language disorders from psychiatric conditions, the aphasias will be summarized here. The reason it is vital to make this distinction is that aphasias almost always involve an injury to the dominant cerebral hemisphere, which requires urgent investigation and treatment. Psychiatric conditions are less medically urgent, and involve a different form of treatment. Aphasias are usually classified as **fluent** or **non-fluent aphasias** on the basis of the flow of speech.

Further distinction is made by using three tests:
- **Comprehension** – tested by the ability to follow simple, and later complex, requests
- **Repetition** – tested with simple and complex phrases
- **Naming** – tested with common and uncommon objects

An alternate system divides aphasias into **receptive** and **expressive** based on the ability to understand and speak. This poses difficulties for non-neurologists because there are frequently features of both in aphasic patients.

**Paraphasias (paraphasic errors)** are a substitution of a letter or word for the intended word. There are four types:
- Related (approximative) – *light* is used instead of *lamp*
- Unrelated (semantic) – *caboose* is used instead of *lamp*
- Literal (phonemic) – *lump* is used instead of *lamp*
- Neologistic (jargon) – *piloknarf* is used instead of *lamp*

**Paraphasias** and **tangential speech** (talking beyond the point and not returning to it) are features of aphasic speech.

# Non-Fluent Aphasias
- Broca's
- Transcortical Motor
- Global

## Broca's Aphasia
Broca's aphasia is also called **motor aphasia, expressive aphasia**, and **anterior aphasia** (Broca's area is anatomically anterior to Wernicke's). It is characterized by the following features:
- Speech is non-fluent
- Comprehension of writing and speech remains intact
- Repetition is impaired

Non-fluent speech has the following characteristics:
- Slower than average (half to one-third the normal rate)
- Abnormal flow with an irregular rhythm
- Frequent extended pauses producing a halting quality
- The amount of speech is decreased, often with missing connecting words (prepositions, conjunctions, pronouns, articles); verb tenses may also be abnormal

These deficits result in **agrammatism**, which is speech or writing that lacks syntax because words are not put in a correct sequence according to the rules of grammar. The choppy communication style is called **telegram** or **telegrahic style**. For example, the following phrase:

*Rapid Psychler produces humorous psychiatric textbooks.*

becomes

*Torpid cycler . . . produces . . . . . publical . . . . avocation . . .*

The agrammatism, halting style, and paraphasias that may be present are also shown above. Articulation is usually poor (**dysarthric speech**).

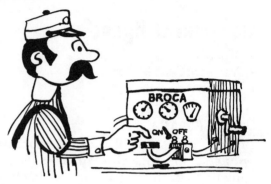

> Broca's = "broken" telegraphic speech

## Transcortical Motor Aphasia

Transcortical motor aphasia differs from Broca's aphasia only in that repetition remains intact. **Echolalia** may be present. Patients cannot engage in conversation or directly name items. Comprehension of written and spoken language remains largely intact.

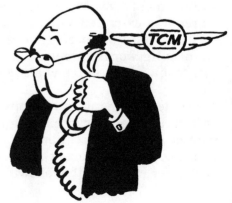

> "Transcortical Motor Ways. . . we comprehend your order and will repeat it back to you."

## Global Aphasia

**Global aphasia** is an extreme non-fluent aphasia that results when the dominant hemisphere is so severely damaged that language function ceases. Patients make few utterances devoid of semantic content. Vascular and traumatic lesions are the most common causes. Extensive physical deficits accompany this severe type of aphasia.

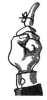

### Non-fluent Aphasia Practice Points

• Most injuries to Broca's area are extensive and damage nearby structures, so that Broca's aphasia is often accompanied by right **hemiparesis** (motor cortex affected) and **homonymous hemianopsia** (a visual field defect)

• The middle cerebral artery supplies this region

• Awareness of these deficits cause a depressive episode

• The frontal lobes are responsible for many higher functions; damage can cause a **frontal lobe syndrome** that affects behavior, emotions, speech, thought form and content, and cause lack of initiative (**abulia**)

# Fluent Aphasias

• Wernicke's
• Transcortical Sensory
• Conduction
• Anomic

Fluent aphasias have the following characteristics:
• Intact articulation and a normal rate of speaking
• Complete sentences with proper syntax
• Speech consists of paraphasias and jargon
• **Neologisms** and words that are used because they sound the same (**clang associations**) are common
• A replacement is substituted for the problematic word, or a description is given of an object, or its use is verbalized instead of the name of the item itself

## Wernicke's Aphasia

Wernicke's aphasia is also called **sensory aphasia**, **receptive aphasia**, and **posterior aphasia**. It is characterized by the following features:
- Fluency remains intact
- Comprehension is impaired
- Repetition is impaired

Wernicke's aphasia contains more paraphasias than does Broca's. If the speech of a patient with Wernicke's aphasia was muffled or blended into the background, it would not sound unusual until you heard the actual semantic content, which is virtually unintelligible. For example:

*Rapid Psychler produces humorous and educational publications.*

   becomes

*Quick pedalers are the make of knowing whatever might not fraught.*

Patients with Wernicke's aphasia are unaware of the nonsensical nature of their speech and may speak continuously.

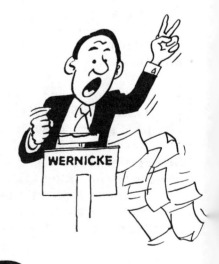

Wernicke's =
"wordy"
speech

WERNICKE

## Transcortical Sensory Aphasia

**Transcortical sensory aphasia** differs from Wernicke's aphasia only in that repetition remains intact. As in transcortical motor aphasia, speech may resemble **echolalia**. Naming and comprehension are impaired, as they are in Wernicke's. There is also a **mixed transcortical aphasia** which features non-fluent speech and impaired comprehension, but intact repetition.

## Conduction Aphasia

Conduction aphasia results from a lesion in the arcuate fasciculus. This causes a fluent aphasia with the following features:
- Intact comprehension
- Impaired repetition
- Impaired naming
- Awareness of speech abnormalities
- Reading aloud is impaired, while reading silently is not

Paraphasias are generally of the literal type (letter substitution), for example:

*Rapid Psychler produces humorous and educational publications.*

becomes

*Rabid Dychler detruses hamorous and educational clubications.*

## Anomnic Aphasia

Anomic aphasia is also called **angular gyrus aphasia, amnestic aphasia, nominal aphasia**, and **dysnomia**. It has the following features:
- Speech remains fluent
- Intact comprehension
- Intact repetition
- Variable presence of paraphasias
- Variable semantic meaning to speech

The speech of patients with anomic aphasia has frequent interruptions while they search for particular words. Generalities such as "thing," "it," "thing-a-ma-jig" occur after pauses. For example:

*Rapid Psychler produces humorous and educational publications.*

becomes

*You know those people, with the bicycle design, they printed it.*

A specific type of anomia is **prosopagnosia**, where patients lack the ability to recognize familiar faces. Other deficits include being unable to name signs, colors, people's names, etc. This condition has an overlap with **benign senescent forgetfulness** and early dementia. These may be ruled in if the following conditions are met:
• Paraphasias are not prominent
• Onset is gradual
• Repetition and comprehension are intact
• Pronunciation remains good
• Localizing neurologic signs are absent

### Fluent Aphasia Practice Points

• The most common language disturbances after closed head injuries are Anomic and Wernicke's aphasias

• Patients can become agitated and even paranoid; the language disturbance and the absence of physical signs can resemble the psychosis of mania or schizophrenia

• The motor strip and Wernicke's area are far enough apart that physical signs are uncommon with fluent aphasias

# II – What Other Qualities of Speech Should Be Considered?

Apart from the primary language disorders, there are other qualities to consider when recording features of a person's speech. The aspects presented in the following section have to do with the "mechanical" aspects of speech production and for this reason are considered separately from disorders of thought process.

## Accent & Dialect

Accent and dialect are terms used interchangeably to describe regional or cultural differences in pronunciation. Accent can be used to refer to the speech of patients who are not native English speakers (e.g. a French or Spanish accent). Dialect can be used to describe regional variations in those who are native anglophones.

There are five major dialects in the U.S. – New York, New England, Southern, Appalachian and Western. In Canada, those from the Atlantic Provinces have a distinct style of speech, while the rest of the country speaks with a "middle American" dialect. In Great Britain, the skill in distinguishing dialect is finely honed. Britons cannot only detect which hamlet someone is from, they can make an educated guess as to whether it the side of the street. Australians, New Zealanders, and South Africans speak with accents which are distinguishable from one another. At one English-speaking film festival, an Australian film needed subtitles!

## Amount of Speech

Amount of speech varies widely in interview situations. Mental health professionals spend years learning how to obtain and organize salient information, leaving patients considerable leeway in what constitutes a "normal" amount of speech (recorded as *responsive, spontaneous, well-spoken, fluent,* or *animated*). Anxious patients provide a lot of extraneous detail through their desire to simply be helpful.

Conversely, other patients feel inhibited and provide sparse answers and offer little information spontaneously.

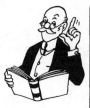

Conditions where the amount of speech can be increased:
• Mania (see **pressure of speech** below)
• Anxiety disorders
• Obsessive compulsive personalities (needless detail)
• Cluster B Personalities (seek to control the interview)
• Temporal lobe epilepsy/partial complex epilepsy (may miss social cues)
• Fluent aphasias

Terms used to describe an increased amount of speech are: *verbose, loquacious, talkative, copious speech, logorrhea, overabundant, or expansive.*

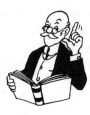

Conditions where the amount of speech can be decreased:
• Depression
• Schizophrenia
• Catatonia
• Avoidant, dependent, and schizoid personalities
• Dementia (can be verbose in early stages)
• Delirium

Terms used to describe a decreased amount of speech are: *paucity of speech, impoverished, laconic, taciturn, single word answers, or minimally responsive.*

At one extreme is **pressure of speech**, where patients are driven to keep talking, and have an increased rate and amount of speech. A key distinguishing factor is that they are not usually interruptible. The other extreme is the absence of speech, called **mutism**, seen in neurologic conditions and extreme forms of psychiatric illnesses.

**Articulation** refers to the clarity with which words are spoken. This is not a disorder of word finding or grammar.

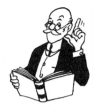

Words can be poorly pronounced due to:
• Slurring (e.g. lithium toxicity, alcohol ingestion)
• Poorly fitting dentures (resembles tardive dyskinesia)
• Missing teeth (**edentulous**)
• Chewing gum
• Central and peripheral neurologic conditions
• Impaired hearing
• Tardive dyskinesia
• Accents from non-native speakers
• Lisps
• Altered level of consciousness
• **Phonation** difficulties caused by decreased resonance of the mouth, nose, or throat

Terms used to describe this are: *garbled, slurred, mumbled, clipped, choppy, unclear,* or *poor diction.*

**Modulation** is the loudness or softness of speech. Some patients are naturally louder when they speak, while others add emphasis at various points in the interview.

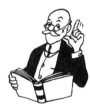

Conditions where patients speak louder than normal include:
• Mania
• Psychosis (of any type)
• Cluster B personality disorders (especially narcissistic and histrionic)
• Dementia
• Delirium
• Hearing impairment or deafness
• Substance intoxication or withdrawal

Conditions where modulation is reduced include:
• Depression
• Medical disorders (e.g. hypothyroidism, diseases of the larynx or recurrent laryngeal nerve, hyperacusis)
• Personality disorders, particularly avoidant and schizoid
• Paranoia (in personalities, delusions or schizophrenia)
• Substance intoxication or withdrawal

# III — What is Prosody?

Prosody is the term that refers to the emotional or affective components of speech. Prosody is used to describe the rhyming meter in poetry. The narrators of "spoken books" provide an excellent example of prosody. Here, one person uses different aspects of speech to: convey action or thought, give each character an identifiable voice, and speak in a manner that keeps listeners interested.

Disorders of prosody are called **aprosodias**. Just as aphasic speech is accompanied by writing difficulties, aprosodias occur with a loss of non-verbal communication. The gestures and facial expressions that constitute the **paralinguistic aspects** of speech are missing. The non-dominant (usually right) hemisphere has the major contribution to prosody.

Patients with aprosodias are unable to detect the emotional aspects of the speech they hear. The difficulties with reception may be more pronounced with posterior non-dominant hemispheric lesions. Anterior lesions are thought to cause greater difficulties with the expressive component. This anterior/posterior pattern is similar to that of aphasias.

Prosody can be tested as follows:
• Have patients say the same phrase under contrasting emo-

tional conditions – e.g. saying, *"I've got to get out of here"* due to (**a**) a boring movie, then (**b**) a fire
• Have patients listen to you say the same phrase with a different affective component
• Review pictures of emotionally charged situations

Prosody can be can be assessed according to the following components:
• *Pitch/intonation/musicality*
• *Spontaneity/latency*
• *Rhythm/cadence*
• *Stress/inflection*

## Pitch

Pitch, as in music, refers to the highness or lowness of the spoken words. Pitch usually varies throughout the course of a sentence. For example, it rises when questions are asked and falls when authoritative statements are made. Pitch also changes with emotional state (e.g. rising with anxiety and falling with depression). Puberty lowers the natural speaking voice of both sexes. In adulthood, pitch changes occur due to throat diseases, smoking, etc. Of interest is that pitch range can be altered by psychiatric illnesses, especially psychosis. *Intonation* and *musicality* are other terms used to describe the animation present in speech. A lack of pitch change can occur as a variant of normal speech.

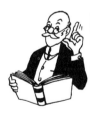

Pitch aprosodias are seen in:
• Obsessive-compulsive or schizoid personalities
• Parkinson's disease or parkinsonism
• Depression and dysthymia
• Nondominant hemispherical lesions and aphasias

Unchanging pitch is described as *monotonous, flat,* or *expressionless.*

## Spontaneity

Spontaneity is the degree of engagement in the interview. Information volunteered without a question being posed is called *spontaneous speech*. **Latency** refers to the time interval in which patients answer questions or connect their sentences. Generally, there is an inverse relationship between the two, i.e. patients who lack spontaneity have an increased latency prior to speaking.

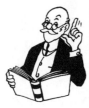

Increased spontaneity and decreased latency occur in:
• Mania
• Anxiety disorders
• Fluent aphasias

Decreased spontaneity and increased latency occur in:
• Depression
• Parkinson's disease or parkinsonism
• Alcohol or substance intoxication
• Non-fluent aphasias, autism, delirium, or dementia

## Rhythm/Cadence

Rhythm, or cadence, varies in normal speech to add emphasis and maintain interest, just as in music. Certain types of rhythm disturbances exist:

• **Stuttering** 307.0
A. Disturbance in the normal fluency and time patterning of speech (inappropriate for the individual's age), characterized by frequent occurrences of the following:
    (1) sound and syllable repetitions
    (2) sound prolongations
    (3) interjections
    (4) broken words
    (5) audible or silent blocking
    (6) circumlocutions

(7) words produced with an excess of physical tension

(8) monosyallabic whole-word repetitions

Diagnostic Criteria are from the DSM-IV.
© American Psychiatric Association, Washington, D.C. 1994
Reprinted with permission.

People are aware that they stutter; a phonetic example is as follows:

Rrrrapid Psychchchler proproproduces huhuhuhumorous

• **Cluttering** is a non-fluent disruption involving bursts of rapid speech containing syntactical errors; the articulation is poor and the speaker is unaware of the speech abnormalities

*Rapid Psychler produces humorous and educational publications.*

becomes

*Rap . . . . . . . . sychpaduce . . . . . . . . antationo . . . . . . . . . libax . . . . . tations*

• **Scanning speech** describes a non-fluent abnormality where there are irregular pauses between syllables, as if each syllable were scanned separately prior to being pronounced; this occurs in multiple sclerosis, chronic alcoholism, and head injuries (especially cerebellar trauma)

| e.g. *Rapid* | *Psych ler* | *pro* | | *du* | *ces* |
|---|---|---|---|---|---|
| *hu mor* | *ous* | *and* | *edu* | *ca* | *tional* |

• Other rhythm disturbances can be seen in psychomotor epilepsy (stacatto or machine-gun-like) and the mumbling, pedantic speech seen in Huntington's chorea

• **Inflection**, or **stress**, adds an extra communicative element to speech, contributing to the **pragmatics** of language.

As an example, consider how the following inflection (indicated by the underlined word) changes the meaning of what is being said:

<u>I'd</u> like to help you out.
(I will help you, instead of someone else helping you)

I'd <u>like</u> to help you out.
(I want to help you, but I can't)

I'd like to <u>help</u> you out.
(I'll help you, but I won't do it for you)

I'd like to help <u>you</u> out.
(I'll help you, but not your friend)

I'd like to help you <u>out</u>.
(Get out! How did you get in?)

Irony and sarcasm (both indispensable elements of language) are added by inflection. Patients with aprosodias miss the finer messages conveyed with stresses in speech. In many instances, non-native speakers, patients with subnormal intelligence and those who are overly concrete in their thinking will also miss the meanings conveyed by inflection. This does not constitute an aprosodia.

### Speech Practice Points

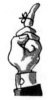

• **Spoonerisms** are a type of paraphasia (closest to a literal or phonemic type) involving a transposition of the first letters or sounds of a word; Spooner (1844 – 1930) is said to have proposed a toast to the "Queer Old Dean" instead of the "Dear Old Queen" (see also p. 144)

• Patients with Broca's aphasia retain their ability to cuss, usually when frustrated by their language difficulties; this indicates there is another locus/aspect of speech control

# Testing of Aphasias

When a patient has speech difficulties, formal testing for aphasia is warranted. A method for testing is as follows:

---

### Screen for Disability
- hearing impairment, cranial nerve lesions, vision impairment
- substance intoxication, withdrawal, etc.

---

---

### Test for Writing Ability
- agraphia is present to some degree in all forms of aphasia
- if intact, there is no aphasia – continue only if an abnormality is present

---

---

### Assess Degree of Fluency
- nonfluent speech is telegraphic (consisting mainly of nouns and verbs)
- fluent speech contains jargon, paraphasias, neologisms
- assess various qualities of speech and prosody

**Fluent**                           **Non-fluent**

---

---

### Assess Degree of Comprehension
- use sequential motor tasks of increasing complexity
- use a series of questions requiring a yes or no answer

**Comprehension Intact**        **Comprehension Impaired**

---

## Assess Ability to Repeat
• start with complex sentences first

**Repetition Intact**　　　　**Repetition Impaired**

## Assess Ability to Name Objects
• start with an object; if unable to answer,
give clues as to its use
• if still unable to answer, give the first syllable
of its name as a clue
• if still unable to answer, offer a list containing the item

## Assess Ability to Read
• test reading silently and aloud
• ask questions to evaluate degree of comprehension
• there are often similar defects in reading and speaking

# Summary

An assessment of speech is integral to the full and accurate assessment of psychiatric illness. As outlined at the beginning of this chapter, several illnesses have specific criteria related to abnormalities of *speech* and *thought process*. The mechanical aspects of speech disorders, quality of speech, and prosody were presented here because they do not strictly have to do with the form or process of thought (covered in later chapters).

While higher mammals have means of communication, humans are unique in their development of syntactical language. Various qualities of speech convey additional information. *How* something is said can be more important than *what* is actually said. An assessment of speech overlaps with a multitude of other mental status parameters: thought, mood & affect, intelligence, cooperation, etc.

Aphasias are language deficits that diminish or remove the ability to express and comprehend ideas. Reading, writing, speaking, naming, repeating, and comprehending can all be affected. The main area for speech is called the **perisylvian region**, encompassing parts of the frontal and temporal lobes. When patients have difficulties communicating, testing for aphasia is warranted. The major types of aphasias and methods to test for them have been outlined.

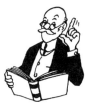

Characteristic speech patterns accompany some mental illnesses:
• Manic patients have an increased amount of speech, which is delivered quickly, and often loudly
• Depressed patients are soft-spoken, slow to answer questions, and often have little to say
• Psychosis can change a patient's voice and other speech characteristics
• Other aspects of speech provide valuable diagnostic clues: e.g. tics, slurred speech, paraphasias, echolalia

# More Spoonerisms

• Our Lord is a shoving leopard.

• It is kisstomery to cuss the bride.

• I believe you're occupewing my pie. May I sew you to another sheet?

• When the soldiers return from France, we will have the hags flung out.

• I keep my icicle well-boiled.

• You have tasted two worms at this school.

• The Navy has an impressive number of cattle ships and bruisers.

• To the headmaster's secretary: "Is the bean dizzy?"

• I don't like to eat parrots and keys.

• It nevers pains, but it roars.

• I tossed my lemper miss thorning.

• If only they would get me low.

• I commended a student for fighting a liar in the kitchen.

• You hissed my mystery lecture.

• I'll take mine in a mere bug.

• Brown lettuce makes a sad ballad

# References

## Books

American Psychiatric Association
**Diagnostic and Statistical Manual of Mental Disorders, 4th Ed.**
American Psychiatric Association, Washington D.C., 1994

D. C. Black
**ILL – Intrepid Linguist Library: Spoonerisms, Sycophants, & Sops**
Dell Publishing, New York, 1988

C. Bowles
**G'Day – Teach Yourself Australian**
Angus & Robertson Publishers, North Ryde, NSW, Australia, 1987

R. Campbell
**Psychiatric Dictionary, 7th Ed.**
Oxford University Press, New York, 1996

H.I. Kaplan & B.J. Sadock, Editors
**Synopsis of Psychiatry, 8th Ed.**
Williams & Wilkins, Baltimore, 1998

D.M. Kaufman
**Clinical Neurology for Psychiatrists, 5th Ed.**
W.B. Saunders, Philadelphia, 2001

R. Lederer
**Get Thee to a Punnery**
Dell Publishing, New York, 1988

H. Mohr
**How to Talk Minnesotan**
Penguin Books, New York, 1987

L. Rolak
**Neurology Secrets**
Hanley & Belfus, Philadelphia, 1993

B.J. Sadock & V.A. Sadock, Editors
**Comprehensive Textbook of Psychiatry, 7th Ed.**
Lippincott, Williams & Wilkins, Philadelphia, 2000

A. Sims
**Symptoms in the Mind, 2nd Ed.**
Saunders, London, England, 1995

E.L. Zuckerman
**The Clinician's Thesaurus, 5th Ed.**
Clinician's Toolbox, The Guilford Press, New York, 2000

## Articles

J.M. Anderson, R. Gilmore, S. Roper, B. Crosson, R.M. Bauer, & S. Nadeau
**Conduction Aphasia and the Arcuate Fasciculus: A Re-Examination of the Wernicke-Geschwind Model**
*Brain Lang.* 70(1): 1 – 12, 1999

R.S. Bernt & A. Caramazza
**How "Regular" Is Sentence Completion in Broca's Aphasia?**
*Brain Lang.* 67(3): 242 – 247, 1999

E.B. Cooper & L.F. De Nil
**Is Stuttering a Speech Disorder?**
*ASHA* 41(2): 10 – 11, 1999

D. Costa & R. Kroll
**Stuttering: An Update for Physicians**
*Canadian Medical Assoc. Journal* 162(13): 1849 – 1855, 2000

D.A. Daly
**Speech Cluttering**
*JAMA* 272(7): 565, 1994

H. Guyard, O. Sabouraud, & J. Gagnepain
**A Procedure to Differentiate Phonological Disturbances in Broca's Aphasia and Wernicke's Aphasia**
*Brain Lang.* 13(1): 19 – 30, 1981

B. Jay
**What Was the Matter With Dr Spooner?**
*Br. Med. J. (Clin. Res. Ed.)* 295(6604): 942 – 3, 1987

N. Helm-Estabrooks & G. Hotz
**Sudden Onset of "Stuttering" in an Adult: Neurogenic or Psychogenic?**
*Semin. Speech Lang.* 19(1): 23 – 29, 1998

V.W. Henderson
**Sigmund Freud and the Diagram-Maker School of Aphasiology**
*Brain Lang.* 43(1): 19 – 41, 1992

R.D. Hunt & D.J. Cohen
**Psychiatric Aspects of Learning Difficulties**
*Pediatric Clinics of North America* 31(2): 471 – 497, 1984

M.D. Kimelman
**Prosody, Linguistic Demands, and Auditory Comprehension in Aphasia**
*Brain Lang.* 69(2): 212 – 221, 1999

H.S. Kirshner & W.G. Webb
**Alexia and Agraphia in Wernicke's Aphasia**
*J. Neurol. Neurosurg. Psychiatry* 45(8): 719 – 724, 1982

M. Lawrence & D.M. Barclay, III
**Stuttering: A Brief Review**
*Am. Fam. Physician* 57(9): 2175 – 2178, 1998

A.F. Leentjens, S.M. Wielaert, F. van Harskamp, & F.W. Wilmink
**Disturbances of Affective Prosody in Patients With Schizophrenia: A Cross Sectional Study**
*J. Neurol. Neurosurg. Psychiatry* 64(3): 375 – 378, 1998

W.W. Lytton & J.C. Brust
**Direct Dyslexia: Preserved Oral Readings of Real Words in Wernicke's Aphasia**
*Brain* 112(Pt. 3): 583 – 594, 1989

O.M. Marx
**Freud and Aphasia: An Historical Analysis**
*American Journal of Psychiatry* 124(6): 815 – 825, 1967

P.J. Mathews, L.K. Obler, & M.L. Albert
**Wernicke and Alzheimer on the Language Disturbances of Dementia and Aphasia**
*Brain Lang.* 46(3): 439 – 462, 1994

L. Miller
**On Aphasia at 100: The Neuropsychodynamic Legacy of Sigmund Freud**
*Psychoanal. Rev.* 78(3): 364 – 378, 1991

M. Payne & W.E. Cooper
**Paralexic Errors in Broca's and Wernicke's Aphasia**
*Neuropsychologia* 23(4): 571 – 574, 1985

T. Plankers
**Speaking in the Claustrum: The Psychodynamics of Stuttering**
*Int. J. Psychoanal.* 80(Pt. 2): 239 – 256, 1999

J.M. Potter
**President's address (abridged): Dr. Spooner and His Dysgraphia**
*Proc. R. Soc. Med.* 69(9): 639 – 648, 1976

M. Rutter
**Developmental Neuropsychiatry: Concepts, Issues, and Prospects**
*J. Clin. Neuropsychology* 4(2): 91 – 115, 1982

S. Waisrub
**Spooner Syndrome (editorial)**
*JAMA* 237(7): 677, 1977

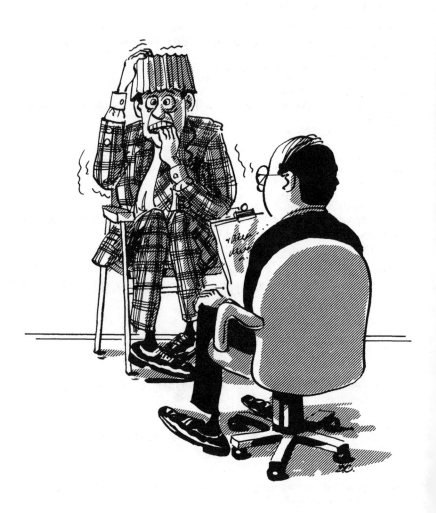

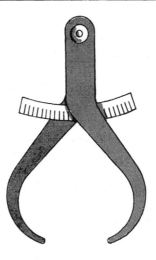

# Chapter 6

# Thought Process

## What Is Thought Process?

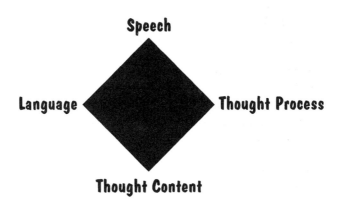

Speech

Language

Thought Process

Thought Content

• **Speech** refers to any form of verbal expression. With aphasias, speech is produced with deficits in fluency, repetition, comprehension, prosody, etc.

• **Language** is the exchange of comprehensible ideas, and describes the communicative value of speech.

• **Thought Content** describes *what* is being talked about (this is covered in detail in the next chapter).

• **Thought Process** or **Thought Form** describes the way in which ideas are produced and organized. This is an assessment of *how* patients are communicating. The degree of connection between ideas, and the flow of thought, are disrupted in many psychiatric illnesses. When this occurs it is referred to as a **(formal) thought disorder**. The way that ideas are linked together is just as important as what the ideas contain. Because thought cannot be accessed directly, it is assessed via speech, writing, and behavior.

# What Is the Diagnostic Significance of Abnormalities in Thought Process?

Because language is encoded thought, the DSM-IV combines the assessment of speech and thought process. The diagnostic criteria involving abnormalities of speech were outlined in the last chapter. Without repeating the individual criteria, the disorders are:
• **Mental Retardation** 31X.X
• **Expressive Language Disorder** 315.31
• **Stuttering** 307.0
• **Autism** 299.00
• **Delirium** 293.0
• **Dementia** 290.X
• **Schizoaffective Disorder** 295.70
• **Schizophreniform Disorder** 295.40

Diagnostic criteria that specifically include thought process disturbances are as follows:

• **Schizophrenia** 295.X
A. (3) Disorganized speech (e.g. frequent derailment or incoherence)

• **Brief Psychotic Disorder** 298.8
A. (3) Disorganized speech (e.g. frequent derailment or incoherence)

• **Manic Episode/Hypomanic Episode** 296.X
B. (4) Flight of ideas or subjective experience that thoughts are racing

• **Schizotypal Personality Disorder** 301.22
(4) Odd thinking and speech (e.g. vague, circumstantial, metaphorical, overelaborate, or stereotyped)

Diagnostic Criteria are from the DSM-IV.
© American Psychiatric Association, Washington, D.C. 1994
Reprinted with permission.

# What Constitutes a Disorder of Thought Process?

The following parameters are used to describe thought process:
• Goal directedness
• Tightness of associations between words, phrases, sentences, and paragraphs
• Rate, pressure, and rhythm of speech
• Idiosyncracy of word usage

Thought process is easiest to assess when patients are given open-ended questions. Here, they must decide:
• What information is important to say
• How directly they answer questions
• When to move on to another topic
• How to move on to another topic, and the degree of connectedness to what was just being discussed

In a closed-ended style of interview, disorders of thought process may not be elicited. However, once it is apparent that a thought disorder is present, greater structure in an interview may be the only way of moving on to new areas. The individual disorders of thought process are:

- **Circumstantiality (Section I)**
- **Tangentiality (II)**
- **Flight of Ideas (III)**
- **Rambling (IV)**
- **Loose Associations (V)**
- **Thought Blocking (VIa)**
- **Thought Derailment (VIb)**
- **Fragmentation (VII)**
- **Verbigeration (VIII)**
- **Jargon (IX)**
- **Word Salad (X)**
- **Incoherence (XI)**

These disorders are listed on the next page, and ranked in approximate order of increasing severity.

# What is a "Normal" Thought Process?

There is considerable variation in how thought is expressed. People also express varying degrees of coherence, detail, and organization at different times. Thought process must be considered in conjunction with other features of the interview. Someone who is anxious may speak quickly and provide extraneous detail. A person who is highly creative may make "stream of consciousness" verbalizations and appear to have disjointed ideas. Some people make great leaps in thinking before verbalizing anything, and the logical connections between their statements may need to be explained. It is valuable to record segments of the interview to illustrate your opinion of the patient's thought process, then, at the end of the interview, make a judgment about her overall ability to communicate her difficulties.

| Process Disturbance | Nature of Disturbance |
|---|---|
| Circumstantiality Tangentiality | • words are completely formed<br>• sentence structure maintained<br>• linkage between ideas remains tight<br>• overinclusive of detail (**circumstantiality**) or do not directly address the point (**tangentiality**) |
| Flight of Ideas | • words and sentences maintained<br>• connection between ideas apparent<br>• frequent shifts in topic<br>• rapid rate of speech |
| Rambling | • clusters of sentences remain goal-directed, but are interspersed with groups that are not goal-directed |
| Loose Associations | • words and sentences maintained<br>• phrases and sentences still properly constructed<br>• connection between ideas is unclear, not obvious, or nonsensical |
| Thought Derailment Thought Blocking | • syntax intact, speech suddenly stops (**blocking**); if it resumes, the topic changes (**derailment**)<br>• may or may not return to previous topic<br>• patients are unaware this is happening |
| Fragmentation | • words remain intact; phrases are disconnected from each other |
| Verbigeration | • repetition of words and phrases |
| Jargon | • syntax intact, speech meaningless |
| Word Salad | • words remain intact; all syntax is lost |
| Incoherence | • words are unintelligible; speech is garbled or dysarthric |

The following are common descriptions of thought process:
- **Tightness of thought**
*well-organized/tangential/loosely connected/incoherent*
- **Flow of speech**
*spontaneous/hesitant/interrupted/halting*
- **Directness of responses**
*informative and relevant/embellished/markedly overinclusive*
- **Flow of ideas**
*logical and with variability/restricted/repetitive*
- **Vocabulary**
*descriptive/restricted/idiosyncratic use of words*
- **Flow of information**
*good exchange/adequate/vague/disorganized*

In order to visualize the various disorders of thought process, the following representation will be used:

**A•B•C•D•E•F•G•H•I•J•K•L•M•N•O•P•Q•R•S•T•U•V•W•X•Y•Z**

- each letter represents a word
- the alphabetical sequence indicates proper syntax
- progression from left to right indicates a logical sequence

The following propaganda statement can be schematized using the above substitution of letters for words.

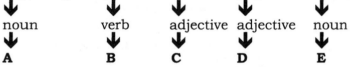

A sentence that doesn't follow the rules of grammar (due to a thought process disorder) might appear as follows:

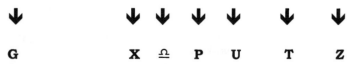

Here, improper syntax is indicated by the non-sequential listing of the letters. Because *hofic* isn't a word, it is represented by a funky symbol (which will be the designation for **neologisms**, explained on p. 165).

## I – Circumstantiality

**Definition:** Circumstantial speech contains an overly detailed amount of information that provides a lot of digressive, extraneous detail in order to give everyone within listening distance a firm grasp on all of the relevant or even quasi-relevant factors so that the point, when reached, is clearly made with substantive evidence. The preceding sentence is an example of circumstantiality. A more direct definition is speech that contains an excessive amount of detail, but does finally address the question.

**Diagrammatic Representation:**

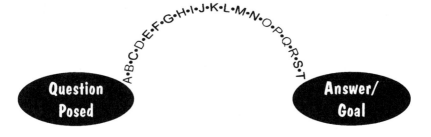

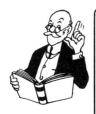

Circumstantiality is most commonly seen in:
• Normal situations; it is endemic in digressive professors, salespeople, politicians, and many lawyers
• Obsessive-compulsive and narcissistic personalities
• Temporal lobe (partial-complex) epilepsy
• Hypomania and anxiety disorders
• Substance ingestion and abuse (e.g. with alcohol, stimulants, etc.)
• Cognitive disorders (e.g. delirium, dementia, and mental retardation)

## II – Tangentiality

**Definition:** Tangential speech can be followed, remains logical, and stays within the "ballpark" of the topic at hand. Proper words and grammar are used. The distinctive factor here is that the person does not arrive at the point or answer the question. Tangentiality helps move conversations along, but in an interview situation it can be a sign of pathology. The severity and frequency of tangential speech needs to be gauged to determine if it impacts on the quality of the interview. Patients in whom tangentiality is not pathological can refocus their replies when asked to do so.

**Diagrammatic Representation:**

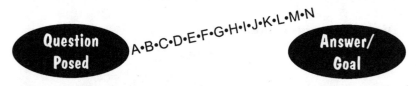

**Example:** *Where did you buy your car?*
*My car has 4 cylinders. It gives me good gas mileage in the city but not much passing power on the highway. I live near a highway and have a garage for my car. I keep it inside even in the summer because sunlight makes the paint fade.*

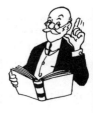

Tangential speech is most often seen in:
• Personality disorders where verbal communication creates or maintains a sense of feeling connected to others (i.e. histrionic and dependent personalities)
• Cognitive disorders such as delirium or dementia
• Hypomania and anxiety disorders
• Substance ingestion and abuse (e.g. alcohol, stimulants, marijuana, etc.)
• Schizophrenia; though other disorders of thought process are more typical for this illness (i.e. loose associations)

## III – Flight of Ideas

**Definition:** Flight of ideas is rapid, non-goal directed speech that "takes off" in a tangential manner. Patients are usually distractible and change topic every sentence or two. Speech remains logical, and the connections between ideas are still recognizable, though this depends on the interviewer's ability to keep up. Patients don't elaborate on their ideas before moving on. Their statements contain proper words and grammar. Flight of ideas differs from tangential speech in that topic changes are more abrupt, more frequent, and often prompted by a word in the previous sentence.

**Diagrammatic Representation:**

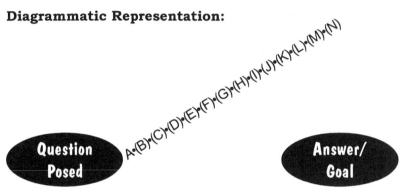

N.B. Brackets are used in this diagram to indicate that there are connections between ideas, though this may not be obvious to the interviewer (contrast this with loose associations).

**Example:** *Name the Seven Dwarfs.*
**Direct Answer:** *Bashful, Doc, Dopey, Grumpy, Happy, Sleepy, Sneezy.*
**Flight of Ideas:** *Happily, I don't think on such a small level. Small things come in good packages. I cut myself opening my mail yesterday, it still stings. I got stung by a bee last summer, but it's only fair, since I eat honey. I have breakfast every morning because it is the most important meal of the day. I like to eat three squares when I can, but not out of the can. Cans keep food around for years, but not if you take the label off. I bought a labeling machine, and now everything in my house has a proper name. I like to address my property on a first name basis. Ah, the joys of ownership.*

An examination of these sentences reveals discernible connections, with a word acting as the focus for the next statement. Note also the abrupt and frequent change in topics.

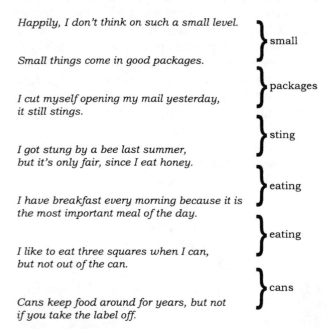

*Happily, I don't think on such a small level.*

} small

*Small things come in good packages.*

} packages

*I cut myself opening my mail yesterday, it still stings.*

} sting

*I got stung by a bee last summer, but it's only fair, since I eat honey.*

} eating

*I have breakfast every morning because it is the most important meal of the day.*

} eating

*I like to eat three squares when I can, but not out of the can.*

} cans

*Cans keep food around for years, but not if you take the label off.*

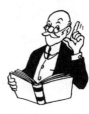

Flight of ideas is most commonly seen in:
• Mania and hypomania; flight of ideas with pressured speech is one of the cardinal signs of a manic episode
• In severe mania, patients speak in an uninterruptable monologue and head off on irrelevant tangents
• Patients often pick up on something around them to start their flight of thought; in this example, "happily" was used as a partial answer to the question, since Happy is one of the Seven Dwarfs ☺
• Flight of ideas can also be seen in psychotic disorders (e.g. schizophrenia, brief psychotic disorder, drug induced psychosis), delirium, and dementia

## IV – Rambling Speech

Rambling speech is composed of clusters of related, goal-directed sentences, which then become interspersed with statements that are not logically connected. It is characteristic of a medical or "organic" brain disorders (often alcohol related). Rambling is not as severe as loosening of associations, but lacks the connections seen in flight of ideas.

## V – Loose Associations

**Definition:** Association refers to the logical connection or "tightness" between ideas. In loose associations, a disintegration of meaningful connections between ideas occurs. Proper words, phrases, and sentences are still used. Eugene Bleuler coined the term schizophrenia to refer to a schism (divide) between thought, emotion, and behavior. He outlined four terms starting with the letter 'A' as **cardinal symptoms of schizophrenia**: affective flattening, autism, ambivalence, and associational disturbances.

**Example:**

If the example paragraph that illustrated flight of ideas is used, but every second sentence deleted (with some further editing), the following series of statements remain:

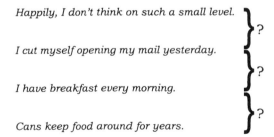

*Happily, I don't think on such a small level.* ⎫ ?

*I cut myself opening my mail yesterday.* ⎬ ?

*I have breakfast every morning.* ⎭ ?

*Cans keep food around for years.*

There is no logical connection between these sentences. Loosening of associations is characteristic of the thought process in schizophrenia and other psychotic disorders. However, mania can become so severe that the connections between ideas become lost.

# A Comparison of Thought Process Disorders

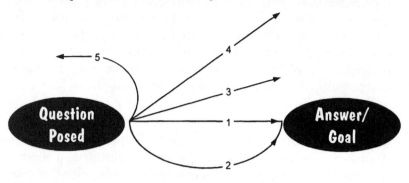

**1.** Goal-directed, logical thought addresses the point, and answers the question directly.

**2.** Circumstantial thought contains a mass of digressions, subsidiary clauses, and "talking around" the point. People are often aware of their wordiness and that their style of thinking impedes or delays reaching the goal.

**3.** Tangential thought is not goal-directed, though it starts out being relevant and generally stays in the vicinity of the topic. The point or question is not ultimately addressed, which distinguishes this from circumstantiality. If the thought process does not reach the goal and is overly detailed, it can be described as both tangential and circumstantial.

**4.** Flight of ideas takes off more quickly and radically than tangential speech. Rapid, uncensored associations are made due to increased distractibility and the pressure to keep talking. This is a form of accelerated speech.

**5.** Loosening of associations is the disruption of meaningful connections between words and phrases. Transitions are not based on logical connections between ideas.

## VIa Thought Blocking & VIb Thought Derailment

**Definition:** Thought blocking is the sudden involuntary interruption of thought (and speech) before an idea has been completed. It is not the same experience as requiring more time to formulate an idea, or being too emotionally overwhelmed to continue speaking. After a block has occurred, patient cannot recall what they were talking about. A similar interruption in thinking and movement occurs during petit mal (absence) seizures. Derailment occurs when speech begins after a short pause (a few seconds), but about another topic. Patients are unaware of the switch in topic. Derailment is the same phenomenon as loose associations. Speech is fluent and grammatically correct with these process disorders.

**Diagrammatic Representation:**

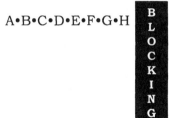
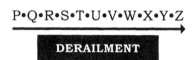

A•B•C•D•E•F•G•H

BLOCKING

P•Q•R•S•T•U•V•W•X•Y•Z

DERAILMENT

**Example:** *How about those Orioles?*
*They're the team this year! They've made some important changes. . . . . I've got to catch a midnight train to Georgia.*

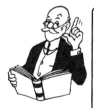

- Thought blocking is one of the negative symptoms of schizophrenia and is considered a form of **alogia**
- Thought derailment is one of the positive symptoms of schizophrenia and is considered one of the factors contributing to a **(formal) thought disorder**
- Delirious patients can also demonstrate these signs

## VII – Fragmentation

**Definition:** Fragmentation is the loss of meaningful connections between words and phrases. The speech lacks focus and does not bring about closure. It consists of phrases that are unrelated in meaning. The phrases themselves still have proper syntax and are composed of understandable words. This type of abnormality is similar to **Broca's aphasia** in its broken delivery. However, in fragmentation, the speech contains the connecting words, articulation is intact, and pauses are not notably long (recall these are features of Broca's aphasia).

**Diagrammatic Representation:**
A•B•C•D•E . . . I•J•K . . . O•P•Q•R•S•T . . .Y•Z

**Example:**
*I have to . . . . what is my . . . gone today . . . .near and far . . all or nothing at all . . flip, flop, and fly.*

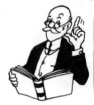

• Fragmentation is not specific for any particular illness, but can be seen in psychotic disorders, mood disorders with psychotic features, dementia, delirium, etc.

## VIII – Verbigeration

**Definition:** Also known as **palilalia**, this is the automatic repetition of words or sounds. Similar to behavioral stereotypies, verbigeration is considered to be a stereotypy of language

**Diagrammatic Representation:**
A•B•C•C•C•C . . . . B•C•C•C•C . . . .

**Example: *Where did you park your car?***
*I parked it, it, it, it . . . . . parked it, it, it, it*

Verbigeration is most commonly seen in catatonia (due to psychotic or mood disorders, and organic brain syndromes).

## IX – Jargon

**Definition:** Jargon, also called **jargon agrammatism**, **double-talk**, or **driveling**, is composed of speech that has lost its communicative value. Syntax is preserved, and speech remains fluent. This is the type of speech that is typical of **Wernicke's aphasia**. The repetition of stock phrases (perseveration) or syllables (verbigeration) is not prominent.

**Diagrammatic Representation:**
A•C•D•C . . . U•T•W•O . . . P•E•X•D•U•R•P•L•E . . .

**Example: *What was McMaster Medical School like?***
*In verbatim oval often inside making sudden. When system phones, try delayed transparency. Principles fourth at one.*

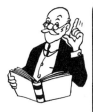

Jargon is most commonly seen as a feature of:
• Any of the causes of Wernicke's aphasia (e.g. strokes, tumors, head injuries, etc.)
• Chronic psychotic conditions with a severe course

## X – Word Salad

**Definition:** Word salad is an extreme form of loose associations, to the point where words have no connection to one another. It is as if a sentence was placed in a food processor and the diced-up words were tossed in a bowl. The speech in word salad is incomprehensible, and resembles the incoherence of **global aphasia**. Articulation in word salad remains intact, delivery is usually fluent, and prosody of speech is present. Word salad differs from fragmentation in that there is no connection between individual words (recall the *phrases* and *sentences* were unconnected in fragmentation). Word salad differs from jargon in that there is no preservation of syntax, though the speech in both thought disorders is equally meaningless.

**Diagrammatic Representation:**
A•X•Q•D•B•E•B•O•P•A•O•L•S•U•X•P•O•R•V•T•X•X•W•V•T•Z

**Example: *What are KFC's secret herbs and spices?***
*at, to, but, not, when, if, that, my, never, fuller, clip, original*

Word salad is most commonly seen in:
• Chronic schizophrenia with a severe course
• Advanced dementias, and severe delirium

## XI – Incoherence

Incoherent speech contains words that are unintelligible. The person's speech is garbled or dysarthric.

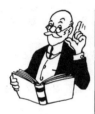

Incoherence can be caused by:
• Severe dysarthria causing indecipherable mumbling
• Extensive numbers of made-up words (**neologisms** – see p. 165)
• Private use of words (words that exist but are used in an idiosyncratic way – see p. 167)
• Severe loosening of associations (p. 159)

# Other Thought Process Disorders

• **Clang Associations (Section XII)**
• **Echolalia (XIII)**
• **Neologisms (XIV)**
• **Non sequiturs (XV)**
• **Private Use of Words (XVI)**
• **Pressure of Speech (XVII)**
• **Puns (XVIII)**
• **Rate (XIX)**
• **Rhythm (XX)**

## XII – Clang Associations

Clang associations are made on the basis of sound, not syntax or logical flow. This most frequently occurs with rhyming the last word in a sentence. In some cases, this is considered a type of **phonemic** or **literal paraphasia** where patients are compelled to substitute a word that sounds similar to one they just used.

**Example:**
*I have to go, you know. To and fro before the snow starts to blow.*

Clang associations are most commonly seen in mania, but also occur in aphasias, schizophrenia, and dementias.

## XIII – Echolalia

Echolalia has been mentioned earlier in the *Behavior Chapter* (see p. 64, 80). It is the automatic repetition of someone else's speech. Echolalia is distinguished from **perseveration** in that the words repeated are the interviewer's (not the patient's as in perseveration). Echolalia is distinguished from **palilalia (verbigeration)** in that whole phrases and sentences are repeated, not just the last word or syllable.

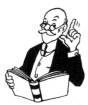

Echolalia is seen in:
• Catatonia
• Transcortical motor aphasias
• Transcortical sensory aphasias
• Dementias

## XIV – Neologisms

Neologisms are words or phrases made up by patients, and that have meanings just for them (idiosyncratic). Neologisms may be formed by the improper use of the sound of words or other perceptual abnormalities. They are also called **jargon paraphasias**. In psychiatric disorders, neologisms occur in a syntactically correct place in a patient's speech, as if they were words the interviewer wasn't familiar with. Ask about unfamiliar terms; you will either detect a neologism or learn a new word. Additionally, neologisms sound as if they could be words. For example, which in the following list are actual words?

- jolmet
- meltom
- rocer
- jingo
- monad
- regulus

The words on the left side are neologisms. The created word has a meaning that only the patient understands. Jolmet might be the border surrounding a sheet of stamps; meltom could be the ground on an electrical plug. No sense can be made from these words by breaking them down into their components. For example, *phonesia* is the act of dialing a number and forgetting whom you were calling, this is an understandable amalgamation (phone + amnesia = phonesia). Terms like these were developed, collected, and published by the comedian Rich Hall (1984). He called them **sniglets** (defined as a word that doesn't exist, but should).

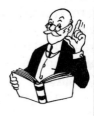

Neologisms can appear in any of the disorders of thought form listed in this chapter. They are most commonly seen in schizophrenia, but can occur in any type of psychotic disorder, dementia, and a number of the aphasias. Patients are not generally aware that their speech contains neologisms.

## XV – Non-sequiturs

Non-sequitur is Latin for *does not follow*. It has the same word root as sequence. Non-sequiturs occur as a function of normal speech and thought. If someone gets an idea or is suddenly reminded of something (e.g. got milk?), he or she will make a verbalization that is quite apart from what was just being discussed. The reply itself demonstrates proper grammar and syntax, and is not otherwise remarkable except for being off topic.

Non-sequiturs can also be a sign of pathology. Generally, they are said to occur whenever the answer is unrelated to

the question, whether interpreted literally or abstractly.
**Example:** *What is the capital of France?*

1. Paris
2. The franc
3. The letter F
4. Wine

Which of the following answers is a non-sequitur? At first glance, only (1) may seen correct. However, since *capital* can also refer to money and capital letters, only (4) is an unrelated response.

Non-sequiturs can be seen as part of several abnormalities of thought form:
• Circumstantial speech
• Tangential speech
• Loose associations
• Flight of ideas
• Derailment (with a short period of blocking)

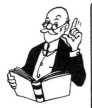

Non-sequiturs are non-specific signs of illness, but are reported to be more common in:
• Schizophrenia
• Dementias
• Aphasias
• Various types of brain injuries

## XVI — Private Use of Words

This is the incorrect use of an existing word. Syntax remains correct, but the word is used out of context. It is also called a **literal** or **semantic paraphasia**. The word substituted for the correct one is unrelated either in sound or function.

**Example:** *Yesterday I visited my friend gerund.*

Gerund is a word, but its use here is of a private nature. It was not substituted for Gerrard, which might have been either a **related (approximative)** or **literal (phonemic)** paraphasias (see also p. 127).

## XVII — Pressure of Speech (Pressure of Thought)

A rapid rate of speech is a variant of normal, and is frequently seen when patients are anxious. Pressured speech has a rapid rate with an uninterruptible, intrusive quality, as if patients are compelled to keep talking. This is also called **pressure of ideas** or **thought pressure**.

**Diagrammatic Representation**:
• At an average rate of speech, this sentence takes about 4 seconds to read.

*Rapid Psychler produces humorous and educational publications.*

• When speech is pressured, reading time is about 2 seconds, and patients will keep going (and going).

*Rapid Psychler produces humorous and educational publications.*

Pressure of speech is one of the principal signs of manic or hypomanic episodes, and is accompanied by the sensation of **racing thoughts**. The combination is expressed verbally as **flight of ideas**. These features can also occur in anxiety states, use of stimulants, and hyperthyroidism.

## XVIII — Puns

A pun is a play on words made humorous by involving double meanings or similar-sounding words.

**Example:**
• Santa's helpers are subordinate clauses.
• Buddhist to a hot dog vendor: "*Make me one with everything.*"

Continual punning can be a disorder of thought process where patients are compelled to use words for their sounds or alternate meanings (such as homonyms). In flight of ideas, the connections between words or ideas may be based on their multiple or abstract meanings.

## XIX – Rate of Speech (Rate of Thought)

The rate of speech (and thought) can vary widely in psychiatric illnesses. Rate tends to vary with amount of speech and loudness. In mania, patients speak quickly, have a lot to say, and say it loudly. Depressed patients speak in the opposite manner.

Increased rate of speech needs to be distinguished from pressure of speech. Patients who have a rapid rate of speech are: interruptible, do not appear compelled to keep speaking, and may be anxious or have medical illnesses. When asked to do so, they are able to slow down their rate of speech.

## XX – Rhythm

This was presented in the *Prosody Section* of Chapter 5.

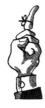

## Thought Process Practice Points

• Distinguishing word salad from Wernicke's aphasia can be very difficult
• If the associations between someone's thoughts seem loosened, point out the shift in topic and ask what the connection was between the two ideas
• Patients demonstrate loosening of associations when writing as well as speaking
• Although loose associations are considered a cardinal sign of schizophrenia, they are also seen in cognitive disorders (delirium and dementias), mood disorders (especially severe mania or psychotic depression), and drug intoxication or withdrawal states
• **Thought insertion** or **thought withdrawal** (defined in the chapter on *Thought Content*) can affect the process of thought by increasing or decreasing (respectively) the number of ideas to express
• **Condensation** is a disorder of thought process in which several concepts are expressed in a unified form; this occurs mainly in schizophrenia and substance abuse

# Psychiatry vs. Neurology

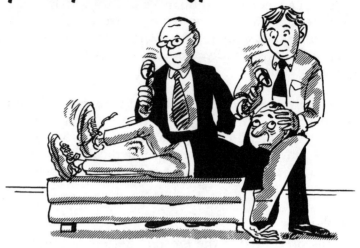

| Psychspeak | | Neurospeak |
|---|---|---|
| Driveling speech | ←→ | Jargon agrammatism |
| Neologisms | ←→ | Phonemic paraphasias |
| Private use of words | ←→ | Semantic paraphasias |
| Verbigeration | ←→ | Palilalia |

## Thought Process Disorder vs. Aphasia

A thought process disorder generally doesn't interfere with:
- Reading
- Naming
- Writing
- Repeating
- Copying

Patients may, however, be too disorganized to fully participate in the above activities. In thought process disorders,
neologisms are symbolic (replace a noun or verb), repeated,
and used in a syntactically correct way. In aphasias, they
can replace any word (non-symbolic), are not repeated, and
occur randomly. Aphasias cause the deletion of connecting
words (articles, prepositions, conjunctions, etc.), so speech
consists mainly of nouns and verbs. Patients with thought
disorders generally speak fluently with preserved syntax and
prosody.

# Summary

A formal thought disorder is one of the cardinal signs of psychosis, with the other being perceptual abnormalities. Thought can be disordered because of its content or because of how it is organized (process). Thought can only be assessed indirectly via speech, sign language, or writing. The form or process of thought involves as assessment of the following parameters:
• Goal directedness of thought
• Tightness of associations between words, phrases, sentences, and paragraphs
• Rate, pressure, and rhythm of speech
• Idiosyncracy of word usage

Speech can occur in complete sentences with good articulation and proper syntax even though a patient is psychotic. It is the flow and production of thought that reveals the impairment. Patients are generally unaware of their thought processes and cannot conceal these disorders as they might hallucinations or delusions.

Disorders of thought process show a wide range of variability, from moderate overinclusiveness to the meaningless production of words. In some disorders, patients use words based on their sound instead of their meaning. While certain types of thought process disorders have conditions they are most often associated with, there is no abnormality pathognomonic for a specific psychiatric illness.

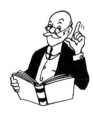

Important conditions to investigate in patients with thought process disorders are:
• Epilepsy (especially temporal lobe/partial-complex)
• Dementias
• Degenerative neurologic conditions
• Substance abuse, dependence, and withdrawal
• Strokes (cerebrovascular accidents)
• Mental retardation

# Malapropisms

A malapropism is the unintentional choice of a word that alters (or contradicts) the meaning of a statement. They are named after the character *Mrs. Malaprop* from Sheridan's comedy called *The Rivals*. For example, she referred to another character as the "pineapple of politeness" when she meant to say the "pinnacle." Other humorous substitutions were the word "illiterate" for "obliterate," and "ineffectual" for "intellectual." Here are some others:

• Homer wrote the *Oddity*, in which Penelope was the last hardship that Ulysses endured on his journey.

• Adults enjoy adultery more than infants enjoy infancy.

• Julius Caesar extinguished himself on the battlefields of Gaul.

• Mr. and Mrs. Bobbiwash request the honor of your presents at the marriage of their daughter. . .

• Rome wasn't burned in a day.

• Am I my brother's brother?

• The flooding was so bad they had to evaporate the city.

• Socrates died from an overdose of wedlock.

• Gravity was invented by Isaac Apple.

• The package was sent by partial post.

• Hamlet's son was named Piglet.

• I musterded my courage and set forth on a quest. . .

# References

## Books

American Psychiatric Association
**Diagnostic and Statistical Manual of Mental Disorders, 4th Ed.**
American Psychiatric Association, Washington D.C., 1994

R. Campbell
**Psychiatric Dictionary, 7th Ed.**
Oxford University Press, New York, 1996

R. Hall
**Sniglets**
Macmillan Publishing Co., New York, 1984

H.I. Kaplan & B.J. Sadock, Editors
**Synopsis of Psychiatry, 8th Ed.**
Williams & Wilkins, Baltimore, 1998

D.M. Kaufman
**Clinical Neurology for Psychiatrists, 5th Ed.**
W.B. Saunders, Philadelphia, 2001

L. Rolak
**Neurology Secrets**
Hanley & Belfus, Philadelphia, 1993

B.J. Sadock & V.A. Sadock, Editors
**Comprehensive Textbook of Psychiatry, 7th Ed.**
Lippincott, Williams & Wilkins, Philadelphia, 2000

A. Sims
**Symptoms in the Mind, 2nd Ed.**
Saunders, London, England, 1995

M.A. Taylor
**The Neuropsychiatric Mental Status Exam**
PMA Publishing Corp. New York, 1981

E.L. Zuckerman
**The Clinician's Thesaurus, 5th Ed.**
Clinician's Toolbox, The Guilford Press, New York, 2000

# Articles

B. Butterworth
**Hesitation and the Production of Verbal Paraphasias and Neologisms in Jargon Aphasia**
*Brain Lang.* 8(2): 133 – 161, 1979

D. Caplan, L. Kellar, & S. Locke
**Inflection of Neologisms in Aphasia**
*Brain* 95(1): 169 – 172, 1972

A. Crider
**Perseveration in Schizophrenia**
*Schizophrenia Bull.* 23(1): 63 – 74, 1997

D.V. Forrest
**New Words and Neologisms – With a Thesaurus of Coinages by a Schizophrenic Savant**
*Psychiatry* 32(1): 44 – 73, 1969

E. Goldberg
**Varieties of Perseveration: A Comparison of Two Taxonomies**
*J. Clin. Exp. Neuropsychology* 8(6): 710 – 726

G. Hotz & N. Helm-Estabrooks
**Perseveration Part I: A Review**
*Brain Inj.* 9(2): 151 – 159, 1995

G. Hotz & N. Helm-Estabrooks
**Perseveration Part II: A Study of Perseveration in Closed Head Injury**
*Brain Inj.* 9(2): 161 – 172, 1995

V.C. Jampala, M.A. Taylor, & R. Abrams
**The Diagnostic Implications of Formal Thought Disorder in Mania and Schizophrenia: A Reassessment**
*American Journal of Psychiatry* 146(4): 459–63, 1989

R. Joseph
**Frontal Lobe Psychopathology: Mania, Depression, Confabulation, Catatonia, Perseveration, Obsessive Compulsions, and Schizophrenia**
*Psychiatry* 62(2): 138 – 172, 1999

W.T. LeVine & R.L. Conrad
**The Classification of Schizophrenic Neologisms**
*Psychiatry* 42(2): 177 – 181, 1979

L.G. Lippman & M.L. Dunn
**Contextual Connections Within Puns: Effects on Perceived Humor and Memory**
*J. Gen. Psychology* 127(2): 185 – 197, 2000

W.R. McLeod
**Loose Associations: Straight and Crooked Thinking and the Group of Schizophrenias.**
*Aust N Z J Psychiatry* 12(4): 221 – 31, 1978

J.M. Roberts
**Echolalia and Comprehension in Autistic Children**
*J. Autism Dev. Disorders* 19(2): 271 – 281, 1989

F.B. Rogers
**Primitive Thought Process and Mental Illness**
*NJ Med.* 90 (12): 923 – 924, 1993

J. Sandon & M.L. Albert
**Varieties of Perseveration**
*Neuropsychologia* 22(6): 715 – 732, 1984

A. Siegel, M. Harrow, F.E. Reilly, & G.J. Tucker
**Loose Associations and Disordered Speech Patterns in Chronic Schizophrenia**
*J. Nerv. Ment. Dis.* 162(2): 105 – 112, 1976

J. Volden & C. Lord
**Neologisms and Idiosyncratic Language in Autistic Speakers**
*J. Autism Dev. Disorders* 21(2): 109 – 130, 1991

J. Willis-Shore, J.H. Poole, H. Skinner, L. Benioff, & S. Vinogradov
**Two Commonly Used Indices of Thought Disorder**
*Schizophrenia Research* 42(3): 261–2, 2000

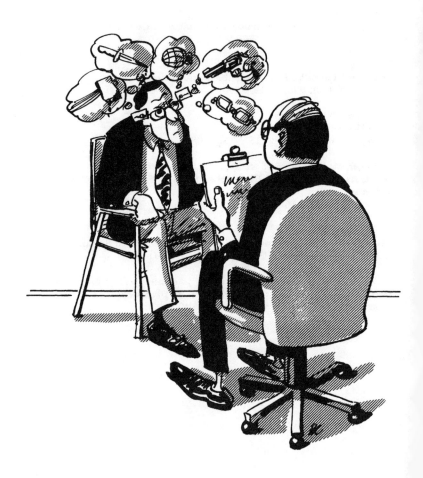

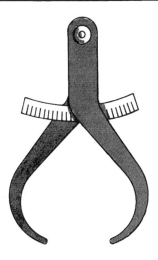

# Chapter 7

# Thought Content

## What Is Thought Content?

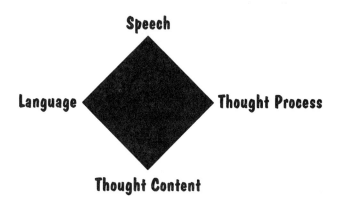

Thought content refers to *what* patients talk about in the body of the interview. While it may be tempting to say, "Ms. C.Y. answered the questions I asked her," an interview is guided by the content of the answers given, with lines questioning being refined by the information patients provide.

One of the key reasons the beginning of an interview is left unstructured is to allow an assessment of thought content. Special attention should be given to what patients talk about spontaneously, elaborate on, and what themes develop as they speak. This acts as a type of *projective test* because patients talk about what is important to them, and "project" their concerns in the interview. As stressors or symptoms are elicited, exploration along the lines of who, what, where, when, why, and how help guide the flow of relevant material while allowing patients the chance to continue speaking in a relatively unrestricted manner. Interviews that consist of a closed-ended or laundry-list approach restrict the flow of spontaneous information.

# What Is the Diagnostic Significance of Abnormalities in Thought Content?

Abnormalities of thought content are integral in the diagnosis of many mental illnesses.

• **Schizophrenia** 295.X
• **Brief Psychotic Disorder** 298.8
• **Schizophreniform Disorder** 295.40
• **Schizoaffective Disorder** 295.70
A. (1) Delusions

• **Delusional Disorder** 297.1
A. Non-bizarre delusions

• **Shared Psychotic Disorder (folie à deux)** 297.3
A. A delusion develops in an individual in the context of a close relationship with another person who has an established delusion

• **Major Depressive Episode** 296.X
A. (7) . . . excessive or inappropriate guilt (which may be delusional). . .

• **Manic Episode/Hypomanic Episode** 296.X
B. (1) Inflated self-esteem or grandiosity

• **Specific Phobia** 300.29
A. Marked and persistent fear that is excessive or unreasonable, cued by the presence or anticipation of a specific object or situation.

• **Social Phobia** 300.23
A. A marked and persistent fear of one or more social or performance situations in which the person is exposed to unfamiliar people or to possible scrutiny by others. . .

• **Obsessive-Compulsive Disorder** 300.3
A. *Obsessions:*
(1) Recurrent and persistent thoughts, impulses, or images that are experienced, at some time during the disturbance, as intrusive and inappropriate and that cause marked anxiety or distress
(2) The thoughts, impulses, or images are not simply excessive worries about real-life problems
(4) The person recognizes that the obsessional thoughts, impulses, or images are a product of his or her own mind
*Compulsions:*
(1) Repetitive behaviors or mental acts that the person feels driven to perform in response to an obsession, or according to rules that must be applied rigidly

• **Posttraumatic Stress Disorder** 309.81
B. (1) Recurrent and intrusive distressing recollections of the event, including images, thoughts, or perceptions

• **Hypochondriasis** 300.7
A. Preoccupation with fears of having, or the idea that one has, a serious disease based on the person's misinterpretation of bodily symptoms

• **Paranoid Personality Disorder** 301.0
A. (1) Suspects, without sufficient basis, that others are exploiting, harming, or deceiving him or her
(2) Is preoccupied with unjustified doubts about the loyalty of trustworthiness of friends or associates
(7) Has recurrent suspicions, without justification, regarding the fidelity of spouse or sexual partner

• **Schizotypal Personality Disorder** 301.22
A. (1) Ideas of reference (excluding delusions of reference)
(2) Odd beliefs or magical thinking that influences behavior and is inconsistent with subcultural norms
(4) Odd thinking and speech
(5) Suspiciousness or paranoid ideation

• **Borderline Personality Disorder** 301.83
A. (9) Transient, stress-related paranoid ideation. . .

• **Antisocial Personality Disorder** 301.7
A. (7) Lack of remorse, as indicated by being indifferent to or rationalizing having hurt, mistreated, or stolen from another

• **Narcissistic Personality Disorder** 301.81
A. (1) Has a grandiose sense of self-importance
(2) Is preoccupied with fantasies of unlimited success, power, brilliance, beauty, or love
(3) Believes that he or she is "special" and unique and can only be understood by, or should associate with, other special or high status people (or institutions)
(5) Has a sense of entitlement
(8) Is often envious of others or believes that others are envious of him or her

• **Avoidant Personality Disorder** 301.82
A. (4) Is preoccupied with being criticized or rejected in social situations

• **Dependent Personality Disorder** 301.6
A. (8) Is unrealistically preoccupied with fears of being left

to take care of himself or herself

**• Obsessive-Compulsive Personality Disorder** 301.4
A. (1) Is preoccupied with details, rules, lists, order, organization, or schedules to the extent that the major point of the activity is lost
(4) Is overconscientious, scrupulous, and inflexible about matters of morality, ethics, or values
(8) Shows rigidity and stubbornness

Diagnostic Criteria are from the DSM-IV.
© American Psychiatric Association, Washington, D.C. 1994
Reprinted with permission.

# What Constitutes a Disorder of Thought Content?

Thought content is considered abnormal when it contains any of the following elements:

**• Delusions (Section I)**
      Persecutory (Paranoid)
      Grandiose
      Jealous
      Erotomanic
      Somatic
      Passivity and Control
      Other Delusions
      Culture-Bound Syndromes
      Mood Congruence & Ego Syntonicity

**• Overvalued Ideas (II)**
**• Obsessions (III)**
**• Phobias (IV)**
**• Suicidal Thoughts (Chapter 8)**
**• Homicidal Thoughts (Chapter 8)**

To paraphrase a famous quote, *the ebb and flow of thoughts have a direct effect on emotional health.* Patients experiencing delusions, obsessions, or phobias often seek attention because their lives, or the lives of those around them, are significantly disrupted. On the other hand, some patients are adept at concealing such experiences and make them difficult to elicit, especially in a first interview. The degree of awareness of having abnormal thoughts (called **insight**) varies widely. Impaired or absent insight is usually a sign of a more serious disturbance and/or worse prognosis. The abnormalities of thought presented here can evoke a wide range of emotional responses in patients.

Because of the seriousness of suicidal and homicidal thoughts, they are presented in the next chapter.

# I — Delusions

Delusions are one of the cardinal symptoms of serious mental illness, though they are not specific to a particular condition. Delusions have been reported in over fifty psychiatric and general medical conditions.

The word itself comes from the Latin *delirare,* which means lunacy. Literally translated, the word means, "to become unhinged," "to go out of the furrow," or "to deviate from a straight line" [using the roots *de* (from) and *lira* (furrow or track)]. Though delusion and delirium have the same word root, they describe conditions which are quite different.

A delusion is defined as a fixed, false belief that:
• Is inconsistent with cultural or subcultural norms
• Is inappropriate for the person's level of education
• Is not altered with proof to the contrary (incorrigibility)
• Preoccupies the patient to such a great extent that he or she finds it difficult to avoid thinking or speaking about it
• Is not resisted by the patient
• Ranges from implausible to impossible
• Places the patient at the center of events
• Is a self-evident truth to the person (subjective certainty)

The content of delusions ranges from **fragmented** to **systematized**, and from situations that are possible (**non-bizarre**) to those that are impossible (**bizarre**). In cases where a patient appears to have a discrete, plausible, but false belief (e.g. someone is reading my mail), it may only be possible to establish if this is a delusion with additional (corollary) information. Cultural differences can also account for "unusual" ideas, and it is behooves us to investigate this possibility. In order to distinguish a delusion from other abnormalities of thought content, it is crucial to establish that it is indeed *fixed*. Someone who is confabulating (or who is being deliberately misleading) will change some part of the history when asked to repeat the details.

## How Do Delusions Start?

In order for delusions to develop, a combination of predisposing factors needs to be present. Examples include:
• Impairment of brain functioning
• A personality disorder (causing a distortion of reality)
• An inability to manage stress which impacts on a genetic vulnerability (diathesis) to decompensate; this is called the **stress-diathesis model** of mental illness

Specific factors that are thought to be operative are:
• **Delusional intuition (autochthonous delusions)** describes the sudden arrival of an idea which automatically becomes a belief; this is similar to a "eureka" experience which comes "out of the blue," and illustrates the self-evident aspect of a delusion in that if a patient believes it, it must be true ("Make it so.")
• **Delusional perception** refers to the abnormal significance ascribed to a real stimulus; for example, a patient hears an air-conditioner start and assumes she is about to be exposed to poison gas (note: this occurs in someone who was not previously paranoid)
• **Delusional atmosphere/delusional mood** is the experience where the environment appears altered so everything seems unusual, ominous, or even threatening; the surroundings seem peculiar and a significant event is felt to be immi-

nent; frequently patients are apprehensive until an understanding (though arbitrary and false) of the situation can be reached

• **Delusional memory/retrospective delusions** refers to the faulty recollection of memories in a way that adds "proof" to current beliefs

Delusions that start *de novo* as a result of the above (or other factors) are called **primary delusions**. **Secondary delusions** arise out of a mood state, perceptual abnormality (including sensory deprivation or impairment), social factors, or any pre-existing psychopathology.

Delusions often contain a *kernel of truth* or are based on a *key experience*. The subsequent handling of this experience is overly personalized, extended, and held to such an extreme level of conviction that it is not amenable to logic. For example, a patient who suffers from delusional infestation with parasites may initially have had lice. Another patient who claims to have a romantic connection with a movie star may have met that person, but then extends this connection into an erotomanic delusion (see p. 192).

Delusional patients have an altered process of reasoning. **Apophony** (from the Greek *to become manifest*) is the phenomenon in which arbitrary or false ideas are considered fact without adequate proof. Events and objects become imbued with a personal, autistic significance (also called the **residuum**). Apophony is also used to refer to the attribution of new meanings for psychological events (like delusional perception or delusional atmosphere outlined on the previous page).

Delusional patients also make sweeping inferences based on small amounts of information (called **generalization**). They do not use their knowledge or experience to modify their beliefs.

**Social Attribution Theory** posits that delusional patients excessively ascribe negative events to external factors. A patient who passes through a radar trap (without speeding) is convinced that it was arranged so the police could monitor his actions. Conversely, positive events are thought to occur purely for internal reasons (e.g. a patient wins a lottery because she has a divine connection, and this is a reward for her continued efforts).

Delusions become a psychological compromise that makes sense of the internal chaos and external reality with which patients must contend. This process is called **consolidation**. This is the central principle in the theory of **adaptation**, which posits that symptoms are formed in mental illnesses as a means of survival. The content of delusions is not random, but a highly personalized representation of the patient's inner world.

## What Is the Psychodynamic Understanding of Delusions?

Delusions serve important psychological functions for patients in whom they occur. Delusions can be understood in terms of fulfilling an unconscious wish or a psychological need. One of the best explanations of delusions is that they allow a person to project onto the environment specific feelings (such as hate) that are unacceptable to him on a conscious level.

Historical information about delusional patients often reveals experiences with hostility in early relationships. This becomes internalized as a model for future relationships. In adulthood, this hostility becomes projected onto the external world, a process which helps satisfy internal emotional needs, but results in false convictions about the environment.

Delusions are maintained because they help bolster the low self-esteem of patients. In a primitive way, delusions provide meaning to the lives of those who suffer from them. Patients who were previously isolated, hopeless, or felt they had little purpose in life now have something to rally around.

Common delusional themes can be related to **Erickson's Life Cycle Stages**:

| Stage | Central Issue | Theme of Delusion |
|---|---|---|
| • Basic Trust vs. Basic Mistrust | Safety | Paranoia |
| • Autonomy vs. Shame & Doubt | Bodily Functions | Somatization |
| • Initiative vs. Guilt | Achievement | Grandiosity |
| • Industry vs. Inferiority | Achievement | Grandiosity |
| • Identity vs. Role Diffusion | Love | Jealousy & Erotomania |
| • Intimacy vs. Isolation | Love | Jealousy & Erotomania |

## How Do I Ask About Delusions?

Formulating questions about delusions constitutes one of the most difficult tasks during an interview. As opposed to patients with phobias or obsessions, delusional patients usually don't recognize that they are ill. Asking, "So, are you delusional?" probably won't work, making more refined means necessary.

### 1. Watch for themes during the interview:
Despite the complexity of mental illnesses, most delusions fall into a small number of themes (paranoid, somatic, grandiose, jealous, etc.).

### 2. Questions to help detect the presence of delusions:
• *"What's been on your mind recently?"*
• *"Do you spend a lot of time thinking about one or two things?"*
• *"Do you have some ideas that you hold very strongly?"*
• *"Do others frequently disagree with your views on things?"*
• *"When you aren't busy with something, what do you think about?"*
• *"What are the things that are most important to you?"*

Because delusions dominate thinking (and also mood and behavior to a large extent), these questions are likely to reveal some aspect of delusional thinking if it is present. When patients mention something that could be of a delusional nature, respond with curiosity. An interested, conversational manner will elicit more information.

**3. Questions to examine (potentially) delusional material:**
• *"I'm interested in what you just said – tell me more."*
• *"How do you know this is the case?"*
• *"How did all this start?"*
• *"Why would someone want to do this to you?"*
• *"What's happened so far?"*
• *"How do you account for what has taken place?"*

Irrespective of interviewing skill, delusions can't always be elicited. Patients who have some awareness that others don't share their ideas (preserved insight), or who have been hospitalized because of delusions, may conceal their thoughts.

## How Do I Deal With Delusions Once They Are Expressed?

It is important to bear in mind that delusions represent reality to patients who experience them. Your reactions (verbal and behavioral) have a significant degree of influence over what patients will share. As mentioned, an inquisitive approach that investigates the extent of the delusional thinking is optimal. Novice interviewers often make one of two mistakes (some make both) when uncovering delusional material:
• Adopting a nonchalant, lackluster demeanor, as if not to frighten the patient by showing too much interest
• Sitting bolt upright with a widened stare, sharpened pencil, and demonstrating an unprecedented level of interest in the interview

Guidelines for handling delusions are as follows:
• Don't interrogate patients – a rapid-fire approach will usually miss delusions in the first place; an undue degree of

interest or change in interviewing style may have a special, idiosyncratic meaning for the patient (e.g. you become part of the delusion because of your interest)
• Don't argue with patients – no delusion has been cured by logic or providing any degree of proof to the contrary; it can be very tempting to "enlighten" patients or point out the obvious contradictions or weaknesses in their understanding of events
• Empathize with patients to preserve rapport and facilitate the sharing of more information
• Tactfully avoid being the arbiter of reality and telling patients whether or not you agree with them
• If pressed to render an opinion, try something like:
  *"I'm keeping an open mind."*
  *"I can't decide without more information."*
  *"My job is to understand what your views are."*

## Ia – Persecutory (Paranoid) Delusions

Paranoia, literally translated from Greek, means, "a mind beside itself." These are the most common delusions, regardless of which disorder the patient has. Paranoia exists on a spectrum in psychiatric illnesses:

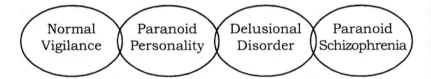

| Normal Vigilance | Paranoid Personality | Delusional Disorder | Paranoid Schizophrenia |

**Projection** is the main ego defense involved in paranoia. In persecutory delusions, an internal threat is substituted with an external one. An external agency (individual or group) is accused of acting against the patient. Patients often have a knack of making the projections "fit" the group being accused (e.g. fear of being "framed" by a group of criminals). Paranoid patients are hypervigilant, and miss little that goes on around them. Their difficulties arise out of the automatic assumption that others are conspiring against them (also called **delusional misinterpretation**).

**Paranoid Themes**
- Being followed
- Being monitored (tape recorded, videotaped, etc.)
- Having things stolen, particularly while the patient is away from home
- Being poisoned or drugged
- Having one's reputation ruined or integrity maligned
- Prejudice, slights, obstruction from long-term goals
- **Querulous paranoia** is the continual involvement of the legal system to remedy perceived injustices
- Repeated difficulties with authority figures
- Criticism of those seen as weaker or needy
- Searching intensively to confirm suspicions to the exclusion of more reasonable conclusions

## 1b – Grandiose Delusions/Delusions of Grandeur

Grandiose delusions involve impossible levels of wealth, fame, power, physical ability, etc. The achievements extend beyond the range of human achievement to include supernatural powers or omnipotence. Patients will tell you, sometimes in the same breath, about their accumulated billions, close relationships with the rich and famous, and plans for the global takeover of several businesses.

Grandiose delusions bear a similarity to persecutory delusions in that everything that happens around the patient must have something to do with that person. This is called **self-referential grandiosity**.

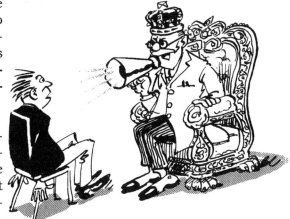

In some instances, patients have the expectation that they are in training for a secret mission. In this sense, their beliefs are some-what opposite the persecutory type in that the patient is now *involved* as a clandestine operative.

In psychiatric conditions, grandiose delusions are seen in schizophrenia and mania. The narcissistic personality disorder has an overlap with the self-aggrandizing aspects of these delusions. However, narcissistic personalities are not delusional, and consider themselves capable of feats within the realm of human achievement. Differentiation of narcissism from the non-bizarre delusions in a delusional disorder may be more difficult.

**Grandiose Themes**
• Entitlement and privilege
• Ability to endow people or machines with special powers
• Religion or royalty are often involved
• May make attempts to contact famous people
• Distorted perception of limits of abilities
• Has a great but unrecognized talent
• Takes credit for one or several remarkable discoveries

## Ic — Delusions of Jealousy
This is generally considered to be the unfounded conviction that one's spouse or loved one is being unfaithful. However, the term **delusion of infidelity** is more specific to this condition. **Morbid** or **malignant jealousy** can be used to describe situations where jealousy is the predominant content without the sexual component.

What makes it difficult to distinguish a delusion from justified jealousy is that infidelity is usually a discreet process. It can be almost impossible for the accused person to prove his or her fidelity. Ironically, continued accusations can actually drive a partner into another relationship. In a sense, this makes the *crime fit the punishment* through the process of **projective identification**. Here, patients induce others to behave in a way that justifies their suspicions. This can also be thought of as a *self-fulfilling prophecy*. Additionally, the accused partner is often attractive or outgoing, which adds substance to the claims of infidelity.

This delusion frequently starts with the patient projecting his or her libidinal wishes. He or she may desire another lover, and by projecting these (unacceptable) urges outward, blames the spouse/partner for harboring them. The patient may have been promiscuous in the past, and automatically assumes that his current partner will stray. Another common finding is that the patient is overly dependent on the partner, and may wish for complete possession of that person.

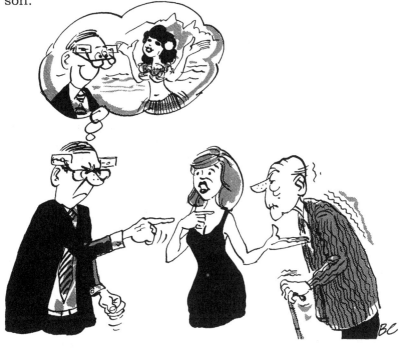

Delusions of jealousy can occur in males when they become impotent or have homosexual urges for the men with whom their partner is supposedly involved. Delusional jealousy is also seen in alcohol abusers and after head injuries. It is notoriously difficult to treat, often remaining stable for years. This delusion is among the most likely to cause patients to take action against the partner and/or others involved.

## Id – Erotomanic Delusions

In erotomania, patients are convinced that someone is secretly in love with them. The object of this delusion is often a famous, rich, or powerful person. It occurs more frequently in women, and has been called "old maid's insanity." Other terms for the condition are **de Clérambault's syndrome** and **psychose passionelle**.

Patients with this delusion can be extreme nuisances to public figures. They will devote extraordinary energy and many hours of time to get the attention of the object of their desires. Erotomanic patients may commit crimes such as break & enter, kidnapping, blackmail, or even make false accusations of sexual assault or paternity in order to make contact with the person.

Affected individuals arbitrarily assign significance to unremarkable events as a sign that their target still loves them. For example, if a political figure wears a blue suit when giving a speech, it is a clear indication to the delusional patient that a bond exists. **Paradoxical conduct** refers to the situation where all efforts to deny a romantic link are interpreted by the patient as further proof that a secret connection exists.

There is some debate regarding the course of erotomanic delusions, and the level of danger for the person involved (the object of the delusion). Some authors report erotomania to be short-lived, and as an actual relationship becomes less and less likely with time, patients seek other attachments. Other authors report that this delusion cannot only continue for years, but there have been instances where patients commit suicide and/or homicide upon confronting the person to whom they are attracted.

A related delusion, called the **phantom lover syndrome**, is the conviction of being loved by someone who doesn't exist, but is identified as an "ordinary person."

## le – Somatic Delusions

Somatic delusions involve illness or bodily functions. **Monosymptomatic hypochondriacal delusions** (take a breath before you say this out loud) are encapsulated beliefs patients have about certain aspects of their bodies. The most common varieties are:

• **Delusions of odor** – patients are convinced they have a foul smell about them that cannot be removed; bad breath (halitosis) or body odor are the most common foci for delusions; patients do not experience consistently unpleasant smells (apart from their beliefs about their own bodies) and do not have olfactory hallucinations

• **Delusions of infestation/dermatozoic delusions** – these usually involve micro-organisms (germs, microbes, parasites) or small but visible infectious agents that inhabit the internal organs or skin; snakes, rodents, and insects are frequently described as the source of the infestation

• **Delusions of appearance (body dysmorphism)** – involve an exaggerated or entirely fabricated physical defect; patients are convinced they are disfigured and that this is immediately obvious to any observer

Somatic delusions can range from possible (a blood infection) to bizarre (a missing heart). Again, they are often centered around an actual, but mild, illness or discomfort. **Hypochondriasis**, **body dysmorphic disorder**, and **conversion disorder** have an overlap with this condition but are distinguishable in that patients do not hold their ideas to a delusional level of intensity in these conditions. Somatic delusions are most commonly seen in depression and schizophrenia. However, other psychotic disorders, alcohol and cocaine withdrawal, partial-complex epilepsy, and strokes can also be accompanied by these convictions. Frequently, patients will have seen many physicians and "doctor shop" to find someone who believes them and is willing to exhaustively investigate their symptoms.

## If — Delusions of Passivity or Control

Kurt Schneider proposed that particular symptoms were of pragmatic value in diagnosing schizophrenia (called **pathognomonic findings**). He enumerated eleven specific findings and called these **first-rank symptoms**. There are also second-rank symptoms, which Schneider thought could be used on their own to diagnose schizophrenia.

Of the eleven symptoms, eight involve delusions that cause the patient to feel under the control of external forces and respond passively (**passivity experiences**). The others are hallucinations and are covered in the *Perception Chapter*.

### Experiences of Thought Control
**1. Thought Broadcasting** – patients experience their thoughts as being automatically broadcast to others, or lost to the external world (as if by television or radio)
**2. Thought Insertion** – thoughts are placed into the patient's head from an outside source
**3. Thought Withdrawal** – thoughts are removed or stolen from the patient's head before they can be expressed

### Experiences of Influence
**4. Insertion of Sensation/Somatic passivity** – submission to an external controlling force
**5. Insertion of Feelings** – made or forced feelings
**6. Insertion of Impulses** – submission to an impulse
**7. Insertion of an Outside Will** – passivity of volition

### 8. Delusional Perception
This is the attribution of a false (delusional) meaning to an ordinary event (covered on p. 183 – 184).

**First-rank symptoms** remain an important component of many diagnostic systems for schizophrenia, but they have not been found to be sensitive or specific for the diagnosis.

## Ig – Other Delusions

Despite their great variety, delusions fall into a relatively compact set of themes. As indicated earlier, delusions often relate to early developmental needs, issues, struggles, and milestones.

Common themes involve: nonexistence, one's body, self, and the outside world. Delusions are given the suffix "mania" to denote an exaggerated interest in, or preference for something, but also implying a behavior or action. Other aspects of thought content are given the suffix "philia" indicating a disposition towards something. For example, *pyromania* refers to fire setting and *pyrophilia* refers to an excessive interest in fires.

### Some Common Delusions
• **Animal Metamorphosis** – cat (galeanthropy), dog (cynanthropy), wolf (lycanthropy)
• **Cacodaemonomania** – poisoned by an evil spirit
• **Caesarmania** – delusion of grandiose ability (or inventing a garlic-laden salad)
• **Capgras' Syndrome** – an impostor has replaced someone significant to the patient and has an identical appearance; also called negative misidentification (e.g. "It looks like my wife, but I know that it is not her.")
• **Delusion of Reference** – ascribing personal meaning to common events; often involves the TV, newspapers, or radio as having special messages just for the patient, but can include idiosyncratic associations (a bird flew by, therefore my car is low on oil); if held to a lesser degree of conviction, these are called **ideas of reference**
• **Doppelganger** – having a double
• **Dorian Gray** – the person stays the same age while everyone else ages
• **Enosimania** – guilt, unworthiness for having committed some catastrophic deed
• **Folie à deux** – a delusion is transferred from a psychotic person to a recipient who accepts the belief
• **Folie induite** – transfer of a delusion to someone who is

already psychotic; a delusion added to a pre-existing one
• **Fregoli's Syndrome** – a persecutor impersonates people the patient sees; also called positive misidentification (e.g. "They may look different, but I know these people are my enemies in disguise.")
• **Incubus** – a demonic lover
• **Intermetamorphosis** – a familiar person (usually a persecutor) and a misidentified stranger share both physical and psychological attributes
• **Magical Thinking** – believing that an event will occur simply by wishing it so, as if by magic
• **Messianic** – being God (also called **theomania**)
• **Mignon** – being of royal lineage
• **Nihilism** – nonexistence; loss of organs, body or everything; damnation; sense of death or disintegration; also called **Cotard's syndrome**
• **Phantom Boarder** – unwelcome delusional house guests
• **Poverty** – loss of all wealth and property
• **Reduplicative Paramnesia** – thinking that people, places or body parts have been duplicated (**heutoscopy** is also the delusion of having a double)
• **Wahnstimmung** (German) – delusions of persecution

## Ih – Culture-Bound Syndromes
A sampling of delusions from other cultures . . .
• **Brain Fag** – belief that the brain can suffer fatigue from overuse (particularly after exams)
• **Koro** – belief the penis or vulva will recede into the body and cause death (differentiate this from **kuru** which is a slow virus infection causing neurologic degeneration)
• **Rootwork/mal puesto** – belief that one can subject others, or be subjected to, hexes, spells, or curses
• **Taijin kyofusho** – the belief that one's body or its parts and functions are offensive to others
• **Windigo** – delusion that one can be transformed into a giant monster that eats human flesh
• **Zar** – delusional possession by a spirit

## Ii – Mood Congruence & Ego Syntonicity

The terms **mood-congruent** and **mood-incongruent** are applied to delusions and hallucinations (psychotic features) that complicate mood disorders.

Common themes in depression are: guilt, worthlessness, death, failure, hopelessness, punishment, illness, etc. If the content of delusions in depressed patients forms along these lines, the term **mood-congruent** is applied.

In manic episodes, mood-congruent delusions follow the themes of: power, brilliance, wealth, longevity, achievement, special relationships or connections, knowledge, etc.

Manic patients with delusions of nihilism, poverty, or inadequacy have **mood-incongruent delusions**, as would depressed patients with delusions of grandeur, omnipotence, or relationships with famous people.

Mood-incongruent psychotic features represent a distinct subtype of mood disorder, and their presence has treatment and prognostic implications that are presented in the *Affect & Mood Chapter*.

The term **ego-syntonic** is used to refer to symptoms that are not foreign or distressing to patients. Patients do not experience delusional thoughts as disturbing. The delusional beliefs become accepted as reality, and are therefore ego-syntonic. For example, paranoid patients are not disturbed by their continual thoughts of persecution. Instead, they accept that the world is this way and are vigilant for evidence to confirm that they are being conspired against, etc.

Ego-syntonicity is central to the definition of a personality disorder. Here, a patient's attitudes and actions are not subjectively distressing. Instead, problems are created for those who interact with the patient. Similarly, because a delusional patient doesn't challenge his or her convictions, it is those around the patient who suffer the consequences.

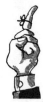

### Delusion-Related Practice Points

• Movies/plays that contain delusional themes are: *Cat People* (galeanthropy); *Unfaithfully Yours,* and *Othello* (delusion of infidelity); *Invasion of the Body Snatchers* (Capgras); *Rosemary's Baby* (cacodaemonomania)

• Many attempts have been made to relate the theme of a delusion to a specific illness – for example, nihilistic delusions to depression or thought broadcasting to schizophrenia; while certain illnesses are more commonly linked to specific delusions, this association is not reliable enough to be an indication of diagnosis

• **Systematization** refers to the degree to which delusions are organized; chronically psychotic patients can develop elaborate delusional systems that remain stable over time and incorporate new parameters into the *scheme* or *matrix* of the delusion

• Systematized delusions are most often seen in illnesses with a chronic psychotic component; fleeting or unstable delusions are more typical of organic cognitive disorders

# II – Overvalued Ideas

An overvalued idea differs from a delusion in that:
• It is less firmly held
• The content is less absurd
• It is not systematized

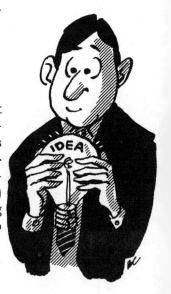

Beliefs become *overvalued* in that they preoccupy the patient's thinking and alter his behavior. Examples of overvalued ideas are **superstitions** or **magical thinking**. A superstitious (as opposed to delusional) patient will concede that walking under a ladder isn't really likely to change his luck.

# III – Obsessions

An obsession is a thought, impulse, or image that is:
• Recurrent and persistent
• Unwanted (called **ego-alien** or **ego-dystonic**)
• Not simply an exaggerated degree of concern over current problems
• Recognized as a product of the patient's own mind; obsessions are generated from *within* as opposed to from *without* (as in **thought insertion**)
• Not able to be controlled by the person's will
• Recognized as absurd and irrational (preserved insight)
• Resisted, at least at some point to some degree
• Accompanied by a sense of *anxious dread*
• Usually paired with a compulsion to decrease anxiety

## Obsessive Themes

Like delusions, obsessions tend to fall into a relatively small number of themes:

| Theme | Obsession |
|---|---|
| Cleanliness | Contamination |
| Order | Symmetry, Precision |
| Sex & Aggression | Assault, Sexual Assault, Homicide, Insults |
| Doubt | Safety, Catastrophe, Unworthiness |

Another scheme for classifying obsessions is as follows:
• **Intellectual Obsessions** – involve philosophical or metaphysical questions surrounding life, the universe & everything; destiny; curved space; gravity waves, etc.
• **Inhibiting Obsessions** – doubts or prohibitions about actions which may be harmful to others; the patient may become withdrawn or isolated to ensure such actions do not occur
• **Impulsive Obsessions** – urges to steal, collect (hoard), count (**arithomania**)

## How Do I Ask About Obsessions?

Obsessions are recognized by patients as being absurd and distressing, yet they are not expressed as prominently in interviews as are delusions. Suggestions for questions are:
• *"Do you experience repetitive thoughts that you can't stop? Do they feel like your own thoughts?"*
• *"Are you ever forced to think something against your will?"*

Another approach is to ask specific questions involving the major themes of obsessions:
• *"Do you have intrusive thoughts about. . . (contamination, hurting someone, having to count something, etc.)?"*

## How Do Obsessions Begin?

Obsessions tend to fall within a small number of themes, with aggression, cleanliness, and order being the most prominent. In Freud's psychosexual stages of development, these are the issues that dominate the **anal phase**. Control and autonomy are the key outcomes from this stage. Freud linked obsessive behaviors to difficulties during the anal stage of development, and defined the **anal triad** as consisting of parsimoniousness, orderliness, and obstinacy (mnemonic – P.O.O.).

Toilet training is usually the first intrusion of socialization into an infant's otherwise unrestrained existence. Achieving continence involves submitting to parental expectations on demand, and then being judged on the outcome. When children fail at the task, overambitious or demanding parents evoke feelings of being bad and dirty. Issues of cleanliness, timeliness, stubbornness, and control can reasonably be seen as linked to this stage of development. Failing to produce on schedule, with an immediate perception of disappointment, arouses feelings of anger and aggression. **Ambivalence** develops as a result of the simultaneous existence of longing (love) and aggressive wishes (hate). This conflict of opposing emotions paralyzes the patient with doubt and indecision, and can result in the **doing-undoing** pattern seen with obsessions and compulsions. **Magical**

**thinking** is also a component of obsessive-compulsive disorder (OCD) in that the obsession is given great power, and is deemed to have more of a connection to events than is realistic. For example, having thoughts of a disaster does not make it occur. The ego defenses are used to modify the expression of unfulfilled dependency wishes, or strong feelings (anger) directed at caregivers are:

• **Isolation (of affect)** separates or strips an idea from its accompanying feeling or affect. This is the predominant defense contributing to the obsessive component. An idea is made conscious, but the feelings are kept within the unconscious. When this defense is used to a lesser degree, three others mechanisms may be used:
    **Intellectualization** – excessive use of abstract thinking
    **Moralization** – morality isolates contradictory feelings
    **Rationalization** – justifying unacceptable attitudes

• **Undoing** involves an action, either verbalization or behavior, that symbolically makes amends for conflicts, stresses, or unacceptable wishes. This is the predominant defense contributing to the compulsive component.

• **Reaction Formation** transforms an impulse into a diametrically opposed thought, feeling or behavior. This is frequently seen as a "counterdependent" attitude in which patients (primarily with obsessive-compulsive personalities) eradicate dependency on anyone. Similarly, maintaining a calm exterior guards against the awareness of angry feelings. For example, orderliness is a reaction formation against the childhood desire to play with feces or to make a mess.

• **Displacement** redirects feelings from a conflict or stressor onto a symbolically related, but less threatening, person or object. "Kicking the dog" or "shooting the messenger" are examples of this defense.

Anger or aggression towards caregivers becomes unconsciously forbidden, so substitutes (the dog or the messenger) become targets for these feelings. This is also the preger) become targets for these feelings. This is also the predominant defense in the formation of a **phobia**. While the presumed etiology of OCD and OCPD (defined below) are blended here, a comparison of their features is as follows:

## OCD vs. Obsessive-Compulsive Personality Disorder (OCPD)

While similar in name, these are phenomenologically distinct conditions. Key features that help distinguish between the two are:

| Feature | OCD | OCPD |
|---|---|---|
| Central Concept | Recurrent, intrusive thoughts and/or behaviors/mental acts | Enduring preoccupation with perfection, orderliness, and interpersonal control |
| Subjective Experience | Ego-dystonic; recognizes irrationality of mental events and behavior | Ego-syntonic until close relationships are affected or defenses break down |
| Impact on daily routine | Time consuming; interferes with ability to function | Defends traits and methods as being effective and justified by productivity |
| Mentation | Aware of forced nature of thoughts, recognizes them as a product of own mind; resists compulsions | Thoughts lack quality of intrusiveness; behavior occurs automatically, most processes remain unconscious |
| Mani-festations | Often involves themes | Pervasive throughout |
| Anxiety | Marked; anxious dread | Not usually evident |
| Etiology | Growing evidence for genetic factors | Psychosocial influences predominate |

OCD and OCPD were initially formulated as a single disorder, hence the similarity in name. There are conflicting opinions about the degree to which OCPD exists prior to the onset of OCD. Currently, there is more evidence against this association. OCD is associated with other Cluster C personality disorders (most often avoidant and dependent) more frequently than with OCPD.

## Obsession-Related Practice Points

• **Preoccupations** are another component of thought content; they differ from obsessions in that they are a willful return to thinking about a topic

• **Ruminations** are another term for intellectual obsessions; here, people "chew" (mull over) their "cud" (thoughts) but achieve no resolution; there is an unnecessary quality (both in time and intensity) to this form of thinking, which is a manifestation of ambivalence

• Compulsions can also be mental acts, and considered as components of thought content, e.g. praying, counting, or repeating words silently

• Although obsessions or compulsions can be present alone, in the vast majority of patients, both are present

• Another way to elicit obsessional thoughts is to ask about common compulsive behaviors: counting, checking, cleaning, touching, ordering, arranging, etc.; if these behaviors are present, ask what motivates these actions

• Although OCD is ego-dystonic, patients frequently take years to come to psychiatric attention; it may be that patients recognize the absurd nature of obsessions and have difficulty sharing them

• Many patients see other specialists for problems related to the sequelae of their compulsions – skin, gum, and joint problems are especially common

• The people at the *Obsessive-Compulsive Foundation* must be saluted for their sense of humor – these are actual badges they have had printed:

•*Compulsive people do it over and over.*
• *What if?*
• *Every member counts!*

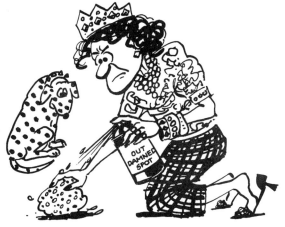

# IV – Everything You Always Wanted to Know About Phobias (but were afraid to ask)

Phobias are marked and persistent fears that are:
• Viewed by the patient as excessive and unreasonable (phobias are **ego-dystonic**; patients have preserved insight)
• Circumscribed (the person has clearly demarcated objects or situations that are feared)
• Invariably accompanied by a sense of anxiety upon exposure or the thought of exposure to the object(s) or situation(s)
• Capable of causing sufficient distress that patients go to great lengths to avoid the anxiety-provoking stimulus
• Of generally benign objects or situations; for example, fears of a rabid doberman or a dangerous neighborhood can be understood; fears of tomatoes or numbers cannot

The DSM-IV contains the categories of **specific phobias** and **social phobias**, the components of which can be remembered with the following mnemonic:

## "ASP & BOAS"*

**A**nimal type – e.g. killer chihuahuas or goldfish
**S**ituational type – e.g. bridges, tunnels, flying, driving, etc.
**P**eople (social phobia) – e.g. public speaking

**B**lood/Injection – e.g. seeing blood or having procedures
**O**ther – used when other categories simply won't do
**A**goraphobia – avoidance of places where escape or getting help are difficult
**S**urroundings – elements in the natural environment such as storms, water, heights, etc.

---

* For those unfamiliar with reptilian suborder *ophidia*, an asp is a venomous snake (viper) and also makes an excellent Scrabble® word; this mnemonic is helpful because snakes are a common phobia (even for Indiana Jones).

## Agoraphobia

**Agoraphobia** is a condition that deserves special mention. The word is derived from Greek and means "fear of the marketplace." The DSM-IV defines it as:

*Anxiety about being in places or situations from which escape might be difficult (or embarrassing) or in which help may not be available in the event of having an unexpected or situationally predisposed Panic Attack or panic-like symptoms. (DSM-IV, p. 396)*

Agoraphobia is a common phobia and the one that causes the greatest impairment of social and occupational functioning. In the DSM-IV, agoraphobia is considered in conjunction with panic disorder. Generally, patients who experience repeated panic attacks become "phobic" of the places where attacks occur, or where help or escape are difficult to arrange. Patients who have a moderate to severe course of panic disorder frequently have at least some degree of agoraphobia.

Patients with agoraphobia curtail their activities significantly. They make constant demands on friends and family members to accompany them on outings. Agoraphobic patients frequently need to be seated near the exit on a bus or in a movie theater. Their continual demands can lead to strained relationships. Patients can become housebound if others cannot carry out their requests, or if the illness becomes too severe. Agoraphobia is frequently complicated by other phobias, obsessions, and overvalued ideas. Additionally, depressive disorders and substance abuse often complicate the lives of agoraphobics.

Agoraphobia is coded in the DSM-IV in two ways:
• Panic Disorder with Agoraphobia  300.21
• Agoraphobia Without History of Panic Disorder  300.22

## How Do I Ask About Phobias?

Phobias are not usually difficult to ask about because they are ego-dystonic and patients recognize them as troublesome. Unless patients have agoraphobia, or fear something in the room, they are not likely to be anxious (due to the phobia) during the interview. Phobias may well be the most common psychiatric condition, with estimates of prevalence ranging as high as 25% of the population. The presence of phobias can also be inferred through behavior. For example, someone who avoids the public acceptance of an award may have a social phobia or agoraphobia. Suggestions for questions to explore the presence of phobias are as follows:

### Specific Phobias
• *"Do you have strong fears about certain objects or situations?"*
• *"Are there objects or situations that make you intensely anxious if you cannot avoid them?"*
• *"Do you make special efforts to avoid certain objects or situations?"*

### Social Phobias
• *"Do you have strong or persistent fears about being humiliated in public?"*
• *"Do you have strong or persistent fears that you will do something embarrassing in front of strangers?"*

### Agoraphobia
• *"Do you require special arrangements to be made for you to feel comfortable when you are outside your home?"*
• *"Do you have such a strong sense of anxiety that someone must be with you before you can leave your house?"*
• *"To what degree do you limit your activities because of anxiety?"*

## How Do Phobias Begin?
A phobia is the end result of a long chain of (theoretical) events. Herr Freud and his contribution to **ego psychology** provided an understanding of how phobias start.

Freud incorporated his early findings into what became known as the **structural theory**, introduced with the publication of *The Ego and the Id* in 1923. This model has a *tripartite* structure containing the **id, ego,** and **superego**.

Present from birth, the **id** is completely unconscious and seeks gratification of instinctual (mainly sexual and aggressive) drives. The **superego** forms from an identification with the same-sex parent at the resolution of the **oedipal conflict**. It suppresses instinctual aims and serves as the moral conscience, dictating both what *should* and *should not* be done. The superego is largely unconscious, but has a conscious element. Ego functions are explained on p. 324 – 6.

The fundamental concept in ego psychology is that of *conflict* among these three agencies. The **id, ego,** and **superego** battle for expression and discharge of sexual and aggressive drives. This conflict produces anxiety, specifically called **signal anxiety**. This anxiety alerts the ego that a **defense mechanism** is required, conceptualized as follows:

The id seeks expression of an impulse

The superego prohibits the impulse from being expressed

This conflict produces signal anxiety
↓
An ego defense is unconsciously recruited
to decrease the anxiety
↓
A neurotic symptom (phobia) is formed

The following ego defenses are involved in the development of phobias:
• **Displacement** – here, the sexual or aggressive conflict is transferred from the person who evokes it to an unconnected, irrelevant object or situation; this new stimulus becomes associated with strong feelings (marked anxiety) simply because of its presence
• **Symbolization** – this is similar to displacement except that the phobic object or situation is symbolically connected with the conflict; as in the classic **stimulus-response**

**theory**, a neutral stimulus (the phobic object) can be paired with an anxiety-provoking experience, resulting in a permanent emotional association of the two.

The classic struggle associated with phobias was **castration anxiety**, which develops out of a child's oedipal conflict (in boys, sexual urges towards the mother and aggressive urges towards the father). The phobic stimulus may be unconnected with castration anxiety (the ego defense of **displacement**) or more directly associated (the ego defense of **symbolization**). For example, the fear of father can be displaced onto/symbolized by wristwatches (because he wore one on his spanking hand). Other anxieties are also recognized as stemming from these early experiences – e.g. agoraphobia as an adult version of **separation anxiety**.

## Fear vs. Anxiety

**Anxiety** is a sense of uneasiness or distress (having mental and physical components), and is a reaction to unreal or imagined dangers. **Fear** is a similar reaction, but to known or actual dangers. The German word **angst** (meaning *fear*) was mistranslated as *anxiety* in Freud's early writing. Some psychiatric literature doesn't distinguish between the two because fear can have a repressed, unconscious aspect.

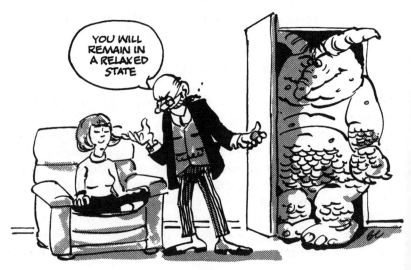

# Summary

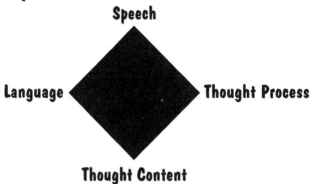

**Speech**

**Language** ◄ ► **Thought Process**

**Thought Content**

• Delusions are fixed, false beliefs that are ego-syntonic and become accepted as reality by patients who experience them. Delusions can be of a bizarre nature (physically impossible) or non-bizarre (possible though unlikely). These beliefs often dominate the thinking of patients, and, being a cardinal sign of psychosis, are the most serious of the disorders of thought content.

• Obsessions are unwanted, persistent, intrusive thoughts that are ego-dystonic. Patients recognize them as originating from their own minds (in **thought insertion**, patients perceive the ideas as coming from elsewhere).

• Phobias are exaggerated fears (as recognized by the patient) of neutral objects or situations. Unless patients are anticipating or actually confronting the object/situation, phobias are not intrusive thoughts.

• Perceptual abnormalities are discussed in Chapter 10. However, disorders of perception can contribute to abnormalities of thought content. A patient who hallucinates about the Four Horsemen of the Apocalypse may well have persisting fears of persecution, which could be of delusional intensity. Abnormal perceptions may provide the "kernel" of truth or actual experience, which the delusion is built around.

# Phobias – New & Unusual

- **Anginaphobia** – fear of narrowness
- **Anuptophobia** – fear of staying single
- **Cherophobia** – fear of good news
- **Dementophobia** – fear of insanity
- **Ergophobia** – fear of work
- **Gelophobia** – fear of laughing
- **Genuphobia** – fear of knees
- **Glossophobia** – fear of talking
- **Gymnophobia** – fear of naked bodies
- **Herpetophobia** – fear of lizards
- **Iatrophobia** – fear of doctors
- **Kainophobia** – fear of newness
- **Kenophobia** – fear of empty spaces
- **Kleptophobia** – fear of stealing
- **Logophobia** – fear of words
- **Methyphobia** – fear of alcohol
- **Mnemonophobia** – fear of memories
- **Musophobia** – fear of mice
- **Myxophobia** – fear of slime
- **Neopharmaphobia** – fear of new drugs
- **Osmophobia** – fear of smells
- **Panphobia** – fear of everything
- **Pentheraphobia** – fear of mother-in-law
- **Phobophobia** – fear of fear itself
- **Polyphobia** – fear of many things
- **Psychophobia** – fear of the mind
- **Sinistrophobia** – fear of things "of the left"/left-handed
- **Sitophobia** – fear of food or eating
- **Sophophobia** – fear of learning

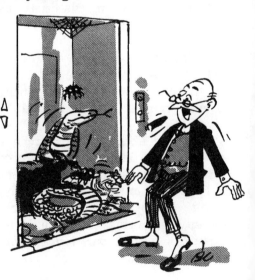

# References

## Books

American Psychiatric Association
**Diagnostic and Statistical Manual of Mental Disorders, 4th Ed.**
American Psychiatric Association, Washington D.C., 1994

R. Campbell
**Psychiatric Dictionary, 7th Ed.**
Oxford University Press, New York, 1996

R. Doctor & A. Khan
**The Encyclopedia of Phobias, Fears and Anxieties**
Facts on File, Inc., New York, 1989

P.A. Garety & D.R. Hemsley
**Delusions: Investigations into the Psychology of Delusional Reasoning**
Maudsley Monographs, No. 36
Oxford University Press, Inc., New York, 1994

H.I. Kaplan & B.J. Sadock, Editors
**Synopsis of Psychiatry, 8th Ed.**
Williams & Wilkins, Baltimore, 1998

D.M. Kaufman
**Clinical Neurology for Psychiatrists, 5th Ed.**
W.B. Saunders, Philadelphia, 2001

E. Othmer & S.C. Othmer
**The Clinical Interview Using DSM-IV**
American Psychiatric Press Inc., Washington D.C., 1994

L. Rolak
**Neurology Secrets**
Hanley & Belfus, Philadelphia, 1993

B.J. Sadock & V.A. Sadock, Editors
**Comprehensive Textbook of Psychiatry, 7th Ed.**
Lippincott, Williams & Wilkins, Philadelphia, 2000

A. Sims
**Symptoms in the Mind, 2nd Ed.**
Saunders, London, England, 1995

M.A. Taylor
**The Neuropsychiatric Mental Status Exam**
PMA Publishing Corp. New York, 1981

E.L. Zuckerman
**The Clinician's Thesaurus, 5th Ed.**
Clinician's Toolbox, The Guilford Press, New York, 2000

# Articles
## Delusions

P.S. Appelbaum, P.C. Robbins, & L.H. Roth
**Dimensional Approach to Delusions: Comparison Across Types and Diagnoses**
*American Journal of Psychiatry* 156(12): 1938 – 1943, 1999

P.B. Baker, B.L. Cook, & G. Winokur
**Delusional Infestation: The Interface of Delusions and Hallucinations**
*Psychiatric Clinics of North America* 18(2): 345 – 361, 1995

B. Bowins & G. Shugar
**Delusions and Self-Esteem**
*Canadian Journal of Psychiatry* 43(2): 154 – 158, 1998

T.E. Feinberg, L.A. Eaton, D.M. Roane, & J.T. Giacino
**Multiple Fregoli Delusions After Traumatic Brain Injury**
*Cortex* 35(3): 373 – 387, 1999

I. Fukunishi
**Five Cases of Delusions Associated With Renal Anemia (letter)**
*Psychosomatics* 38(6): 591 – 592, 1997

A.D. Gaines
**Culture-Specific Delusions: Sense and Nonsense in Cultural Context**
*Psychiatric Clinics of North America* 18(2): 281 – 301, 1995

J.P. Hwang, S.J. Tsai, C.H. Yang, K.M. Liu, & J.F. Lirng
**Persecutory Delusions in Dementia**
*J. Clin. Psychiatry* 60(8): 550 – 553, 1999

C. Jones, R.D. Griffiths, & G. Humphris
**A Case of Capgras Delusion Following Critical Illness**
*Intensive Care Med.* 25(10): 1183 – 1184, 1999

R. Kemp, S. Chua, P. McKenna, & A. David
**Reasoning and Delusions**
*British Journal of Psychiatry* 170: 398 – 405, 1997

T.C. Manschreck
**Pathogenesis of Delusions**
*Psychiatric Clinics of North America* 18(2): 213 – 229, 1995

T.C. Manschreck
**Delusional Disorder: The Recognition and Management of Paranoia**
*J. Clin. Psychiatry* (suppl. 3): 32 – 38, 1996

I. McGilchrist & J. Cutting
**Somatic Delusions in Schizophrenia and Affective Psychosis**
*British Journal of Psychiatry* 167(3): 350 – 361, 1995

M.J. Seder
**Understanding Delusions**
*Psychiatric Clinics of North America* 18(2): 251 – 262, 1995

S.F. Zomer, R.F. De Wit, J.E. Van Bronswijk, G. Nabarro, & W.A. Van Vloten
**Delusions of Parasitosis: A Psychiatric Disorder to be Treated by Dermatologists?**
*British Journal of Dermatology* 138(6): 1030 – 1032, 1998

## Obsessions

M.J. Kozak & E.B. Foa
**Obsessions, Overvalued Ideas, and Delusions in Obsessive-Compulsive Disorder**
*Behav. Res. Ther.* 32(3): 343 – 353, 1994

S. Rachman
**A Cognitive Theory of Obsessions: Elaboration**
*Behav. Res. Ther.* 36(4): 385 – 401, 1998

D.C. Rettwe, S.E. Swedo, H.L. Leonard, M.C. Lenane, & J.L. Rappoport
**Obsessions and Compulsions Across Time in 79 Children and Adolescents With Obsessive-Compulsive Disorder**
*J. Am. Acad. Child Adolescent Psychiatry* 31(6): 1050 – 1056, 1992

## Overvalued Ideas

F. Neziroglu, D. McKay, J.A. Yaryura-Tobias, K.P. Stevens, & J. Todaro
**The Overvalued Ideas Scale: Development, Reliability, and Validity in Obsessive-Compulsive Disorder**
*Behav. Res. Ther.* 37(9): 881 – 902, 1999

## Phobias

G.C. Curtis, W.J. Magee, W.W. Eaton, H.U. Wittchen, & R.C. Kessler
**Specific Fears and Phobias: Epidemiology and Classification**
*British Journal of Psychiatry* 173: 212 – 217, 1998

N.J. King, G. Eleonora, & T.H. Ollendick
**Etiology of Childhood Phobias: Current Status of Rachmann's Three Pathways Theory**
*Behav. Res. Ther.* 36(3): 297 – 309, 1998

S.J. Thorpe & P.M. Salkovskis
**Phobic Beliefs: Do Cognitive Factors Play a Role in Specific Phobias?**
*Behav. Res. Ther.* 33(7): 805 – 816, 1995

S.J. Thorpe & P.M. Salkovskis
**Studies On the Role of Disgust in the Acquisition and Maintenance of Specific Phobias**
*Behav. Res. Ther.* 36(9): 877 – 893, 1998

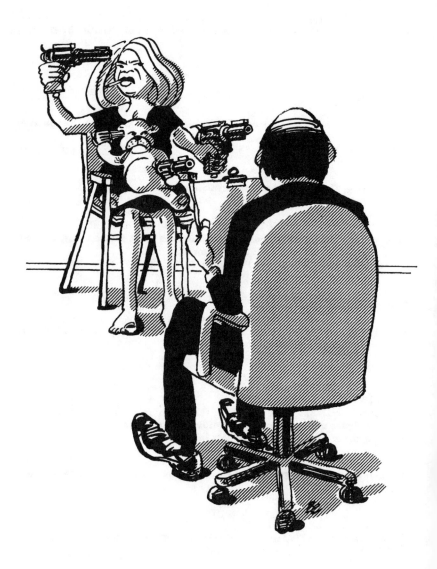

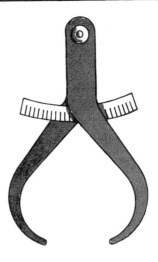

# Chapter 8

# Suicidal & Homicidal Ideation

While these topics technically belong in the *Thought Content Chapter*, their seriousness warrants a separate presentation. Suicidal or homicidal ideation is virtually universal in being grounds for involuntary committal. It is widely reported that the majority of people who commit suicide suffer from a diagnosable mental disorder. Conversely, most violent crime is not perpetrated by people who are mentally ill. The provision for civil commitment on the grounds of being a potential harm to others is meant to detain those who have a *defect in reasoning*, and who cannot be considered to be criminally responsible for their actions (i.e. are unable to appreciate the wrongfulness of their conduct). Frequently, such patients have a formal thought disorder, such as perceptual aberrations (e.g. hallucinations) or paranoid delusions. Patients who have plans to harm someone as a result of a mental illness require protection, as do their intended victims.

# What is the Diagnostic Significance of Suicidal Ideation?

• **Major Depressive Episode** 296.X
A. (9) Recurrent thoughts of death (not just fear of dying), recurrent suicidal ideation without a specific plan, or a suicide attempt or a specific plan for committing suicide

• **Posttraumatic Stress Disorder** 309.81
C. (7) Sense of a foreshortened future (e.g., does not expect to have a career, marriage, children, or a normal life span)

• **Borderline Personality Disorder** 301.83
A. (5) Recurrent suicidal behavior, gestures, or threats, or self-mutilating behavior

The above list consists of diagnostic criteria that clearly specify thoughts of self harm. The criteria for schizophrenia, bipolar disorder, obsessive-compulsive disorder, and substance dependence do not contain explicit wording to this effect, though patients with these conditions have comparatively high rates of suicide.

# What is the Diagnostic Significance of Homicidal Ideation?

• **Antisocial Personality Disorder** 301.7
A. (7) Lack of remorse, as indicated by being indifferent to or rationalizing having hurt, mistreated, or stolen from another

• **Intermittent Explosive Disorder** 312.34
A. Several discrete episodes of failure to resist aggressive impulses that result in serious assaultive acts or destruction of property

• **Sexual Masochism** 302.83
A. Over a period of at least 6 months, recurrent, intense sexually arousing fantasies, sexual urges, or behaviors involving the act (real, not simulated) . . . of being humiliated, beaten, bound or otherwise made to suffer

• **Sexual Sadism** 302.84
. . . the psychological or physical suffering (including humiliation) of the victim is sexually exciting to the person
Diagnostic Criteria are from the DSM-IV
© American Psychiatric Association, Washington, D.C. 1994
Reprinted with permission.

# Suicidal and Homicidal Ideation

- **Suicide Assessment (Section I)**
- **What Are the Risk Factors For Suicide? (II)**
- **What Are the Psychological Factors Operative in Suicidal Ideation? (III)**
- **How Do I Ask About Thoughts of Suicide? (IV)**
- **Are There Ways of Measuring the Potential Risk for Suicide? (V)**
- **Why Is It Sometimes Difficult to Interview, Or Deal With, Suicidal Patients? (VI)**
- **Which Countertransference Reactions Are Common? (VII)**
- **Which Conditions are Most Frequently Associated With Violence? (VIII)**
- **Why Do Patients Become Violent? (IX)**
- **How Do I Ask About Violent Intentions? (X)**
- **Psychiatric Patients and the Legal System (XI)**

- **Are There Methods For Predicting Dangerousness? (XII)**
- **What Are the Legal Issues in Dealing With Violent Patients? (XIII)**
- **How Do I Protect Myself In Interviews? (XIV)**

# I – Suicide Assessment

Many studies have been conducted to delineate the risk factors for completed suicide (these are listed in the next section). Unfortunately, the application of these risk factors alone does not provide an accurate prediction of the suicidal risk for any particular individual. A patient having few, or even none, of the established risk factors may well go on to commit suicide. Suicide assessment, like conducting an interview and MSE, is a blend of knowledge, experience, style, and training. Shea (1999) makes the cogent point that suicide assessment consists of three separate tasks:

- Gathering information related to suicide risk factors
- Gathering information about a patient's suicidal ideation and planning
- Clinical decision making using the above data bases

Interviewing, and ultimately being responsible for treating suicidal patients, is a daunting task, and one that causes considerable stress in mental health professionals. Despite its seriousness, suicidal ideation should be explored in the same manner as any other symptom. Caregivers will deal with suicidal patients effectively when they have the benefit of experience, and of knowledge.

This chapter addresses two main areas of suicide assessment: a cataloguing of risk factors, and a brief psychodynamic explanation about why some patients become suicidal. The "how" of suicide assessment is an area which readers are strongly encouraged to familiarize themselves with various assessment strategies as described in Shea's highly readable and useful book, *The Practical Art of Suicide Assessment*.

# II – What Are the Risk Factors For Suicide?

Key risk factors to consider in assessing suicidal risk are:

## "SOS MADE PLAIN FOR A DR."

**S**ex (gender)
**O**ccupational status
**S**tress level

**M**ental illness
**A**ge
**D**rug abuse (chemical dependency)
**E**ffects of medication (side effects)

**P**recipitants
**L**ethality of method
**A**ntidepressants
**I**solation
**N**ote written (or a will left)

**F**amily history
**O**rganic conditions – chronic medical illness
**R**elationships (**DIRs**)

**A**kathisia

**D**ates (anniversary reaction)
**R**epeated attempts

## Sex (Gender)

In all age ranges, males commit suicide more frequently than females. The ratio varies from a factor of 2:1 to almost 10:1 depending on the age group and race. Two factors help explain the gender discrepancy. As outlined in the 'L' (lethality of method) section, males use more lethal methods. In the time it takes to die of an overdose, asphyxiation, or drowning, a rescue attempt can be made. Only seconds to minutes are available with more lethal means. Males have a higher prevalence of chemical dependency. In North America, the ratio of males to females with alcohol problems is at least 4:1. In other areas of the world it is considerably higher. Depression is more prevalent in females by a factor of about 2:1, and is strongly correlated with completed suicide. Schizophrenia is widely regarded to have a later onset and milder course in females. It is thought that estrogen serves a protective function in schizophrenia. Given that estrogen patches have been used to treat severe post-partum depression, it may be that the course of mood disorders is somewhat different on a gender basis as well.

## Occupational Status

Having an occupation is in general a protective factor. Higher **socioeconomic status (SES)** is associated with higher risk (though a recent change in SES is also a risk factor). A possible explanation is that a higher SES entails a greater degree of responsibility. If things go awry, affected individuals may face consequences from many avenues (family, legal, financial, etc.). Professionals, and in particular physicians, have suicide rates above national averages. Recent studies have indicated that female physicians have rates triple the national average for women over age 25.

## Stress Level

Stress can push people to the point that suicide is seen as an escape. In our individualized and technological society, the cumulative weight of moderate stressors can be too much for some people. Holmes & Rahe (1967) developed a stress scale, which assigned a specific value of life change units (**LCU**) to particular events. This scale was revised by Miller & Rahe (1997). The major factors considered are: death of a spouse or family member, divorce, serious medical illness, leaving work, marriage, and change in family situation.

## Mental Illness

Mental Illness is the strongest risk factor associated with suicide. Over 90% of those who take their own lives have a diagnosable mental condition at their time of death. The presence of a mental illness is estimated to increase the risk of committing suicide tenfold. The majority of patients who commit suicide have seen a physician within six months of their death, and frequently within one month. Other studies have found that a high percentage of patients who took their lives had been given a prescription for a psychotropic medication. Among psychiatric disorders, mood disorders and alcohol abuse (respectively) are the conditions that have the highest association with suicide.

**Mood Disorders**
Mood disorders are thought to be present in at least half, and potentially up to three-quarters, of those who commit suicide. It has also been estimated that 15% of those with mood disorders will go on to take their own lives. Within the spectrum of mood disorders, the diagnoses that result in the highest morbidity are:
• Depression with psychotic features
• Bipolar mixed states (the co-existence of manic and depressive symptoms; of particular concern is that the energy of mania can cause patients to act on the suicidal thoughts brought about by depression)

It has not been conclusively shown that there is a difference in the suicide rates of unipolar and bipolar patients. The risk of self-harm is greatest at the beginning or end of a mood disturbance. The period just after discharge is associated with increased risk for an attempt. Among patients who die by suicide, mood disorders are more common among the elderly, while personality disorders and chemical dependence are more common in the younger groups. Insomnia, anhedonia, and poor concentration are the three most common symptoms associated with suicide risk.

**Schizophrenia**
Schizophrenia is the third most common psychiatric diagnosis among those who have committed suicide. It is estimated that 10% of those with this condition may take their lives. Within this diagnosis, the risk is higher:

• Among young males, and relatively early in the course of the illness
• In those with high premorbid achievement and high personal expectations
• After the recovery from a psychotic episode, during the postpsychotic depressive disorder of schizophrenia (*DSM-IV, p. 711*)
• In those with an awareness of the overall prognosis
• In those with the additional risk factors of social isolation and substance abuse

Command hallucinations or persecutory delusions have not been strongly correlated with suicide potential.

**Personality Disorders**
Personality disorders are also frequently correlated with suicide (in particular, the antisocial and borderline personalities from Cluster B). Suicide is three times more common in prison populations. Personality disorders are associated with substance abuse, impulsivity, and poor social integration and adjustment. Paranoid personalities may harm themselves or others as a way of pre-empting what they perceive to be an inevitable attack.

**Anxiety Disorders**
Anxiety disorders have been found to have an association with suicide risk. In particular, posttraumatic stress disorder and the presence of panic attacks (which can complicate a variety of disorders), and obsessive-compulsive disorder all increase the risk of suicide.

# Age
This is a factor because certain age groups have higher rates of completed suicide. As a general rule, suicidal risk increases with age. This trend becomes established in men starting at about age 45 and climbs continually, with a peak at age 75. Women have a later onset, starting around age 55, and exhibit a less dramatic rise. The elderly have a suicide rate triple that of younger people, and commit one-

quarter of all suicides while encompassing only one-tenth of the population. There is an important exception to this trend. The suicide rate among males aged 15 – 24 years is disproportionately high (especially among whites). In this age group, suicide is consistently reported to be either the second or third most common cause of death (with accidents and homicide being the other causes). While no clear reason has been established, it has been suggested that the prevalence of alcohol and drug abuse is a significant factor. Peer pressure and exposure to media depictions of suicide are also thought to be influential factors.

## Drug Abuse

Drug use/abuse is highly correlated with suicidal actions. It has been estimated that the presence of chemical dependency increases the risk of completed suicide by five times that of someone who is not using drugs. The lethality of the drugs used needs to be taken into consideration – those with the greatest potential to cause death are:

- Amphetamines
- Barbiturates
- Cocaine
- Opioids

It is important to ask about both prescription and non-prescription drug use, though all but cocaine from the above list can be obtained from a physician. Cocaine is still used medically as a vasoconstrictor, but is only available in aqueous form in hospitals. The risk for completed suicide increases dramatically when patients combine drugs of abuse (including alcohol). Some patients use certain drugs to modulate or prolong highs, and then switch to another set to avoid the dysphoria of "crashes." The presence of the following factors increases the risk of suicide:

- Early age of first use
- Chronic use
- Past overdoses
- Male gender
- Family history of substance abuse

### Alcohol

Alcohol deserves special mention because it is the substance most often associated with acts of violence. Ethanol use can lead to problems during intoxication or withdrawal states. Ethanol causes disinhibition, removing the self-restraint that would otherwise be present. The combination of impaired judgment with lowered inhibition can lead to dire consequences. Emergency departments often have intoxicated patients who are combative or self-destructive, yet are entirely different when sober. Alcohol increases the toxicity of substances that are co-ingested. Unlike opioids and benzodiazepines, there is no readily available agent to reverse its effects. Ethanol use can also be a consequence of other factors. Patients with mood disorders or anxiety disorders appear to be particularly likely to imbibe. Alcohol use obscures accurate statistics on suicide. Accidents involving single motor vehicles or pedestrians may well be suicides, but the use of alcohol makes the issue of intention less clear. Deaths by drowning, overdose, falling, etc. similarly raise the question of *suicide vs. accident.*

## Effects of Medication (Side Effects)

The presence and severity of adverse effects to medication should be considered. Some psychiatric medications can lower quality of life by:
• Causing weight gain
• Diminishing the interest for, and ability to engage in, sexual relations
• Causing at least mild difficulties in cognitive functions

## Precipitants

Acutely distressing events increase the risk of suicide. The presence of *loss* is the key precipitant leading to suicidal behavior. This can be a perceived or actual loss of love, esteem, wealth, health, fame, etc. The most common event leading to the wish to die is a disturbance in an interpersonal relationship (**DIR**).

Searching for the "final straw" is a valuable endeavor when assessing suicidal patients. It is important to understand *why* the patient made an attempt, or is considering suicide, *at this point in time.* There is almost always an explanation

for why patients do not want to go on living. Most people at least transiently consider suicide at some point during their lives. Traumatic events like the death of a spouse, child, or parent frequently cause the surviving parties to consider whether their own lives are worth continuing.
• 20% of adults have had persistent thoughts of suicide over a two-week period
• 10% of adults have made a plan as to how they would commit suicide
• 3% of adults have made an attempt at suicide

In situations where a precipitant is not obvious, consideration of other factors may help shed some light:
• In some cases, people react to a *symbolic loss* rather than an actual one; exploring the meaning of apparently minor losses can help identify the source of the precipitant
• People may not be consciously aware of what influences them (e.g. watching a movie or hearing a song can bring about associations that evoke painful memories)

## Lethality of Method

Lethality of the method is another factor that bears on the risk of suicide. In general, the more lethal the means, the more likely it will be carried out. Males tend to use violent methods, such as firearms, knives, jumping, and hanging. Females are more likely to take overdoses, drown, or asphyxiate themselves. In particular, the availability of firearms has been shown to have an impact on the suicide rate.

## Antidepressants

Antidepressants can factor into the assessment of suicidality. There is a typical recovery sequence of depressive symptoms (assuming efficacy and compliance):

With **tricyclic antidepressants (TCAs)** –
• Insomnia and appetite may improve within 7 days

With **selective-serotonin reuptake inhibitors (SSRIs)** –
• Energy and interest may improve within 7 days

The overall recovery tends to follow a pattern of vegetative symptoms recovering first, then cognitive functions, and lastly, mood symptoms and suicidal thoughts. This can put patients in a situation where their energy returns while they are still having thoughts of self-harm.

## Isolation

Social isolation refers to a sense of *unconnectedness* with others, regardless of marital status or occupation. Suicide rates are higher for people who live alone. Before considering this as a risk factor, it is important to know if someone wants to live alone, and if not, how great a departure this is from desired living arrangements.

Relationships, to a large degree, are protective against self-harm. However, someone may be married, living with a partner, or involved in a relationship and still feel isolated. The *quality* of a relationship is a key factor to ask about when evaluating someone's suicidal risk.

Cultural factors also impact on the degree of isolation patients might feel. Certain regions have consistently high rates (Eastern Europe, Scandinavia, Japan). Significantly lower rates are seen in Ireland, the Mediterranean, and the Middle East. The U.S. and Canada have rates in the middle of this range (10 to 15 per 100,000 people per year).

Within certain countries, rates vary according to demographic features such as race, religion, urban/rural location, immigration, and SES. Some consistently reported demographic findings are:
• Whites have higher rates of suicide than blacks
• Protestants have higher rates than Catholics or Muslims
• Rates are higher in cities than in rural areas
• Immigrants have higher rates of suicide than average for their new country
• Higher SES carries an increased risk

It has been proposed that there is a greater sense of belonging and cohesion in groups with lower suicide rates. Also, social isolation can be the result of other factors (e.g. alcohol or drug abuse, personality difficulties, etc.).

## Notes and Will Changes

Notes, and changes to a will indicate that planning was involved in the attempt, which is correlated with an increased risk of completion. Patients who wish to "tidy up their affairs" may have wills created or altered. While the contents of a will are confidential, many patients make reference to their wills, or to changes in them, prior to a suicide attempt. Some patients also purchase burial plots or give away their possessions. Generally, notes are left either to tell others what the person thought of them, or as a plea to those left behind to understand why the suicide occurred. Notes are not always conspicuously placed. They may be mailed or concealed so they are not prematurely discovered.

## Family History

Another important factor is family history. There are studies that demonstrate a genetic inheritance independent of other major risk factors (mood disorders, schizophrenia, and alcoholism).

Twin studies have shown a higher concordance rate for suicide in monozygotic (MZ) twins than dizygotic (DZ) twins. Additionally, adoption studies have found increased rates of completed suicide among the biological relatives of adopted away offspring, furthering speculation about a genetic contribution.

### Identification

Patients, particularly under the age of ten, who lost a parent to suicide are at an increased risk themselves through the process of **identification** with the deceased. These occurrences seem to break the "taboo" of suicide in families. This is one of the ways that the tragedy of suicide perpetuates itself.

## Organic Conditions

Organic (general medical) conditions are risk factors because of their seriousness or chronicity. This is also one of the reasons why suicide is more frequent in the elderly.

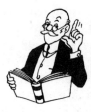

Medical conditions associated with increased risk of suicide are as follows:

**Central Nervous System**
- Dementias
- Epilepsy
- Degenerative conditions
- Head injuries
- Strokes

**Cancer**
- Particularly those that grow quickly or are advanced at the time of discovery

**Musculoskeletal**
- Amputations
- Paralysis
- Chronic pain

**Cardiovascular**
- Unstable angina

**Gastrointestinal**
- Peptic ulcer
- Porphyria
- Inflammatory bowel disease
- Cirrhosis

**Renal**
- Dialysis dependence

**Endocrine**
- Cushing's disease

**HIV seropositivity** or **AIDS**
- Especially with encephalopathy

**Progressive Autoimmune Disorders**

# Relationships
## (Disturbances of Interpersonal Relationships – DIRs)

Disruptions in meaningful relationships provide perhaps the best answer as to *why* people want to take their lives. DIRs are one of the most common, if not the major cause, of visits to emergency rooms for psychiatric/emotional reasons. DIRs refer to:

• The threat of rejection or abandonment
• Loss of approval, acceptance, affection, or attachment

To understand why DIRs can cause someone to consider suicide, it is helpful to review some of the psychology of self-destructive behavior. Freud thought suicidal urges stemmed from frustrations that developed during childhood. Everyone carries an internalized representation of their caretakers (usually parents). This is what is referred to as an **introjected object** (in psychodynamic theories *object* meaning *person*). In situations where parents were, or were perceived to be, harsh, depriving, distant, etc., a strong sense of being abandoned develops. Strong feelings, even *murderous wishes*, accompany this sense of being unwanted. Later in life, this conflict is aroused again when people don't feel loved by those close to them. DIRs reawaken strong feelings on both conscious and unconscious levels. Since Freud's initial ideas, much work has gone into understanding early experiences and their effect on relationships later in life.

One school of thought, pioneered by John Bowlby, is called **attachment theory**. The central concept in attachment theory is that close, positive attachments are a fundamental human need. The quality of early attachments to caretakers largely determines the success of future relationships. Deprivation of early attachments, with the loss (or threatened loss) of positive attachments to caretakers, creates a vulnerability resulting in a range of adverse psychological reactions. The outcome of these reactions can be a diverse array of emotional conditions, including personality disorders, substance abuse, or recurrent thoughts of wanting to commit suicide.

Source: John Mount, MD, 1995

# Causation of Psychological Symptoms

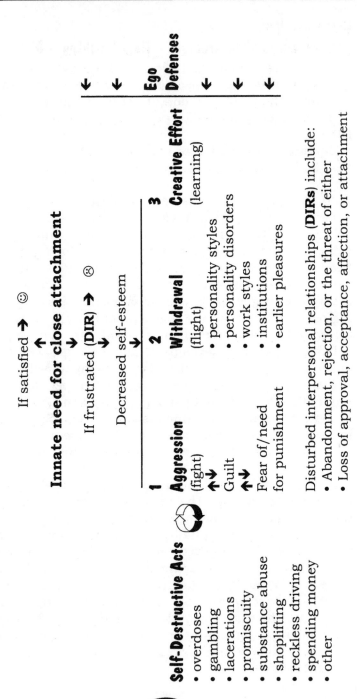

If satisfied → ☺

**Innate need for close attachment**

If frustrated (**DIR**) → ☹

Decreased self-esteem

| 1 | 2 | 3 |
|---|---|---|
| **Aggression** | **Withdrawal** | **Creative Effort** |
| (fight) | (flight) | (learning) |
| Guilt | • personality styles | |
| | • personality disorders | |
| Fear of/need | • work styles | |
| for punishment | • institutions | |
| | • earlier pleasures | |

**Ego Defenses** ↓ ↓ ↓ ↓ ↓

**Self-Destructive Acts**
- overdoses
- gambling
- lacerations
- promiscuity
- substance abuse
- shoplifting
- reckless driving
- spending money
- other

Disturbed interpersonal relationships (**DIRs**) include:
- Abandonment, rejection, or the threat of either
- Loss of approval, acceptance, affection, or attachment

If the innate need for attachment is satisfied by pleasurable interpersonal relationships (**PIRs**), normal development ensues. If the innate need for attachment is frustrated by **DIRs**, the drop in self-esteem brings about one of three consequences.

**1.** The **fight response** involves aggression. Anger can be used destructively against the person, causing the emergence of suicidal feelings. Anger directed at others brings about a potent sense of guilt, along with its unconscious analog – the fear of, or need for, punishment.

**2.** Withdrawing, or the **flight response**, can involve:
• Building interpersonal walls to diminish emotional pain
• Developing work habits that compensate for other deficiencies, often called an "institutional" work style
• Regressing to the need for earlier means of gratification where others aren't needed (often "oral" habits like smoking, drinking alcohol, or excessive food consumption)

**3.** The energy generated by strong emotions can be channeled into creative efforts. This involves both learning about one's source of frustration, and developing an adaptive outlet for it (e.g. music, sports, hobbies, etc.).

## Akathisia

Akathisia is a sense of restlessness causing patients to feel the need to keep moving. Some patients have described this as a feeling of "squirreliness." Akathisia most often occurs after the use of antipsychotic medications, though others (such as SSRIs) have been reported as a cause.

Akathisia can be very distressing, and some patients have taken their lives rather than endure this unpleasant feeling. This is most likely to happen when akathisia is misinterpreted as a worsening of the psychosis, depression, or anxiety. Of note, the treatment involves benzodiazepines or a beta-blocker, not the anticholinergic medications that are used to treat extrapyramidal side-effects.

## Dates

Anniversary reactions occur on the dates of major losses. Patients may be unaware of why they are feeling suicidal at a certain point in time. An exploration of dates significant to that person may reveal the cause. Patients who have lost parents to suicide may not only suffer from anniversary reactions, but also be unconsciously involved in a self-destructive process at the same age as the parent who died.

## Repeated Attempts

Repeated attempts at self-harm increase the risk for a completed suicide. A distinction needs to be made between past serious, unsuccessful attempts, and chronic thoughts of suicide or gestures of self-harm. The latter is called **parasuicide** and refers to chronic self-mutilation, persistent thoughts or threats of suicide, or non-lethal attempts:
• Patients that are demographically at higher risk for completed suicide are older males who are socially isolated, use a method of high lethality, and have either a mood disorder or have a chemical dependence problem
• Attempters tend to be younger women who have social connections, use methods that are unlikely to be fatal, and have a personality disorder or adjustment disorder

Women attempt suicide more frequently than men, though men complete more suicides. Most attempts occur in younger age groups, which is the opposite to the picture for completed suicides. Attempts are made impulsively, whereas completed suicides are more often planned and take place in settings with a low chance of discovery. Among attempters, personality disorder has been reported to be the most common diagnosis (especially borderline and antisocial). Despite these distinctions, patients who attempt suicide have a large number of demographic variables and risk factors in common with those who complete suicide. Engaging in any type of self-harm behavior increases the risk of an eventual suicide. Even in cases where it seems obvious that parasuicidal behavior is for secondary gain, unintended complications can occur (such as a lethal combination of medications).

# III – What Are the Psychological Factors Operative in Suicidal Ideation?

Freud postulated that suicidal urges start out as aggressive wishes towards an internal representation of someone to whom the patient is attached (usually a parent). Murderous wishes (or even rage) are then directed against the self. In this way, violence towards the self or others is seen to have a common cause (as demonstrated in the diagram outlining the *Causation of Psychological Symptoms*).

The central focus in the thought processes of suicidal individuals is *hopelessness*. Irrespective of diagnosis, the absence of hope for the future is a key indicator of long-term suicide risk. Other factors that have been seen to have prognostic significance are: guilt, shame, humiliation, and desperation.

Fantasies commonly expressed by suicidal patients involve the following themes:
• Rebirth or reunion with a deceased person
• Escape from situations perceived as hopeless or too painful to endure
• Retaliation or revenge
• Self-punishment or sacrifice
• Atonement or restitution
• A means of gaining or maintaining control in situations where patients are, or see themselves as, powerless

**Anomie** was a term used by Durkheim to refer to a lack of social control; he based his classification of types of suicide on the relationship between suicide and social conditions:
• **Egotistic suicide** occurs due to a lack of integration with society where individuals no longer feel subject to its norms
• **Anomic suicide** involves a perceived lack of "collective order" in a society where one's hopes cannot be realized
• **Altruistic suicide** is committed for the benefit of society

# IV – How Do I Ask About Thoughts of Suicide?

Interviewers often have great hesitation in asking patients about the presence of suicidal thoughts. A common fear is that merely posing such questions will cause patients to become suicidal, or that patients will take it as a suggestion. Although tact and timing are required, neither of the above situations actually occurs. Consider the following excerpt:

**Patient:** *"In the last month, I've lost my wife, my best friend, my job, my truck, and my dog. My life is like a Country & Western song – I just don't know what to do next."*

**Student:** *"Have you considered suicide?"*

**Patient:** *"Do you think that's what I should do?"*

(A better way of phrasing the question might be, *"Has this situation been so difficult for you that you have had thoughts that your life wasn't worthwhile."*)

Patients expect to be asked about suicidal thoughts, and are usually relieved to be able to speak about them. Here are some suggestions on how to ask about suicidal thoughts:

• *"Are there times when your difficulties are too much for you?"*
• *"Do you ever feel like life is too much for you to bear?"*
• *"Have you thought that things would be easier if you weren't around?"*
• *"Have you ever worked out a plan for taking your life? What did you have planned?"*
• *"Do you find your life devoid of happiness or things that interest you? Is this so bad that you wish you could die?"*
• *"Do you have thoughts right at the moment about wanting to take your life? Do you feel suicidal right now?"*
• *"What happened the last time you felt this way?"*

In order to make a sound assessment of suicide risk, it is critical to explore the patient's history of suicidal ideation and actions over time. In this regard, Shea (1999) developed an approach called the *Chronological Assessment of Suicide Events* (**CASE**), which consists of an exploration of:

- Presenting suicidal ideation and behaviors
- Recent suicidal ideation and behaviors (within 8 weeks)
- Past suicidal ideation and behaviors
- Immediate suicidal ideation and behaviors

The CASE approach provides a sensitive, yet thorough, method for helping patients to openly talk about their suicidal thoughts and plans.

# V – Are There Ways of Measuring the Potential Risk for Suicide?

## • Beck Hopelessness Scale

Aaron T. Beck (1974) developed a scale for the presence and extent of hopelessness; this is a self-report questionnaire that includes 20 questions that gauge the extent to which patients have pessimistic views about their future.

## • Scale for Suicidal Ideation & The Suicide Intent Scale

These instruments were also developed by Beck (1974).

## • Risk Estimator Scale for Suicide

Developed by Motto (1985), this system incorporates 15 variables found to be statistically significant in a study that looked at the completed suicides from a group of patients that were depressed and/or had expressed suicidal ideation.

## • Rorschach ("Inkblot") Test

Using criteria developed by Exner (1993) for scoring responses, this test may have a predictive value.

## • Index of Potential Suicide

This may be given as a self-report test or as an interview. There are 50 items that are given a score between 1 and 5. This was developed by Zung (1974), who also developed a depression rating scale.

## • Suicide Probability Scale (SPS)

This instrument developed by Cull & Gill (1986).

## • Reasons for Living Inventory

This is another commonly used self-report scale.

# VI – Why Is It Sometimes Difficult to Interview, Or Deal With, Suicidal Patients?

Assessing and treating suicidal patients is among the most stressful aspects of being a mental health professional. A suicide in psychiatry is the equivalent of a patient dying on the table in surgery. The suicide of a patient has been reported to cause stress in caregivers equal to the loss of a spouse. Suicidal patients bring about certain difficulties and challenges.

Suicidal patients engender strong reactions in people around them, including the professionals who have to treat them. In the case of caregivers, strong **countertransference** feelings may arise [defined by Kernberg (1965) as the total emotional reaction to a patient]. Because we are human, we experience certain feelings in response to our patients. One of the hallmarks of a seasoned interviewer is to recognize and effectively use countertransference instead of denying it, or simply acting on it. Our emotional reactions to patients yield fertile ground for further exploration, and in many ways, are essential for understanding patients.

Patients become suicidal through a complex series of events, especially in situations involving borderline personality disorder. Here, patients have difficulty being alone, experience hostility as their main emotion, and unconsciously engage in sadomasochistic relationships. Suicidal patients use relatively primitive defense mechanisms, which also make them difficult to deal with. This can result in what has been called **countertransference hate** (Maltsberger 1974), defined as a mixture of malice and aversion. These feelings can arise for a variety of reasons:
• As professionals, we have dedicated many years to the pursuit of knowledge and expertise in our field; it can be frustrating to deal with patients who have given up
• Suicidal patients become an emergency, which requires urgent attention; this can cause a major disruption in one's schedule that will likely inconvenience other patients

• The religious or philosophical views of caregivers regarding suicide can differ with those expressed by patients; thoughts of self-harm may be seen as a moral weakness

• Mental health workers derive esteem from seeing their patients recover and do well; it can represent a blow to one's professional or personal esteem to have a patient under your care consider suicide

• Suicidal patients exert a strong pull to do something to help them; an idealistic motivation is to *heal all, know all and love all*, often referred to as a **narcissistic snare**

• Patients can be passive about their intentions and not reveal them until asked directly or repeatedly; some expect interviewers to be able to read minds, which for something as serious as suicide is likely to elicit negative reactions from interviewers

• Patients can remind us of our own unresolved conflicts about suicide (such as losses we have experienced due to suicide, or a turbulent time when we considered it)

• Primitive ego defenses can be used by patients to affirm that they are "bad" and that suicide is the right thing to do; for example, under the right set of circumstances (e.g. provocation), almost any interviewer can become irritated, at which point patients are prone to use this reaction as proof of their worthlessness or undesirability

• Suicidal ideation is often used by malingerers to gain admission to hospital for social reasons; it is always a difficult decision to deny patients admission even if they have clear secondary gain for fabricating suicidal thoughts, and the interviewer has a high index of suspicion of being manipulated

# VII – Which Countertransference Reactions Are Common?

Maltsberger (1974) outlined countertransference reactions:
• **Repression** – interviewers remain unaware of their reactions by acting out their disinterest as daydreaming, restlessness, drowsiness, yawning, clock watching, etc.

• **Turning against the self** – involves feelings of inadequacy about one's abilities and suitability for the job; feelings of incompetence and a desire to be punished can turn the interview into a penance

• **Reaction formation** – turns the feelings of hatred into the opposite, where doctors become too involved in patients' lives, often with fantasies of omnipotence and rescue

• **Projection** – is hatred turned back against the patient, in this situation, one may have the fantasy of wanting to kill the patient, since this impulse is unacceptable, it is projected back onto the patient as if to say, "I don't want to kill you, you want to kill yourself"

• **Distortion** or **denial** – here, the patient is considered hopeless and is often sent away prematurely

## How Do I Deal With These Reactions?
• First, recognize that you are an emotional being, and that you will have strong reactions to patients; denying these reactions can lead to abandonment or sadistic treatment
• Always take the safe route when dealing with suicidal patients; it is much better to arrange for a brief hospital stay than it is to discharge someone likely to attempt suicide
• Arrange for transfer of care
• Arrange supervision to discuss your emotional reactions; use this as an opportunity to learn about the patient and yourself; remember that countertransference gives you first hand experience of how others feel about the patient

## Suicide Practice Points

• Overall, suicide is the 8th leading cause of death; in the U.S. and Canada, over 100 people take their lives every day

• 2 out of every 3 suicide victims are white males

• Many studies have replicated the autopsy finding of diminished central nervous system levels of **serotonin** in violent suicides. This is measured via a serotonin metabolite called **5-HIAA** (serotonin is 5-hydroxytryptamine – 5-HT). Of note in these studies was the violent aspect of suicides. These findings were most strongly correlated with the lethality of the suicide method. Evidence also exists for dysregulation of dopaminergic and noradrenergic systems.

Ritual suicides are part of certain cultures:
• **Hara-kiri** is stabbing the abdomen with a sword (disembowelment), and was a practice of Japanese warriors when they were disgraced; in Star Trek, Klingons do the same thing (called Hegh'bat)
• **Suttee** – a Hindu custom where a wife sacrifices herself on the funeral pyre of her deceased husband
• **Dadaism** was a nihilistic artistic movement that began in Switzerland in 1916 as a consequence of W.W.I; it was based on anarchy and irrationality; several followers arbitrarily committed suicide for the sake of defying society
• **Psychic suicide** occurs when individuals will themselves to death without external means (e.g. a voodoo curse)

• Forgetting to ask about current suicidal ideation is one of the ways of automatically failing an examination
• In examinations, if the patients indicate suicidality, take personal charge of seeing to their safety at the end of the exam (unless the examiners do so); it may be an exam to you, but it is the patient's life
• 8 to 25 attempts are made for each completed suicide
• Despite the efforts of many volunteers, suicide prevention centers have not been shown to lower suicide rates
• Suicide, particularly on an inpatient unit, is one of the most common reasons for malpractice suits

# VIII – Which Conditions are Most Frequently Associated With Violence?

It is important to keep in mind that any patient with any diagnosis can become violent.

The following mnemonic covers the most common conditions associated with an increased risk for violence:

## "MADS & BADS"

**M**ania – at risk due to impulsivity, grandiosity, high energy level, and possible psychotic symptoms

**A**lcohol – due to intoxication (disinhibition) or withdrawal (altered perception, irritability)

**D**ementia – poor judgment, disinhibition

**S**chizophrenia – most common with the paranoid subtype; command hallucinations or delusions also elevate the risk

**B**orderline Personality Disorder – intense anger and unstable emotions can be part of a rage reaction when abandonment is perceived to be taking place

**A**ntisocial Personality Disorder – disregard for the safety of others; sadistic enjoyment of others' suffering

**D**elirium – hallucinations and delusions can cause violence (usually in a disorganized fashion)

**S**ubstance Abuse – intoxication, particularly with hallucinogens and PCP (phencyclidine)

With any diagnosis, the risk for violence can be elevated with the presence of any of the following factors:

## "ARM PAIN"

**A**ltered state of consciousness (e.g. delirium, intoxication)

**R**epeated assaults – history of violence

**M**ale gender

**P**aranoia (schizophrenia, mania, delusional disorder)
**A**ge – more likely to be violent if younger and impulsive
**I**ncompetence – brain injury, mental retardation, psychosis
**N**eurologic disease – Huntington's chorea, dementia

Violence itself is not a DSM-IV diagnosis. It is considered a *Condition That May Be a Focus of Clinical Attention*, and is categorized as *Adult Antisocial Behavior* (V71.01), and describes illegal and/or immoral crimes against society. Confusion can be caused by use of the word *antisocial*, because in this context it refers to acts committed in the absence of a mental disorder, not due to an antisocial personality disorder.

Violence is endemic in North American society, with estimates showing a prevalence up to one-fifth of the population becoming victims. Crime statistics show that most violent crimes are committed:
• Between people that know each other
• Between males, especially with drug involvement
• With handguns (this factor also increases suicide rates)

There are two types of violence that are of concern in interview situations:
• Violence directed towards others
• Violence directed at you, and/or other interviewers

# IX – Why Do Patients Become Violent?

Violence towards others, like that directed at the self, is a complex phenomenon with bio-psycho-social contributions:

## Biological
• Genetic factors exist for many conditions associated with violence (e.g. personality disorders); the XYY chromosome type has been linked into an increased risk of violence, (though a number of studies have been unable to validate this finding)
• Head injuries increase the chance of poor judgment and

diminished impulse control, as does intoxication or withdrawal from alcohol and other substances
• Lowered serotonin levels (measured by the presence of the metabolite 5-HIAA) are associated with a generalized increased risk of violence towards the self or others
• Patients with mental retardation can self-mutilate, and may become aggressive if efforts are made to stop them: **de Lange syndrome** (also known as the Amsterdam type of mental retardation) consists of a number of usually obvious physical abnormalities; **Lesch-Nyhan syndrome** is an autosomal recessive trait causing abnormal purine metabolism

## Sociocultural
• Violence is more common in urban settings, and is particularly endemic in downtown or "inner city" areas
• Debate exists as to whether racial factors exist outside of socioeconomic factors
• Poverty, or at least economic inequality, between perpetrator and victim is frequently cited as a risk factor
• Marital discord increases the likelihood of violent action
• The availability of firearms increases the likelihood of a serious injury or fatal outcome; societies or areas with stricter gun control have lower rates of violent behavior

## Psychological
Irrespective of the contributions from genetic or sociocultural factors, anyone can become violent under certain circumstances. Suicide and murder often have the same root cause. As presented in the sociocultural section, factors that lower esteem, such as poverty or the break-up of a relationship, are common determinants of violent behavior. The figure on the next page illustrates this relationship. One of the results of diminished self-esteem can be the fight response, resulting in a sense of rage which can be variably dealt with:
• Consciously or unconsciously
• By a number of different defense mechanisms
• As action taken against the self or others

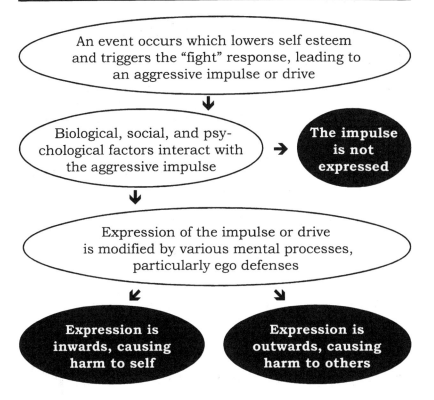

Apter (1989) looked at the use of various ego defenses involved in the above scheme. This study found support for the widely held view that the risk of violence and the risk of suicide are highly correlated. The defenses found to be significant in modulating the expression of violence are:

| Suicide Risk | Violence Risk |
| --- | --- |
| Repression | Denial |
| Regression | Projection and Displacement |

• **Repression** keeps impulses within; **regression** occurs when people are overwhelmed by stressors, and is more often seen in suicidal patients than in violent ones
• **Denial** obscures or obliterates reality; **projection** externalizes the source of a threat; **displacement** redirects intense feelings towards a substitute target

# X — How Do I Ask About Violent Intentions?

Patients may not be open and honest about their intentions. For this reason, the other factors listed in this chapter serve as a guide for the possibility of violence. Additionally, financial or interpersonal stressors are common precipitants for violence. The best predictor of future violent behavior is a history of past violent behavior. Here are sample questions that can be asked:

• *"Have you had thoughts about wanting to get revenge on someone? Did you ever develop a plan?"*
• *"Are you currently having any ideas about wanting to hurt someone? Do you have a particular person in mind?"*
• *"What would you do if you met a person you didn't like?"*
• *"Do you have access to guns, knives, or other weapons?"*
• *"What would it take for you to want to harm or kill someone?"*

# XI — Psychiatric Patients and the Legal System

It is a long-standing perception that the mentally ill are dangerous and prone to committing criminal acts. Teplin (1985) undertook a study of police-citizen contacts. She found that contact between police and people with serious mental disorders made up only 5% of the reported incidents. Calls that involved mentally ill patients were far more likely to be placed because the person was doing something to harm himself or herself instead of others. No correlation between the presence of mental illness and the type of crime committed was found. She concluded that psychiatric patients commit crimes at a level proportionate to their numbers in the population. Other studies have found stronger associations with variables such as age, socioeconomic status, and a prior criminal record.

# XII – Are There Methods For Predicting Dangerousness?

The prediction of future violence encompasses an extensive literature. Such predictions are a common component of forensic assessments, and is information frequently sought in legal proceedings. There is a lively debate between many highly respected clinicians about the ability to accurately predict the likelihood of future harm to others. Test instruments are certainly becoming more refined and valuable. However, much like predicting the weather, longer-term forecasts are bound to be less accurate.

Risk factors can be divided into major categories:
• History of aggressive behavior (e.g. childhood history, record of assaults, etc.)
• Developmental factors (psychopathology in parents, head injury, rebelliousness against authority, etc.)
• Presence of major psychiatric illness
• Personality traits (poor impulse control, inability to examine own behavior, emotional lability, etc.)

The following is a partial list of scales used in the assessment of violence and the prediction of its recurrence:
• Overt Aggression Scale
• Past Feelings and Acts of Violence Scale
• The Multidimensional Anger Inventory
• Buss-Durkee Test
• Bender Gestalt
• Wechsler Memory Scale
• Minnesota Multiphasic Personality Inventory – **MMPI-II** (scored on the *Overcontrolled Hostility Scale*)
• Legal Dangerousness Scale

Projective tests score responses related to violent content, and can make a prediction of potential violence. The two most commonly used tests are the **Rorschach** and the **Thematic Apperception Test** (**TAT**).

# XIII – What Are the Legal Issues in Dealing With Violent Patients?

Confidentiality is one of the hallmarks of the helping professions. Mental health professionals in particular have access to the most personal information about patients. **Confidentiality** is a professional's *obligation* to keep information from third parties. **Privilege** is a patient's *right* to prevent information from being used in legal settings. Medical records can be used in court, and, as such, cannot be kept confidential. Judges have a wide degree of discretion available to them in deciding what evidence to allow. Therapists and/or their records can be subpoenaed.

**CO**nfidentiality = **C**linician's **o**bligation
**PR**ivilege = **P**atient's **r**ight

In 1976, a decision was made in a California court that set the standard for the **duty to warn** third parties when they are in danger. Tatiana Tarasoff was murdered by a man whose romantic gestures she had declined. The perpetrator indicated to his therapist his intention to harm Tarasoff. The therapist informed his supervisor and the police. However, because no serious action had taken place at the time of the warning, no legal action was taken. This decision resulted in two legal implications in treating potentially violent patients. Known as **Tarasoff I & II**, these are legal requirements that therapists have a **duty to warn** and a **duty to protect** potential victims, respectively. Breach of confidentiality is indicated only when there is an *identified victim*, and the potential for harm to them is of a *serious nature*. The American Psychiatric Association guidelines also permit a breach of confidentiality where the suicide of a patient can only be stopped by a psychiatrist notifying the police, and in cases where someone responsible for the safety of others (e.g. airline pilots) is demonstrating markedly impaired judgment.

In such situations, warnings to the potential victim and the police are indicated. Under the *duty to protect* aspect, patients should be managed on an inpatient basis (usually by civil commitment), with increased levels of supervision and restraint (chemical and/or physical). How victims should be warned remains up to clinicians (e.g. a visit, phone call, letter, calling police). Other considerations involve the anxiety caused to the intended victim, and the possibility of that person taking preemptive action. Obtain opinions from colleagues, supervisors, and legal counsel in such situations.

Individual jurisdictions have different rules regarding the ethical disclosure of medical information. The other major exceptions to breaking confidentiality involve:
• Emergencies – in situations that threaten life, limb, or vital organ, it is usually possible to release information
• Civil commitment – the police or legal authorities can be given the information required to detain a patient
• Incapacity – in situations where a patient cannot give consent for the release of information, a substitute decision maker can do so
• Child abuse or reportable medical conditions – notifying agencies that receive information about abused or potentially abused children is something clinicians can do without fear of legal repercussion, even if the abuse is not actually occurring; certain communicable diseases are reportable to public health authorities

## Violence Practice Points
• Proper documentation which records both the information supplied and the decision-making process is essential
• Use your own feelings in the assessment of potentially violent patients, regardless of the absence of risk factors – if you feel uneasy, take precautions
• Medications used to treat "violence" are rationally prescribed to treat underlying conditions; for rapid control of violent outbursts, neuroleptics and benzodiazepines (e.g. lorazepam) are often given

# XIV – How Do I Protect Myself In Interviews?

Estimates of violence against clinicians have shown at least one-third of psychiatrists and psychiatric nurses have been assaulted at least once. For unknown reasons, social workers and psychologists are attacked less frequently. Most attacks occur in emergency rooms or on inpatient units. While this may make outpatient appointments seem appealing, assaults in these settings are usually premeditated and are more likely to involve a weapon.

## In the Emergency Department

A psychiatric interview in the emergency room seeks to answer the question, "Why is the patient here *now*?" The focus is to obtain information that helps determine an appropriate disposition. Before seeing patients, assess the acuteness of the situation so that this remains the patient's emergency, and not yours.

• Attend to your safety first; you can't make an accurate, objective assessment if you are in jeopardy
• Be aware of the security arrangements available and make liberal use of them
• See if the police or security are in attendance or nearby
• Read the emergency record thoroughly
• Skim the patient's hospital file for other information
• Determine how the patient was brought to the hospital (e.g. police, friends, on his or her own); being brought in by others increases the risk of violence
• Find out if the patient is intoxicated, restrained, or being held involuntarily (all of these increase the risk of aggressive acts)
• See if bloodwork has been drawn (e.g. for drug toxicity, medical conditions); is an overdose or head trauma suspected? (both reduce a person's self-restraint)
• See if someone is available to provide collateral history
• See if other staff members have additional information

## When Seeing Patients

• Don't challenge a patient's beliefs, especially when starting the interview; maintain your composure
• Give explanations for your actions; demonstrate openness
• Respect the autonomy of patients
• Stress that thoughts and feelings are to be *verbalized*, not acted upon
• Allow adequate, even ample space for patients

• Sit close to the exit to facilitate your escape if necessary
• Do not block the door should a patient bolt
• Seating arrangements can be discussed with patients
• Introduce others and explain their purpose in the room
• Be attuned to your feelings; don't react with anger or sarcasm

• Do not discuss disposition (i.e. admission or outpatient management) until you have enough information to make a solid decision
• Identify and explore resistance to obtaining cooperation
• Interview rooms should never be locked when in use
• Rooms can be customized for safety – desks bolted down, emergency alarms, unbreakable glass, removal of heavy objects, etc.

• Crisis intervention strategies should be practiced – physical, chemical, non-violent (verbal), etc.
• If necessary, insist that someone else be present (clinical or security staff) in the interview
• Don't act heroically, attend to your safety and comfort
• Do not be influenced by goading from patients, other staff, colleagues, or even supervisors

• If physical restraint becomes necessary avoid participating if adequate personnel are present; remember that you need to preserve rapport with patients, and participating in a restraint procedure will likely ruin this; no matter how psychotic or clouded patients are, they usually remember who was present when they were restrained

# Summary

Suicide is an act of deliberate self-harm that requires immediate intervention. Regardless of cultural, philosophical, or personal views, the evidence to date shows that the overwhelming majority of patients who commit suicide suffer from a major mental disorder at the time of death. Patients need protection, compassion, and assistance during these periods.

Numerous risk factors for suicide were outlined to give interviewers an appreciation of which patients might be at higher risk even before suicidal ideation is asked about.

Questions regarding suicidal thoughts do not cause patients to consider taking their lives, rather, avoiding the topic because of uneasiness leaves suicidal patients undetected. *The absence of expressed thoughts of suicide is not evidence of the absence of suicidal ideation or intent.*

Questions directly assessing suicidal intent *at the time of the interview* are essential to ask. Any degree of positive response requires an immediate inquiry into the presence of a plan, lethality of method, impulse control, etc. Cumulatively, almost 1% of the population commits suicide.

Violence towards the interviewer or others is also a psychiatric emergency. At some point, most clinicians are assaulted in treatment settings or have a patient who expresses the wish to harm someone.

Suicide and homicide represent a significant cause of morbidity and mortality, especially in younger age groups.

Various instruments have been developed to assess the potential for violence to the self or others. The predictive value of such tests is hotly debated in legal settings.

In clinical settings, there is no substitute for a thorough interview and mental status examination.

# References

## Books

American Psychiatric Association
**Diagnostic and Statistical Manual of Mental Disorders, 4th Ed.**
American Psychiatric Association, Washington D.C., 1994

A.T. Beck, D. Schuyler, & I. Herman
*Development of Suicidal Intent Scales,* in
**The Prediction of Suicide**
Charles Press, New York, 1974

J.A. Chiles & K.D. Strosahl
**The Suicidal Patient: Principles of Assessment, Treatment, and Case Management**
American Psychiatric Press, Inc., Washington D.C., 1995

J.G. Cull & W.S. Gill
**Suicide Probability Scale Manual**
Western Psychological Services, Los Angeles, 1986

J.E. Exner
**The Rorschach: A Comprehensive System, 3rd Ed.**
John Wiley & Sons, Inc., New York, 1993

H.I. Kaplan & B.J. Sadock, Editors
**Synopsis of Psychiatry, 8th Ed.**
Williams & Wilkins, Baltimore, 1998

E. Othmer & S.C. Othmer
**The Clinical Interview Using DSM-IV**
American Psychiatric Press Inc., Washington D.C., 1994

B.J. Sadock & V.A. Sadock, Editors
**Comprehensive Textbook of Psychiatry, 7th Ed.**
Lippincott, Williams & Wilkins, Philadelphia, 2000

A. Sims
**Symptoms in the Mind, 2nd Ed.**
Saunders, London, England, 1995

S.C. Shea
**The Practical Art of Suicide Assessment**
John Wiley & Sons, Inc., New York, 1999

W.W.K. Zung
*Index of Potential Suicide: A Rating Scale for Suicide Prevention,* in
**The Prediction of Suicide**
Charles Press, New York 1974

# Articles

A. Apter, R. Plutchik, S. Sevy, M. Korn, S. Brown, & H. van Praag
**Defense Mechanisms in Risk of Suicide and Risk of Violence**
*American Journal. of Psychiatry* 146(8): 1027 – 1031, 1989

X.M. Amador, J.H. Friedman, C. Kasapis, S.A. Yale, & M. Flaum
**Suicidal Behavior in Schizophrenia and its Relationship to Awareness of Illness**
*American Journal of Psychiatry* 153(9): 1185 – 1188, 1996

R.L. Austin, M. Bologna, & H.H. Dodge
**Sex-role Change, Anomie, and Female Suicide: A Test of Alternative Durkheimian Explanations**
*Suicide Life Threat. Behav.* 22(2): 197 – 225, 1992

A.T. Beck, M. Kovacs, & A. Weissman
**Hopelessness and Suicidal Behavior: An Overview**
*JAMA* 234(11): 1146 – 1149, 1975

J.C. Beck, K.A.White, & B. Gage
**Emergency Psychiatric Assessment of Violence**
*American Journal of Psychiatry* 148(11): 1562 – 1565, 1991

S. Blomhoff, S. Seim, & S. Friis
**Can Prediction of Violence Among Psychiatric Inpatients be Improved?**
*Hosp. Community Psychiatry* 41(7): 771 – 775, 1994

R. Borum
**Improving the Clinical Practice of Violence Risk Assessment: Technology, Guidelines, and Training**
*Am. Psychol.* 51(9): 945 – 956, 1996

K.A. Busch, D.C. Clark, J. Fawcett, & H.M. Kravitz
**Clinical Features of Inpatient Suicide**
*Psychiatric Annals* 23: 256 – 262, 1993

M. Deflem
**From Anomie to Anomia and Anomic Depression: A Sociological Critique on the Use of Anomie in Psychiatric Research**
*Soc. Sci. Med.* 29(5): 627 – 634, 1989

R. Feinstein & R. Plutchik
**Violence & Suicide Risk Assessment in the Psychiatric Emergency Room**
*Compr. Psychiatry* 31(4): 337 – 343, 1990

J.E. Exner Jr. & J. Wylie
**Some Rorschach Data Concerning Suicide**
*J. Pers. Assess.* 41(4): 339 – 348, 1977

H.H. Fenn
**Violence: Probability Versus Prediction**
*Hosp. Community Psychiatry* 41(2): 117, 1990

G. Fox
**Risk Assessment: A Systematic Approach to Violence**
*Nurs. Stand.* 12(32): 44 – 47, 1998

E. Frank, L.L. Carpenter, & D.J. Kupfer
**Sex Differences in Recurrent Depression: Are There Any That Are Significant?**
*American Journal of Psychiatry* 145(1): 41 – 45, 1988

R.D. Hare
**Psychopathy as a Risk Factor for Violence**
*Psychiatr. Q.* 70(3): 181 – 197, 1999

R.M.A. Hirschfeld
**Algorithms for the Evaluation and Treatment of Suicidal Patients**
*Primary Psychiatry* 3: 26 – 29, 1996

T.H. Holmes & R.H. Rahe
**The Social Readjustment Rating Scale**
*J. Psychosom. Res.* 11(2): 213 – 218, 1967

D.H. Hughes
**Suicide and Violence Assessment in Psychiatry**
*General Hospital Psychiatry* 18(6): 416 – 421, 1996

O. Kernberg
**Notes on Countertransference**
*J. American Psychoanalytic Association* 13: 38 – 56, 1965

M.I. Krakowski & P. Czobor
**Clinical Symptoms, Neurological Impairment, and Prediction of Violence in Psychiatric Inpatients**
*Hosp. Community Psychiatry* 45(7): 700 – 705, 1994

L. Lamberg
**Prediction of Violence Both Art and Science**
*JAMA* 275(22): 1712, 1996

J.R. Lion
**Pitfalls in the Assessment and Measurement of Violence: A Clinical View**
*J. Neuropsychiatry Clin. Neurosci.* 3(2): S40 – S43, 1991

J.T. Maltsberger & D.H. Buie
**Countertransference Hate in the Treatment of Suicidal Patients**
*Archives of General Psychiatry* 30(5): 625 – 633, 1974

D.E. McNeil & R.L. Binder
**Correlates of Accuracy in the Assessment of Psychiatric Inpatients' Risk of Violence**
*American Journal of Psychiatry* 152(6): 901 – 906, 1995

J.R. Meloy
**The Prediction of Violence in Outpatient Psychotherapy**
*Am. J. Psychother.* 41(1): 38 – 45, 1987

M.A. Miller & R.H. Rahe
**Life Changes Scaling for the 1990's**
*J. Psychosom. Res.* 43(3): 279 – 292, 1997

J. Monahan, H.J. Steadman, P.S. Appelbaum, & P.C. Robbins
**Developing a Clinically Useful Actuarial Tool for Assessing Violence Risk**
*British Journal of Psychiatry* 176: 312 – 319, 2000

J.A. Motto, D.C. Heilbron, & R.P. Juster
**Development of a Clinical Instrument to Estimate Suicide Risk**
*American Journal of Psychiatry* 142(6): 680 – 686, 1985

J. Mount
**Causation of Psychological Symptoms**
Personal Communication, 1985

P. Phillips & S.J. Nasr
**Seclusion and Restraint and Prediction of Violence**
*Am. J. Psychiatry* 140(2): 229 – 232, 1983

R.H. Rahe
**The More Things Change. . .**
*Psychosom. Med.* 56(4): 306 – 307, 1994

M.V. Seeman & M. Lang
**The Role of Estrogens in Schizophrenia Gender Differences**
*Schizophrenia Bulletin* 12(2): 185 – 194, 1990

S.C. Shea
**The Chronological Assessment of Suicide Events: A Practical Interviewing Strategy of Eliciting Suicidal Ideation**
*Journal of Clinical Psychiatry* 59(Suppl. 20): 58 – 72, 1998

G. Sonneck & W. Horn
**Contribution to Suicide Risk Assessment – I: A Simple Method to Predict Crisis After Suicide Attempts (Parasuicides)**
*Crisis* 11(2): 31 – 33, 1990

G. Sonneck & W. Horn
**Contribution to Suicide Risk Assessment – II: On the Practice of Suicide Risk Assessment**
*Crisis* 11(2): 34 – 36, 1990

B. Stanton, R.M. Baldwin, & L. Rachuba
**A Quarter Century of Violence in the United States: An Epidemiologic Assessment**
*Psychiatric Clinics of North America* 20(2): 269 – 282, 1997

S.M. Tatman, A.L. Greene, & L.C. Karr
**Use of the Suicide Probability Scale (SPS) With Adolescents**
*Suicide Life Threat. Behav.* 23(3): 188 – 203, 1993

L. Teplin
**The Criminality of the Mentally III: A Dangerous Misconception**
*American Journal of Psychiatry* 142(5): 593 – 599, 1985

A. Theilgaard
**Aggression and the XYY Personality**
*Int. J. Law Psychiatry* 6(3-4): 413 – 421, 1983

O.J. Thienhaus & M. Piasecki
**Assessment of Psychiatric Patients' Risk of Violence Toward Others**
*Psychiatric Services* 49(9): 1129-30, 1147, 1998

W.W. Zung, H.M. Coppedge, & R.L. Green, Jr.
**Seasonal Variation of Suicide and Depression**
*Arch. Gen. Psychiatry* 30(1): 89 – 91, 1974

# Websites

Training Institute for Suicide Assessment and Clinical Interviewing (Provides detailed information on the CASE Approach)
http://www.suicideassessment.com

The Suicidology Web: Suicide and Parasuicide
http://suicide-parasuicide.rumos.com

American Association of Suicidology
http://www.suicidology.org

American Foundation for Suicide Prevention
http://www.afsp.org

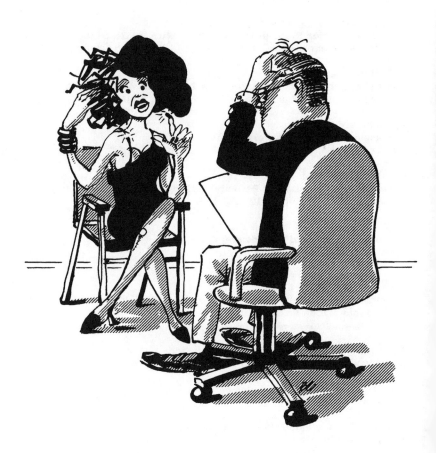

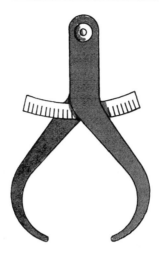

# Chapter 9

# Affect & Mood

## What Are the Factors Involved in Assessing Emotion?

The assessment of emotional states (or disorders) is another of the fundamental domains of the MSE. Disorders of emotion constitute some of the most common and severe illnesses in psychiatry. The components that are assessed are called **affect** and **mood**.

Affect (pronounced with emphasis on the first syllable) refers to the visible, external, or objective manifestations of a patient's emotional state. It is a record of momentary dynamic changes in the expression of emotional responses.

Both internal stimuli (e.g. memories, ideas) and external events (e.g. changes in the environment) can alter affect.

**Mood** is the person's internal feeling state. It is subjective (described by the patient) and refers to the pervasive emotional tone displayed throughout the interview. Mood shifts are less connected to internal or external stimuli than are changes in affect. Mood is considered the "emotional background" whereas affect is the "emotional foreground" of the interview. Affect can be likened to one's degree of satisfaction with the various courses of a meal, while mood is the overall enjoyment of the whole evening.

# What Is the Diagnostic Significance of Affective and Mood Changes?

• **Schizophrenia & Schizoaffective Disorder** 295.X
A. (5) Negative symptoms (e.g. affective flattening)

• **Major Depressive Episode** 296.X
A. (1) depressed mood most of the day. . .
A. (2) markedly diminished interest or pleasure in all activities
A. (6) fatigue or loss of energy nearly every day. . .
A. (7) feelings of worthlessness or excessive or inappropriate guilt. . .

• **Dysthymic Disorder** 300.4
A. Depressed mood most of the day. . .
B. (3) low energy or fatigue
B. (4) low self-esteem
B. (6) feelings of hopelessness

• **Manic Episode & Hypomanic Episode** 296.X
A. A distinct period of abnormally and persistently elevated, expansive, or irritable mood. . .

• **Posttraumatic Stress Disorder** 309.81
C. (5) feelings of detachment or estrangement from others

C. (6) restricted range of affect
D. (2) irritability or outbursts of anger
D. (5) exaggerated startle response

• **Acute Stress Disorder** 308.3
B. (1) a subjective sense of numbing, detachment, or absence of emotional responsiveness

• **Generalized Anxiety Disorder** 300.02
C. (1) restlessness or feeling keyed up or on edge
C. (2) being easily fatigued
C (4) irritability

• **Obsessive-Compulsive Disorder** 300.3
C. The obsessions or compulsions cause marked distress

• **Simple and Social Phobic Disorders** 300.2X
A. Marked and persistent fears. . .
B. Exposure to the phobic stimulus almost invariably provokes an immediate anxiety response. . .
D. The phobic situation is avoided or endured with intense anxiety or distress

• **Intermittent Explosive Disorder** 312.34
A. Several discrete episodes or failure to resist aggressive impulses causing assault or destruction of property

• **Pyromania** 312.33
B. Tension or affective arousal before the act

• **Pathological Gambling** 312.31
A. (4) is restless or irritable when attempting to cut down or stop gambling

• **Schizoid Personality Disorder** 301.20
A. (7) shows emotional coldness, detachment, or flattened affectivity

• **Schizotypal Personality Disorder** 301.22
A. (5) inappropriate or constricted affect

• **Antisocial Personality Disorder**  301.7
A.  (4) irritability and aggressiveness. . .

• **Borderline Personality Disorder**  301.83
A.  (6) affective instability due to a marked reactivity of mood
A.  (7) chronic feelings of emptiness
A.  (8) inappropriate intense feelings of anger or difficulty controlling anger

• **Dependent Personality Disorder**  301.6
A.  (6) feels uncomfortable or helpless when alone . . .

• **Histrionic Personality Disorder**  301.50
A.  (3) displays rapidly shifting and shallow expression of emotions
A.  (6) shows self-dramatization, theatricality and exaggerated expression of emotion

• **Narcissistic Personality Disorder**  301.81
A.  (1) has a grandiose sense of self-importance
A.  (8) is often envious of others. . .
A.  (9) shows arrogant, haughty behaviors or attitudes

• **Post Psychotic Depressive Disorder of Schizophrenia**
(considered a criteria set for further study in Appendix B of the DSM-IV)

This is not intended to be an exhaustive cataloguing of affective and mood criteria from the DSM-IV – there are certainly emotional symptoms seen in other disorders. The purpose of this extended listing is to demonstrate that there is an emotional component to many psychiatric disorders, even if this is not explicitly stated in the diagnostic criteria (e.g. for drug and alcohol use).

Diagnostic Criteria are from the DSM-IV.
© American Psychiatric Association, Washington, D.C. 1994
Reprinted with permission.

# Mood Disorder vs. Affective Disorder

The DSM-IV changed the category of *affective disorders* to *mood disorders*, which is a more accurate description. The emotional disturbances are of a sustained nature and not usually abruptly altered by internal or external stimuli. Hence the rationale for calling them mood disorders.

*Disorders of affect* exist within many of the other conditions listed above. The best example being the Cluster B personality disorders, where emotions can (and do) change rapidly, dramatically, and frequently in response to internal and external cues. A number of other illnesses typically present with wide fluctuations in expressed emotion.

# Describing Affect

Affect can be evaluated along the following parameters:
- **Type/Quality (Section I)**
- **Range/Variability (II)**
- **Degree/Intensity (III)**
- **Stability/Mobility (IV)**
- **Appropriateness (V)**
- **Congruence (VI)**

## I – Type/Quality

Type or quality is the predominant emotion expressed. There are nine principal types of affect:
- Happiness
- Sadness
- Fear/anxiety
- Surprise
- Shame
- Anger
- Interest
- Disgust
- Contentment

## II – Range/Variability

Range refers to the degree to which visible emotions vary throughout the interview. During the assessment, a patient's "normal" affective tone would consist of a combination of a number of the above emotional types or qualities. At some point in the interview, a patient would be expected to smile, frown, appear interested, etc. Since there is no "standard" degree of affect, the term usually used is *"the patient displayed an appropriate range of affect."*

A *narrow* or *restricted* range of affect describes patients who express one or two emotional states. This can be seen in mood disorders (manic patients can have a narrowly high range), schizophrenia, paranoid disorders, partial-complex epilepsy and obsessive-compulsive personalities. A *wide* or *expanded* range, where several emotions are expressed, is seen in Cluster B personality disorders, dementia, delirium, and substance intoxication/withdrawal.

## III – Degree/Intensity

Degree is the extent or intensity to which emotions are expressed. This can also be called **amount** or **amplitude**, and is a measure of the energy expended in conveying feelings. Affective expression occurs along a continuum:

| Low Intensity | Normal | High Intensity |
|---|---|---|
| flattened | appropriate | exaggerated |
| constricted | responsive | dramatic |
| detached | adequate | passionate |

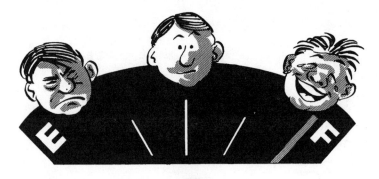

Another way of describing intensity of affect is the *force* of the expression. Much like a good actor conveys depth to a role, intense affect arouses emotional responses in those around the patient.

Patients can have an intense affect with a narrow range (e.g. mania or depression). Conversely, a wide range of expression with low intensity is also seen (e.g. histrionic personalities or delirious patients lack a certain degree of conviction to their affective states). **Blunted affect** is a term often used to describe low or flattened intensity. Sims (1995) uses the term to describe a lack of emotional sensitivity to others.

A flattened intensity of affect can be seen in schizophrenia, conversion disorder (**la belle indifférence**), dementia, and obsessive-compulsive and schizoid personalities. A heightened degree of affect can be seen in mania, narcissistic and borderline personalities, and in anxiety disorders. Depression has a variable presentation: some patients convey intense distress, while others are muted and appear apathetic.

## IV — Stability/Reactivity

Stability refers to the duration of an affective response. Some emotions exist only as long as a facial expression or single tear, others are pervasive throughout the interview. Normally there are shifts in affect during interviews. Such periods are sustained for a few moments and appropriate to the context of the interview. For example: anxiety at the outset, sadness when speaking about recent difficulties, anger at the dog for eating something, happiness when discussing a faster, new computer, etc.

If changes in affect are small or nonexistent (called **fixed** or **immobile**) during the interview, this observation is more a consideration of mood. The term **labile** describes affective changes that occur rapidly and frequently. These changes can take place in either the **intensity** or **range** of affect. For example, a patient may be moved from tears to euphoria within seconds (range), or from mild to intense irritation (degree).

Reactivity of affect refers to the degree to which external factors influence emotional expression. For example, features of the interview process or interviewer can cause emotional reactions in patients. Another aspect of lability is whether or not patients appear to be in *control* of their emotions. In general, patients with mood disorders, substance intoxication or withdrawal, and dementia, have little to no control over their affective state(s). Patients with personality disorders have a greater degree of control.

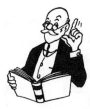

Lability of affect is commonly seen in the following conditions:
• Mania (affect can vary rapidly, e.g. from elated to irritable; expansive to hostile)
• Cluster B personality disorders (this is one of the defining aspects of the histrionic and borderline personalities)
• Delirium and dementia
• Intoxication with drugs or alcohol
• Impulse-control disorders

## V – Appropriateness

Appropriateness is the degree to which visible emotions match thought content. This is also gauged by the degree to which you can empathize with patients.

Affect is either **appropriate** or **inappropriate** to the topic being discussed. For example, a patient who smiles when discussing the death of a parent may be seen as displaying an *inappropriate* affect. If you later learn that this parent was abusive or estranged (and left a large inheritance), then this person's smile is more understandable and the expressed emotion is more *appropriate* to the situation. Inappropriate affect occurs most frequently in schizophrenia, particularly the **disorganized** (historically called the *hebe-*

*phrenic)* **subtype**. Schizophrenia causes people to lose the ability to relate to others, developing a detached, mechanical demeanor. Patients' emotional responses are not what would normally be expected. They may demonstrate what is called a **silly** or **fatuous affect** by: giggling, laughing, grinning, grimacing, rhyming, punning, mocking interviewers, playing with objects, and other child-like actions.

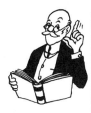

Inappropriate affect is also seen in:
• Malingering – the emotional component of a patient's presentation doesn't "add up" to the verbalized problems
• Substance use – intoxication or withdrawal can cause patients to be inappropriately jovial or unconcerned with medical problems, criminal charges, etc.
• Conversion disorder – **la belle indifférence** describes a distinct lack of concern for reported neurologic deficits
• Depression – when patients have decided to attempt suicide, they can become unconcerned or untroubled by their pre-existing problems
• Delirious or demented patients can seem to be unusually concerned about trivial matters (or the converse)
• Antipsychotic use – affective flattening can occur through the parkinsonian side-effects of these medications

## VI – Congruence
The congruence between affect and the following parameters is important to observe:

### 1. Mood
Affect may or may not be congruent with the mood state a patient reports. For example, patients who describe themselves as depressed would not be expected to smile, joke, and discuss Caribbean cruises. Incongruity may mean ma-

lingering/factitious disorder, the presence of two separate conditions (e.g. mood and personality disorder), substance use, schizoaffective disorder, or a psychotic component to a mood disorder.

## 2. Appearance

Emotional disturbances are often manifested in various aspects of appearance because patients have little time or interest in attending to these points:

*Grooming & Attire* – depressed patients neglect their self-care and are disheveled; they often dress in dark colors. Manic patients dress flamboyantly (often in red) and use poor judgment in picking new looks or styles. Schizophrenic patients may make bizarre alterations and become unkempt.

*Facial expression* is a key component of affective response; unvarying movements are seen in depression and schizophrenia; in mania and personality disorders expressions can be dramatic and exaggerated.

## 3. Behavior

*Posture* indicates interest, self-importance, control etc.; manic, narcissistic, and antisocial patients strut and sit upright; depressed patients slouch and lean on things, etc.

*Body movement/gesticulation* also indicates affective tone; depressed patients move infrequently and slowly; manic patients emphasize their feelings with rapid, exaggerated movements and have trouble containing their activities; hands and lower limbs may give away clues about someone's feelings, keep an eye on the entire body to monitor reactions to questions (sweating, trembling, etc.).

## 4. Speech

Speech conveys information about affective state. *Inflection* provides modulation and emphasis, and makes speech interesting to hear; this is reduced in depression, schizophrenia, or obsessive-compulsive personalities; it is enhanced in mania and cluster B personality disorders.

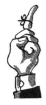

### Affect Practice Points

• It is relatively common for patients to either not be aware or not verbalize their emotional state; in these situations, use your observations to obtain information (e.g. *"Mr. Jones, you looked upset when you described your struggle to keep ahead of your neighbors."*)

• It is also important to inquire about the incongruence between thought content and affect (e.g. *"Mr. Smith, you mentioned that you were going into debt trying to keep up with Mr. Jones, but you smiled when you said this."*)

• Psychotic patients who display silly or inappropriate affect may be responding to internal stimuli, such as hallucinations (i.e. telling them jokes or ridiculing the interviewer) or delusions (e.g. all psychiatrists are cross-dressers)

• Affect originates in the **limbic system** (hippocampus, amygdala, cingulate gyrus, anterior thalamus, mamillary bodies); disease processes (strokes, tumors, multiple sclerosis, meningitis) that occur in these areas can cause affective changes; the hippocampal-amygdala complex is reduced in size in schizophrenia; neurologic disorders affecting the limbic system and basal ganglia commonly present with depression

• Othmer (1994) proposes that affect has 3 functions:

*Self perception* – providing an emotional value judgment

*Communication* – expression of feelings is made known to others

*Motivation* – affect is one of the key elements leading to the initiation of action

# Describing Mood

Mood is evaluated according to the following parameters:
• **Type/Quality (Section VII)**
• **Reactivity (VIII)**
• **Intensity (IX)**
• **Stability/Duration (X)**
• **Pattern (XI)**

## VII – Type/Quality

Quality of mood is the patient's reported emotional state (therefore, you must ask!). The DSM-IV includes the following as pathological mood types:
• Depressed Mood (SectionVIIa)
• Euphoric Mood (VIIb)
• Angry/Irritable Mood (VIIc)
• Anxious Mood (VIId)

### VIIa – Depressed Mood

Depressed mood occurs when patients feel less energetic, hopeful, or capable than what is usual for them. This mood state can be described by any of a number of qualifying terms, such as: *sad, blue, worthless, guilty, flat, hollow, miserable, gloomy, glum, forlorn, morose, troubled, exhausted, somber, brooding, unhappy, subdued, withdrawn,* etc.

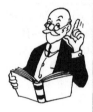

There are a large number of '**d**' words that are used to describe these mood disturbances:

*down, dejected, despondent, demoralized, dysphoric, despairing, dour, dispirited, drained, doleful, downcast, down in the dumps, desperate, defeated, dreary, disappointed, disillusioned, diminished, dissatisfied, disaffected, dysfunctional, disconsolate, disenfranchised, and downhearted*

Because *depression* is used to refer to a mood disorder, a diminished mood state is frequently referred to as **dysphoria**, meaning a state of unhappiness, or feeling ill at ease.

Depressed mood is a diagnostic criterion for the following disorders:
• Depressive disorders
• Bipolar depressions
• Cyclothymia
• Dysthymia
• Adjustment disorder with depressed mood

Transient depressions also occur as a variant of normal mood even when there is no obvious precipitant. The diagnosis of a mood disorder rests on the presence of other features, severity (degree of social and occupational impairment), and duration. Major depressive episodes can be a complication of any other psychiatric condition. The term **double depression** refers to an episode of depression complicating a dysthymic disorder.

The DSM-IV (Appendix B) also contains research criteria for the following proposed conditions: postpsychotic depressive disorder for schizophrenia; minor depressive disorder; recurrent brief depressive disorder; and an alternate set of criteria (Criteria B) for dysthymia.

Depressed mood can be such a long-standing experience for patients that it becomes a character trait. The DSM-IV also lists research criteria for a depressive personality disorder. In the past (DSM-II), the **asthenic personality disorder** was used to refer to patients who exhibit: lassitude, abulia, anhedonia, and the inability to withstand expectable stresses.

Depressed mood is often accompanied by changes in:
• Appearance (decline in self-care)
• Behavior (few spontaneous movements)
• Speech (speak softly; have little to say, etc.)
• Affect (restricted range; variable intensity)
• Thought content (morbid themes)
• Thought form (increased latency of responses)
• Diminished cognitive functioning

**VIIb – Euphoric Mood**
Euphoric mood occurs when patients feel energized, elated or ecstatic. This is of a greater degree than what is experienced when patients are "up" or in a "good mood." Some of the terms used to describe euphoric mood are: *up, flying, grandiose, disinhibited, omnipotent, buoyant, jovial, racing, driven, feeling on top of the world,* and *indestructible.*

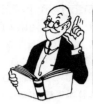

Similar to the 'd' words of depression, there are several 'e' words for euphoria: *energized, elevated, elated, entertaining, exalted, extreme, expansive, extraordinary, ecstatic, effervescent,* and *ebullient*

Euphoric mood is seen in:
• Manic or hypomanic phases of bipolar mood disorders
• Schizophrenia (most often the **disorganized type**)
• Substance abuse (particularly with stimulants)
• Dementia and delirium

There is less empirical support for such conditions as: brief hypomanic disorder, minor manic episode, or a hypomanic personality. When patients are experiencing a dysphoric mood, they frequently seek help. When patients are euphoric, they usually have to be brought for help because of the impact their mood state has had on other people or their social/occupational functioning. Many bipolar patients are "attached" to their highs and value the increased productivity and sense of well-being that accompany them.

Euphoric mood often occurs with changes in:
• Appearance (unusual or bizarre changes)
• Behavior (move rapidly and continuously)
• Speech (speak loudly and have a lot to say)
• Affect (expanded range; labile, intense)
• Thought content (grandiose themes)
• Thought form (flight of ideas; pressure of speech)
• Cognitive functioning (creativity and word association) may be enhanced or diminished because of distractibility

**VIIc – Angry/Irritable Mood**
An angry or irritable mood does not constitute a discrete disorder, but frequently complicates other conditions. Some of the following terms are used to describe these mood states: *annoyed, miffed, pissed off, seething, sharp, disgruntled, cranky, indignant, incensed, bellicose, smoldering, exasperated, furious, ill-tempered, easily provoked,* etc.

**Irritability** is defined as being easily provoked to anger. The DSM-IV lists irritability as one of the three mood states in mania or hypomania. Irritability is usually seen as the mood disorder increases in severity. Anger or irritability can accompany any psychiatric condition and, in isolation, is not of diagnostic significance.

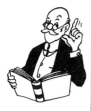

Irritable or angry mood states frequently accompany the following conditions:
• Mania or hypomania
• Cluster B personality disorders
• Intermittent explosive disorder
• Disorders where paranoia is prominent
• Substance use, particularly withdrawal syndromes
• Delirium and dementia
• Head trauma
• Various neurologic conditions
• Temporal lobe (partial-complex) epilepsy, particularly in the **interictal** or **postictal period**

Angry/irritable mood is often accompanied by changes in:
• Appearance (glaring; menacing facial expressions)
• Behavior (muscle tension; threatening movements, posturing)
• Speech (harsh tone of voice)
• Affect (intense; can be restricted or labile)
• Thought content (openly challenging; hostile; sarcastic; demonstrates difficulty with authority; uncooperative)
• Thought form (terse; decreased latency of response)
• Cognition or perception

**VIId – Anxious Mood**
Anxious mood can occur normally, especially if patients are unfamiliar with, or intimated by, interviews. It is also typical for patients to be anxious about such areas as diagnosis, prognosis, and treatment complications. Anxiety is pathological when it is pervasive or present to a degree that it interferes with social or occupational functioning.

Terms used to describe an anxious mood are: *fearful, tense, on edge, worried, nervous, uptight, frazzled, petrified, uneasy, rattled, terrified, paralyzed, scattered,* and *panicky.*

To distinguish anxiety from that seen in anxiety disorders, this mood state is frequently referred to as **apprehension.**

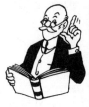

Anxiety is prominently seen in:
- Generalized anxiety disorder
- Phobic disorders
- Obsessive-compulsive disorder
- Posttraumatic stress disorder
- Panic disorder
- Adjustment disorder with a nxiety

Anxiety can complicate any other psychiatric condition and is prominent in a number of general medical conditions (hyperthyroidism, pheochromocytoma, cardiac arrythmias, etc.)

Apprehensive mood is often accompanied by changes in:
- Appearance (widened stare; tense facial expressions)
- Behavior (tremor; quick or jerky movements)
- Speech (tremulous; rapid)
- Affect (intense; restricted)
- Thought content (threatened; impending doom; exaggeration of potential dangers; ruminative, etc.)
- Thought form (decreased latency of response; jumbled, tangential or circumstantial thoughts)
- Cognitive performance (often diminished by anxiety)

## VIII – Reactivity

Reactivity is the degree to which mood is altered by external factors. Mood is mildly altered by events or interactions with others. Manic patients often escalate in mood with stimulation. Depressed patients may feel worse in the morning and have their spirits lift as the day progresses. Similarly, anxious or angry patients have a waxing and waning of their mood under certain conditions.

Historically, depression has been divided into **endogenous** and **reactive** types based on the presence or absence of a (presumed) precipitant. Endogenous depressions were considered to have no precipitant(s). Reference to this distinction is still made in texts and by more "experienced" clinicians. A careful history can usually delineate a precipitant. It may be an event of outwardly minor (but symbolically major) significance. For example, hearing a song on the radio or watching the *Lawrence Welk Show* may bring back memories that serve as a reminder of a lost loved one.

The *endogenous* aspect has been carried forward into a subtype of depression called the **melancholic features specifier**. In this type of depression, there is a lack of mood reactivity to usually pleasurable stimuli. The presence of melancholic features implies a greater likelihood of response to medication or **electroconvulsive therapy (ECT)** than would be expected in patients without such features.

Another subtype of depression called the **atypical features specifier** contains two criteria:
• Mood reactivity, where mood brightens in response to actual or potential positive events
• A long-standing pattern of interpersonal rejection sensitivity (not limited to episodes of mood disturbance) resulting in significant social or occupational impairment

Atypical features are seen more frequently in women and in younger patients. In many cases, only a partial recovery is made from these episodes. Atypical features may indicate that a patient has a bipolar depression or a seasonal pattern (either in the present or future episodes).

## IX – Intensity

Intensity is the degree to which mood is expressed. As with affect, mood has depth, degree, and amplitude. Two patients can experience a depressed mood with a similarly flat affect and restricted range of emotional expression. One patient may appear lethargic, withdrawn, and show little interest in the interview. The other patient may have problems with concentration, lowered self-esteem, and be able to convey the degree to which this episode has interfered with his or her life. The difference between these patients is the depth or intensity of their mood state.

## X – Stability

Stability or duration describes the length of time a mood disturbance exists without significant variation. Mood disorders are required to have a specific minimum time course:

- Major depressive episode          2 weeks
- Manic episode                     1 week
- Dysthymic disorder                2 years
- Cyclothymia                       2 years

The **rapid cycling subtype** of bipolar disorder involves four or more cycles of mania/hypomania and depression within a one-year time span. A cycle is defined as a having either a period of recovery (full or partial) of at least two months' duration from the most recent mood disturbance, or a switch to the opposite mood polarity (e.g. mania to depression).

There is no clear means of distinguishing sustained affect from reactive mood. Certain conditions (e.g. personality disorders, substance abuse) where there is a good deal of variation in the moment-to-moment expression of emotion, can coexist with a mood disorder. To complicate matters, there is a type of bipolar mood disorder called a **mixed state**, in which the criteria for mania and depressive symptoms coexist. The diagram below provides a general guideline:

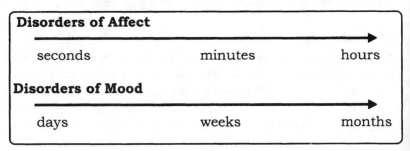

**Disorders of Affect**

seconds          minutes          hours

**Disorders of Mood**

days          weeks          months

# Patterns of Mood Disturbances

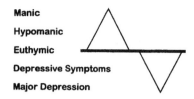

Manic
Hypomanic
Euthymic
Depressive Symptoms
Major Depression

## Bipolar Disorder Type I

• Manic and Depressive Episodes
• Depressive Episodes in some patients are brief or nonexistent
• No separate diagnostic category exists for Unipolar Mania

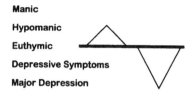

Manic
Hypomanic
Euthymic
Depressive Symptoms
Major Depression

## Bipolar Disorder Type II

• Hypomania with Major Depressive Episodes; the implications of the distinction from Bipolar Type I are still being investigated

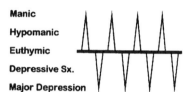

Manic
Hypomanic
Euthymic
Depressive Sx.
Major Depression

## Rapid Cycling Type

• 4 or more episodes of Mania, Hypomania, Mixed, or MDE in 1 year
• Recovery for 2 months between episodes, or a switch to a mood episode of opposite polarity

Manic
Hypomanic
Euthymic
Depressive Sx.
Major Depression

## Cyclothymic Disorder

• Depressive symptoms do not necessarily meet the criteria for a Dysthymic Disorder and are not as severe as an MDE; highs can be hypomanic in intensity

Manic
Hypomanic
Euthymic
Depressive Sx.
Major Depression

## Major Depressive Episode

• Depressive symptoms are of significant duration & severity; usual course is a full recovery, but may have future episodes (the example here shows **recurrent episodes**)

Manic
Hypomanic
Euthymic
Depressive Sx.
Major Depression

## Dysthymic Disorder

• Depressive symptoms are not severe enough for an MDE
• Some patients do develop a coexisting MDE; this is then called a **Double Depression**

# Congruence of Psychotic Symptoms

Psychotic symptoms (delusions and hallucinations) occurring in the context of a mood disorder can be classified as either **mood-congruent** or **mood-incongruent**. Literature reports on the significance of these findings are as follows:

• Kendler (1991) examined four possibilities:
1. **Mood-incongruent psychotic features (MIPF)** do not denote a specific subtype of illness
2. MIPF indicate a distinct subtype of mood disorder
3. MIPF denote a form of schizoaffective disorder
4. MIPF are a type of schizophrenia
Kendler found that the strongest evidence was for the second possibility, with some support for the third.

• Maier (1992) found modest evidence to separate MIPF from schizoaffective disorder
• Coryell (1985) reported that the outcome of depressed patients with MIPF was significantly worse than those with mood-congruent psychotic features
• Tohen (1992) investigated the prognostic significance of MIPF occurring with manic episodes; he found that MIPF predicted a shorter period of remission between mood episodes and a lowered ability to live independently 4 years after the study
• Zemlan (1984) found that patients with MIPF experienced a decrease in psychotic symptoms with lithium, while patients with mood-congruent symptoms did not
• Fennig (1996a) found that the presence of MIPF predicted a poorer GAF rating at 24 months; 15 of 16 patients with MIPF went on to be re-diagnosed with a psychotic disorder (instead of a mood disorder)

Other investigators reported the following:
• Burch (1994) found that the majority of patients had a mixture of mood-congruent and mood-incongruent features, and that the distinction was of no prognostic value
• Fenning (1996b) found little prognostic significance for MIPF

# How Do I Ask About Mood Symptoms?

Mood symptoms are usually distressing to patients and they speak about them readily, or make them apparent early in interviews. Since mood is a subjective phenomenon, patients need to be asked about their emotional state.
- *"How have you been feeling lately?"*
- *"How would you describe your mood right at the moment?"*
- *"I'd like you to rate your mood on a scale from 1 – 10, with one being the worst you've ever felt, and ten as the best. What score would you give yourself right now?"*
- *"How did you feel in response to (. . . some event)?"*

Some patients (particularly obsessive-compulsive person-alities) answer *feeling* questions with *thinking* answers e.g. *"I feel the Orioles will win the World Series,"* or *"I feel like a pizza,"* are not statements of mood.

It may be necessary to point out patient's reactions as a means of eliciting information about mood, e.g. *"You looked very sad when you were talking about being ripped off at the drive-thru. How did you feel at that time?"* As with affect, incongruities between observable signs and reported symptoms need to be explored, e.g. *"You indicated it was difficult for you to miss the Seinfeld re-run last week, but you said this with a smirk on your face."*

Another area fraught with difficulty is being able to distin-guish manic or hypomanic episodes from the elevated mood state that most people experience from time to time. The following questions may help make this distinction:
- *"Was your mood ever so high that friends or family mem-bers thought you needed to get help?"*
- *"Did you get yourself into serious financial or legal trouble, or jeopardize your relationship when your mood was high?"*
- *"Did your mood ever become so elevated that you thought you had some supernatural powers, special connections to important people, or revolutionary ideas?"*

# Rating Scales for Mood Symptoms

## Beck Depression Inventory, 2nd Ed. (BDI-II)
• 21 items are included in this inventory
• The BDI-II is a self-report scale
• The ratings are from 0 – 4 (the higher the number, the worse the symptom)
• The BDI-II takes 5 – 10 minutes to complete
• The BDI-II is a good screening instrument for depression
• Test-retest reliability has not been consistent

## Hamilton Rating Scale for Depression (HAM-D)
• Different versions exist ranging from 17 to 24 items
• The HAM-D is administered and scored by a clinician
• The ratings are from either 0 – 2 or 0 – 4 per item (the higher the number, the worse the symptom)
• Answers to questions and clinical observations are both used to tabulate the score
• The HAM-D takes 15 – 20 minutes to administer
• Test-retest and validity measures are good to excellent
• Medically ill patients and the elderly may have a number of somatic symptoms, which can lead to falsely high scores

## Zung Depression Rating Scale (ZDRS)
• 20 items are rated on this scale
• The ZDRS is a self-report scale
• Items are scored from 1 – 4
• Half of the items are scored positively, the other half negatively; a formula is used to arrive at the final score
• The ZDRS takes 5 – 10 minutes to complete
• Reliability and validity are good
• This scale has not been as extensively studied as the BDI-II or the HAM-D

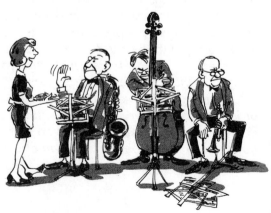

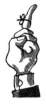

### Mood Practice Points

• **Anhedonia** is the absence of enjoyment from activities that are usually pleasurable

• **Anomie** is an individual's lack of integration into society (real or imagined), leaving few social supports

• **Apathy** is the feeling of a "lack of feeling" characterized by diminished interest, energy and reaction to the environment; such patients are unemotional and listless; apathy has been described as a mood state and can occur with frontal lobe damage, schizophrenia, depression, substance abuse (e.g. sedatives, marijuana)

• **Alexithymia** is the inability to sense and describe mood states; patients are "disconnected" from their feelings and describe them in terms of somatic sensations or behavior; this is seen in schizophrenia, posttraumatic stress disorder, somatoform disorders and strokes

• **Euthymic** is the word used to describe normal mood

• The criteria used to diagnose the dysphoric mood states of depression, cyclothymia, and dysthymia are different

• The distinction between mania and hypomania is made on the basis of degree; if the symptoms are severe enough to interfere with work, relationships, or warrant hospitalization, mania is diagnosed

• Explore what patients mean when they use jargon or simply tell you what their diagnosis is – "depression" can mean quite different things to different people; make further inquiries to make sure you understand what the patient means

## Summary

As Mr. Spock or Data from *Star Trek* can attest, emotions are one of the essential characteristics of what it is to be human. A person's affect and mood reveal what is important to her. Emotions motivate behavior, alter perception, and change thinking. Disorders of emotion are among the most common, and most severe conditions in psychiatry. An assessment of a patient's subjective (mood) and objective (affect) state are required in the MSE.

# References

## Books

American Psychiatric Association
**Diagnostic and Statistical Manual of Mental Disorders, 4th Ed.**
American Psychiatric Association, Washington D.C., 1994

R. Campbell
**Psychiatric Dictionary, 7th Ed.**
Oxford University Press, New York, 1996

F.K. Goodwin & K.R. Jamison
**Manic-Depressive Illness**
Oxford University Press, New York, 1990

E. Othmer & S.C. Othmer
**The Clinical Interview Using DSM-IV**
American Psychiatric Press Inc.; Washington D.C., 1994

B.J. Sadock & V.A. Sadock, Editors
**Comprehensive Textbook of Psychiatry, 7th Ed.**
Lippincott, Williams & Wilkins, Philadelphia, 2000

A. Sims
**Symptoms in the Mind, 2nd Ed.**
Saunders, London, England, 1995

M.A. Taylor
**The Neuropsychiatric Mental Status Exam**
PMA Publishing Corp., New York, 1981

E.L. Zuckerman
**The Clinician's Thesaurus, 5th Ed.**
Clinician's Toolbox, The Guilford Press, New York, 2000

## Articles

A.T. Beck & R.A. Steer
**Beck Depression Inventory-II**
Psychological Corporation, San Antonio, TX

E.A. Burch, R.F. Anton, & W.H. Carson
**Mood Congruent and Incongruent Psychotic Depressions**
*J. Affective Disorders* 31(4): 275 – 280, 1994

W. Coryell & M.T. Tsuang
**Major Depression With Mood-Congruent or Mood-Incongruent Psychotic Features: Outcome After 40 Years**
*American Journal of Psychiatry* 142(4): 479 – 482, 1985

S. Fennig, E.J. Bromet, M.T. Karant, R. Ram, & L. Jandorf
**Mood-Congruent Versus Mood-Incongruent Psychotic Symptoms in First-Admission Patients With Affective Disorder**
*J. Affective Disorders* 37(1): 23 – 29, 1996a

S. Fennig, S. Fennig-Naisberg, & M. Karant
**Mood-Congruent Versus Mood-Incongruent Psychotic Symptoms in Affective Psychotic Disorders**
*Isr. J. Psychiatry* 33(4): 238 – 245, 1996b

P.T. Griffin & D. Kogut
**Validity of Orally Administered Beck and Zung Depression Scales in a State Hospital Setting**
*J. Clin. Psychol.* 44(5): 756 – 759, 1988

M. Hamilton
**A Rating Scale for Depression**
*J. Neurol. Neurosurg. Psychiatry* 23: 56 – 62, 1960

C.L. Hooper & D. Bakish
**An Examination of the Sensitivity of the Six-Item Hamilton Rating Scale for Depression in a Sample of Patients Suffering from Major Depressive Disorder**
*J. Psychiatry Neurosci.* 25(2): 178 – 184, 2000

K.S. Kendler
**Mood-Incongruent Psychotic Affective Illness**
*Archives of General Psychiatry* 48(4): 362 – 369, 1991

S.A. Kerner & K.W. Jacobs
**Correlation Between Scores on the Beck Depression Inventory and the Zung Self-Rating Depression Scale**
*Psychol. Rep.* 53(3 Pt 1): 969 – 970, 1983

W. Maier, D. Lichtermann, J. Minges, R. Heunn, J. Hallmayer, & O. Benkert
**Schizoaffective Disorder and Affective Disorders With Mood-Incongruent Psychotic Features: Keep Separate or Combine?**
*American Journal of Psychiatry* 149(12): 1666 – 1673

M. Tohen, M.T. Tsuang, & D.C. Goodwin
**Prediction of Outcome in Mania by Mood-Congruent or Mood-Incongruent Psychotic Features**
*American Journal of Psychiatry* 149(11): 1580 – 1584, 1992

F.P. Zelman, J. Hirschowitz, & D.L. Garver
**Mood Incongruent Versus Mood-Congruent Psychosis: Differential Antipsychotic Response to Lithium Therapy**
*Psychiatry Res.* 11(4): 317 – 328, 1984

W.W. Zung
**A Self-Rating Depression Scale**
*Archives of General Psychiatry* 12: 63 – 70, 1965

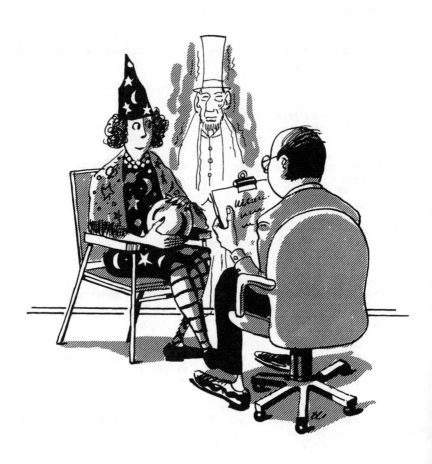

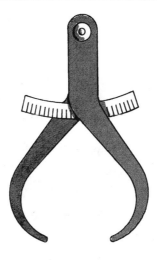

# Chapter 10

# Perception

## What Is Perception?

Perception is the process of experiencing the environment and recognizing or making sense of the stimuli received. Information is received via the five senses: sight, hearing, touch, taste, and smell. An object in the environment causes a **sensation** which, upon interpretation by the brain, becomes a **perception**. Disorders of perception in psychiatry pertain to false associations or the *de novo* arrival of a percept without a stimulus. While imagination can bring about perceptions in any sensory modality, there is normally no difficulty in distinguishing this from real stimuli. As a result of certain mental illnesses, patients are not able to distinguish perceptual aberrations from reality.

The pathway of events leading to the perception of real or imaged stimuli is as follows:

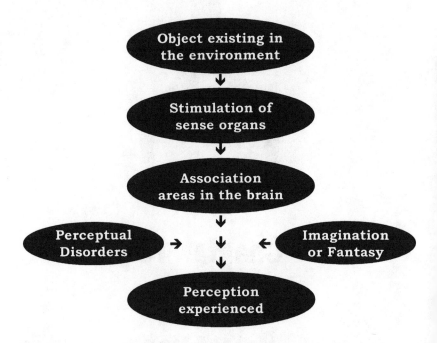

# What is the Diagnostic Significance of Perceptual Abnormalities?

• **Delirium (of any etiology)** 293.0
B.   . . .the development of a perceptual disturbance . . .

• **Schizophrenia & Schizoaffective Disorder**  295.X
A.  (2) Hallucinations

• **Brief Psychotic Disorder**  298.8
A.  (2) Hallucinations

• **Delusional Disorder**  297.1
B.   . . .tactile and olfactory hallucinations may be present if they are related to the delusional theme

• **Mood-Congruent/Incongruent Psychotic Features** (delusions or hallucinations) can complicate mood disorders

• **Panic Disorder** 300.X
A. (9) derealization or depersonalization

• **Acute Stress Disorder** 308.3
B. (1) a subjective sense of numbing, detachment, or absence of emotional responsiveness
B. (2) a reduction in awareness of the surroundings
B. (3) derealization
B. (4) depersonalization

• **Posttraumatic Stress Disorder** 309.81
B. (1) recurrent and intrusive distressing recollections of the event, including images, thoughts or perceptions . . .
B. (3) acting or feeling as if the traumatic event were recurring (. . .including illusions, hallucinations and dissociative flashback episodes. . .)
C (5) feelings of detachment or estrangement from others

• **Hypochondriasis** 300.7
A. Preoccupation with fears of having, or the idea that one has, a serious disease based on the person's misinterpretation of bodily symptoms

• **Factitious Disorder with Predominantly Psychological Symptoms** 312.34

• **Depersonalization Disorder** 300.6
A. Persistent or recurrent experiences of feeling detached from, and as if one is an outside observer of, one's mental processes or body

• **Schizotypal Personality Disorder** 301.22
A. (3) unusual perceptual experiences, including bodily illusions

• **Histrionic Personality Disorder** 301.50
A. (7) is suggestible, i.e. easily influenced by others

• **Borderline Personality Disorder** 301.83

A. (9) transient stress-related paranoid ideation or severe dissociative symptoms

Diagnostic Criteria are from the DSM-IV.
© American Psychiatric Association, Washington, D.C. 1994
Reprinted with permission.

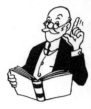

General medical conditions with a high like-lihood of causing perceptual abnormalities:
• Dementia (of any etiology)
• Temporal lobe (partial-complex) epilepsy
• Migraine headaches
• Brain tumors
• Narcolepsy
• Thalamic/peduncular lesions
• Substance intoxication or withdrawal

# What Are the Various Aspects of Perception?

Disorders of perception occur in the following forms:

• **Hallucinations (Section I)**
• **Illusions (II)**
• **Disturbances of Self and Environment (III)**
> Depersonalization
> Derealization
• **Disturbances of Quality or Size (IV)**
> Micropsia
> Macropsia
> Dysmegalopsia
• **Disturbances in the Intensity of Perception (V)**
> Hyperacusis
> Visual hyperaesthesia
• **Disturbances of Experience (VI)**
> Déjà vu
> Jamais vu

# I – Hallucinations

Hallucinations are perceptions that occur when there is no actual stimulus present. They are the most severe of the disorders of perception. Additional features of hallucinations are that they:
• Occur in all sensory modalities
• Can be simple or complex
• Seem as vivid as real experiences
• Occur spontaneously and are beyond the will or control of the patient
• Are often intrusive (as are obsessions)
• Are internal experiences attributed to external sources
• Occur simultaneously with real stimuli
• Serve some psychological function for patients, and often reveal information of psychodynamic relevance

Hallucinations are given the following terms for the sensory modalities in which they occur:

| Sense | Name of hallucination |
|-------|----------------------|
| • sight | visual |
| • sound | auditory |
| • smell | olfactory |
| • taste | gustatory |
| • touch | tactile |

Hallucinations occur on a continuum of intensity. Brief, poorly formed experiences are called **incomplete**, **unformed**, or **elementary hallucinations**. Examples are: flashes of light, whispered sounds, faint odors or tastes, or the sensation of being gently touched.

**Functional hallucinations** require another stimulus or percept to be present first. For example, hearing the opera singer Lorenzo Panzarotti sing about pasta every time the shower runs. In a functional hallucination, he would only be heard when the water was running, and his singing would not simply be a misinterpretation of the sound of running water. Patients with these hallucinations can still discern the sound of the shower. Additionally, the hallucination and original stimulus occur in the same sensory modality (i.e., the running water causes an auditory hallucination, not a visual one of Panzarotti consuming pasta).

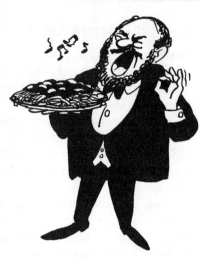

Some patients experience hallucinations in one form that is triggered by a stimulus from in a different sensory modality. These are called **reflex hallucinations**. Using the above example, a running shower would produce gustatory hallucinations of a rich spaghetti sauce or the tactile hallucination of oodles of noodles.

## Ia – Auditory Hallucinations

**Auditory hallucinations** are the most common type occurring in psychiatric conditions. In general, these occur as distinctly heard voices that speak clearly formed words, sentences, or even have conversations. In organic conditions, they are more like **elementary hallucinations**, involving sounds such as ringing, grating, or humming, and are often indistinct.

Auditory hallucinations are most commonly reported in psychotic illnesses and are one of the cardinal symptoms of schizophrenia. They are also part of the criteria for schizophreniform disorder, schizoaffective disorder, brief psychotic disorder, and psychotic disorders due to general medical conditions.

Schneider's first-rank symptoms were covered initially in the chapter on *Thought Content*. Seven of the eleven were delusions, and one was **delusional perception** (the attribution of a false or delusional meaning to an ordinary event).

The remaining three were auditory hallucinations:

• **Audible thoughts**, where patients hear their thoughts said out loud, as if they were echoes. In some situations, patients will speak to those around them about what they presumably heard, as patients expect that others also experienced these audible thoughts. In other instances, patients will hear voices commenting on what they just thought, or were about to think.

• **Voices arguing or discussing** (or both). Here, two or more hallucinatory voices speak about the patient in the third person. These discussions or arguments pertain to the patient (i.e. they are not hallucinatory television shows), and are often critical or derogatory.

• **Voices giving a running commentary** is similar to the above experience. Again, these comments center on the patient and are usually focused on an activity. For example, auditory hallucinations of this nature often comment on actions just before/after or during the event.

The DSM-IV includes these first-rank symptoms as being highly characteristic of schizophrenia. In general, *two* of the following symptoms are required to make the diagnosis:
• Delusions
• Hallucinations
• Disorganized speech
• Grossly disorganized or catatonic behavior
• Negative symptoms

However, only one of these criteria is needed if:
• The delusions are of a bizarre nature
• Hallucinations consist of a voice keeping up a running commentary on the person's behavior or thoughts, or two or more voices conversing with each other

Diagnostic Criteria are from the DSM-IV.
© American Psychiatric Association, Washington, D.C. 1994
Reprinted with permission.

This is as far as the DSM-IV goes in making any symptom *pathognomonic* for a particular illness. There are still time factors, associated functional impairments, and important exclusion factors involved in diagnosing schizophrenia.

Patients are usually able to describe their "voices" in some detail. They are aware of the gender of the hallucinatory speaker and whether or not they know the voice. Often it is someone they are acquainted with, or someone who has passed away. In some instances, patients are instructed or ordered by a voice to perform an act; this experience is called a **command hallucination**. The repetitive nature of these commands can be too much to bear and patients, in time, feel compelled to follow the instructions.

The classical description of auditory hallucinations is that they are experienced as originating "outside" the person's head, as if the source is a completely separate entity. This is in contrast to obsessions, which are recognized being from "within" the patient's mind. Some patients are more insightful, and are aware the voices are a product of their own mind. Auditory hallucinations are usually derogatory and critical of patients. Carrying around this cacophony of insulting, belittling comments is one of the tortures of certain mental illness (e.g. schizophrenia). Fortunately, hallucinations are one of the **positive symptoms** (i.e. they are *added to* the clinical picture), and are among the most responsive to antipsychotic medication.

Auditory hallucinations can be of sounds other than voices. Commonly, this includes: machine-like sounds, music, animal vocalizations, or other sounds of nature.

Mood disorders can also be complicated by delusions and hallucinations. In psychotic depression or mania, the mood disturbance is present initially, and the psychotic features develop as the condition worsens. Interestingly, patients who were congenitally deaf and later developed schizophrenia report the same type of auditory hallucinations as those with unimpaired hearing.

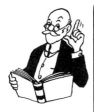

Auditory hallucinations in organic conditions tend not to be as distinct, or have as long a duration as those in psychiatric illnesses. Important medical conditions to consider are:
• Delirium
• Dementia
• Temporal lobe (partial complex) epilepsy
• Migraine headaches (especially of the basilar artery)
• Salicylate (ASA) toxicity
• Ménières disease
• Antibiotic administration (e.g. streptomycin)
• Sensory deprivation (hearing loss)
• Poorly adjusted hearing aids (may be able to hear the voices of people speaking from distances beyond the normal range of hearing)
• Lesions of the temporal/parietal region (e.g. strokes, tumors, herpes encephalitis)
• Vascular lesions of the pons
• Cerebellopontine angle tumors
• Acoustic neuromas (occur in neurofibromatosis)

## Ib — Visual Hallucinations

Visual hallucinations are the second most prevalent type encountered in psychiatric illnesses. It is more common to have visual and auditory hallucinations occurring together than it is to have visual hallucinations alone. One such combination includes auditory hallucinations with partial or inferred visual hallucinations. For example, a patient who hears a voice coming from a coat rack may "see" the arms gesturing as the sound was heard. Isolated visual hallucinations should prompt an investigation for a medical condition or the effects of substance use.

When visual hallucinations occur exclusively in a psychiatric condition, they are almost always due to a psychotic disorder.

Visual hallucinations can be simple or complex. They can be as brief as a "vision" or as involved as having a visit from Abe Lincoln. In occipital lobe infarction, psychedelic and geometric shapes are formed.

In **peduncular hallucinosis**, complex shapes are formed and tend to occur in the evening. Frequently, patients have concomitant disturbances in their sleep-wake cycle and at times enjoy the interesting variety of images.

**Extracampine hallucinations** involve experiencing (seeing, hearing, etc.) other people beyond the normal human sensory range (i.e. being able to look out the window and see someone many miles away).

Visual hallucinations can also form, or be part of, delusional thinking. A patient who experiences a raging Viking leaping out of her hospital closet may develop delusions of persecution. Paranoid patients commonly "see" their persecutors in various public places or just outside their homes. In the delusion of an **imaginary companion**, or a double (**doppelganger**), or a **phantom boarder**, patients may actually claim to have seen such an entity. In **reduplicative paramnesia**, patients both believe they have, and claim to see, duplicated body parts.

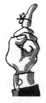

## Visual Hallucination Practice Points

• **Oneiroid states** (from Greek, meaning dream) occur in schizophrenia and delirium. Patients experience vivid hallucinations, which can range from terrifying to engrossing. Oneiroid states can become an "alternate" or "dream world" where patients keep track of this state and reality at the same time.

• The **Charles Bonnet syndrome** is a rare condition consisting of formed, complex, repetitive, visual hallucinations (that are recognized as such); there are no symptoms of other psychiatric conditions, no clouding of consciousness, and no hallucinations in other sensory modalities.

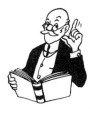

The medical differential diagnosis for visual hallucinations is as follows:
- **Release hallucinations** occur after damage to lesions along the hemispheric part of the visual pathways, involving the temporal, parietal, or occipital lobes; these often occur with visual field defects
- **Palinopsia** is the persistence of a visual image after it is removed, this occurs with occipital lobe lesions
- **Ictal hallucinosis** can occur during seizures, and may contain images of past events
- **Anton's syndrome** (cortical blindness ) occurs with lesions of the cortical visual center; patients deny their blindness and confabulate visual images; this is often accompantied by a strong emotional component
- Migraine headaches occur with scotomas consisting of graying of the visual field, blurring of the center of vision, flashing zig-zag lines, crescents of brilliant colors, or distortion of objects; these images can last up to twenty minutes
- The aura of a classic migraine can cause visual hallucinations without going on to cause a headache
- Dementias,  Pick's disease, etc.
- Huntington's chorea
- Eye problems – injury, retinal detachment, recent surgery, etc.
- Narcolepsy
- Substance intoxication or withdrawal

## Ic – Olfactory Hallucinations

Olfactory hallucinations are far less common than auditory or visual types, and their presence (along with gustatory and tactile hallucinations) warrants a medical investigation.

Olfactory hallucinations can occur in:
• Patients with psychotic disorders
• Patients with co-existing psychiatric disorders and partial-complex epilepsy
• Patients with comorbid psychiatric and other general medical problems

Unfortunately, olfactory hallucinations rarely involve fragrances like rose petals. The most common smells are described as burning rubber, rotting garbage, or very strong body odors. These smells are often of personal relevance to patients.

Smell is the sense most closely linked to memory, and olfactory hallucinations are often accompanied by strong emotions. The olfactory association areas are in the frontal lobes and limbic system (hypothalamus and amygdala).

In some cases, olfactory hallucinations accompany those in other modalities or delusions. For example, the raging Viking who came out of the closet may have had a particular scent about him in addition to sounds he made, etc. Patients who have somatic delusions ("I'm rotting inside") can hallucinate certain accompanying smells. For example, paranoid patients who believe they are being subjected to poison gases can hallucinate the smell of a noxious substance being piped in through their heating or airconditioning.

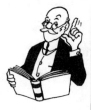

Olfactory hallucinations occur in the following medical conditions:
• Temporal lobe (partial-complex) epilepsy – often form the **aura** of a seizure, particularly if the focus is in the uncus (**uncinate seizures**)
• Migraine headaches (as part of aura), but overall they are more common in partical-complex epilepsy
• Diseases involving the frontal lobes or limbic system

## Id – Gustatory Hallucinations

Gustatory hallucinations are the least common type, and occur in the same types of medical conditions as olfactory hallucinations. Patients who believe they are being poisoned may experience unusual tastes. Like olfactory hallucinations, these are rarely pleasant, and are often described as metallic, acid, bitter, or some bizarre combination of tastes. Psychotropic medication can have an effect on taste sensation. *Lithium* (metallic), *zopiclone* (metallic) and *disulfiram* (garlic-like) are common examples.

## Ie – Somatic Hallucinations

Somatic hallucinations consist of three types:

**1. Tactile hallucinations** involve disorders of bodily sensation. Examples include
• **formication** (from Latin, meaning ant; mind you don't substitute the 'm') which is the sensation of ants or other insects crawling on the skin
• **haptic** – such as being touched by a phantom
• **hygric** – which involves shifts in fluid (*"All my lymph is in my head"*)
• **thermal** (*"My head is on fire"*)

**2. Kinesthetic hallucinations** are sensations of moving body parts such as joint position, body rotation, etc.

**3. Cenesthetic** or **visceral hallucinations** are those involving internal organs (*"My spleen has aligned itself along the axis of the equator"*).

As with other types of hallucinations, these are most common in psychotic conditions and are seen in medically ill patients who have epilepsy or migraine headaches. These hallucinations are often paired with either **somatic delusions** or **delusions of control**. Because delusions are often based on a kernel of truth, psychotic patients may be describing actual perceptions in a distorted or bizarre fashion.

## Other Hallucinations

**Hypnagogic hallucinations** occur while falling asleep, **hypnopompic hallucinations** occur while awakening. These types of experiences occur in a large percentage of the population and, in isolation, are not considered pathological. They can also occur during periods of illness when dehydration, or fever occurs, or when sedating medications are given.

Hypnagogic and hypnopompic hallucinations are usually visual, but can be auditory or tactile. While the duration is brief, they can occur as complex hallucinations.

Hypnagogic and hypnopompic hallucinations occur in **narcolepsy.** Narcolepsy is a condition involving irresistible sleep attacks that:
• Cause **cataplexy**, the sudden and complete loss of muscle tone (differentiate this from **catalepsy**)
• Often occur at times of intense emotional expression
• Have sleep-onset REM periods (these start within 10 minutes of falling asleep instead of the normal 90 min.)
• Cause excessive daytime somnolence

Most adults have had the experience of hearing their names called, only to find that there was no one there. Other brief, familiar sounds (footsteps, doors closing) are also commonly experienced, and are not considered to be pathological.

Bereavement is the reaction to, and grieving process endured, after the death of a loved one. This period is often filled with "hallucinatory" experiences of the deceased person (such as seeing the person in a crowd).

Three other factors can affect perception and lead to hallucinations where no mental illness exists:
• People who have vivid imaginations
• People who are especially impressionable
• Sensory deprivation

# II – Illusions

An illusion is a *misperception* of an existing stimulus. Such percepts are exaggerated, distorted, or altered so that they appear as something different to the person, but remain within that sensory modality. For example, an object which is seen does not become transformed into a sound. As with hallucinations, illusions occur in each of the five senses.

Illusory experiences are affected by the following factors:
• The need to make sense of the environment; here, illusions "fill in the blanks" left by inattention or uncertainty; for example, people may misread a word or be oblivious to a spelling mistake because they "knew what was meant" in the passage
• Emotional state or expectation influences perception; a person who is frightened by walking alone at night is more likely to see a menacing figure in the shadows than if he was walking in daylight with a friend
• **Pareidolia** is a type of imagery that persists after looking at an object (usually a pattern); the illusion and real stimulus exist simultaneously, but the pareidolic illusion is recognized as unreal; a common example of this is seeing faces or shapes in clouds

The DSM-IV only mentions illusions as a criterion in one disorder (schizotypal personality disorder). Most major texts provide scant information on the significance of illusions. They are mentioned most frequently in relation to substance intoxication or withdrawal. It may be that these conditions divert a patient's attention so that misperceptions of the environment become more likely.

Another factor, which has not been formally established, is the significance of the *degree of distortion*. For example, is a person more ill if she misperceives as a person a cardboard or a mannequin?

# III – Disturbances of Self & Environment

**Depersonalization** is a change in the perception of self where the individual feels *as if* he or she has become unreal. **Derealization** is a change in the awareness or the perception of the external world.

It may be difficult to make a clear distinction between the two disturbances because patients often feel themselves blending into the surroundings during an episode of depersonalization.

These conditions have the following associated features:
• They are unpleasant, often causing anxiety or dysphoria
• Patients are aware that these experiences are unreal (as opposed to the experience during dissociation)
• Typical descriptions involve: leaving one's body or somehow being outside of one's self, *"looking down at myself from the ceiling"* or *"watching myself in a movie"*

Descriptions of inadequacy are frequently reported. Patients feel as if they have become barren, deficient, or incompetent. Often there is a distortion of the passage of time, which feels either accelerated or slowed down.

These experiences are common among psychologically healthy people. An estimated 40% of the population may be intermittently affected. It has been suggested that this is an automatic mechanism triggered by stressful situations.

In the DSM-IV, there is a distinct condition called **depersonalization disorder**.

Depersonalization also occurs in schizophrenia, mood disorders, and anxiety disorders, particularly **agoraphobia**. Depersonalization also occurs among personality-disordered patients who lack a strong sense of self (weak ego boundaries), feel incomplete, or are notably insecure. This is most commonly seen in borderline, histrionic, and schizotypal personalities.

# IV – Disturbances of Quality or Size

While these terms technically are illusions, they are often referred to separately and are included for the sake of completeness.

• **Micropsia** is the distortion of seeing things as being smaller than their actual size (like looking backwards through a set of binoculars)
• **Macropsia** is the distortion of objects seeming larger than their actual size; collectively, micropsia and macropsia are referred to as **metamorphosia**
• **Dysmegalopsia** is the perception of seeing one side of an object as being larger than the other (something like the faces in a Picasso painting)

• **Lilliputian hallucinations** involve seeing little creatures, that may also be experienced as speaking to, or walking on, the patient (and causing tactile sensations). The word comes from the celebrated work by Jonathan Swift called *Gulliver's Travels* (written in 1726). In the land of Lilliput, Gulliver is a giant. Lilliputian is also used to describe small-mindedness or being petty. Later in his travels, Gulliver happens upon a land of giants, called Brobdingnag. The terms *gargantuan* or *brobdingnagian* may be used by erudite people as a synonym of macropsia. *Alice in Wonderland* (Lewis Carroll) and *Pickwick Papers* (Charles Dickens) also contain accounts of metamorphosia.

# V – Disturbances in the Intensity of Perception

In these alterations of perception, sensory input is either accentuated or diminished in intensity. For example, **hyperacusis** occurs when sounds are experienced as being louder than they actually occur (**hypoacusis** is the opposite). Smell, touch, taste, and sight (called **visual hyperaesthesia** when enhanced) can all be similarly affected.

# VI – Disturbances of Experience

**Déjà vu** is a French term meaning "already seen" or "there's nothing new in that." It is used to denote a feeling of familiarity to situations that are novel.

**Jamais vu** means "never seen," and is applied to situations that are familiar but strike the person as something they have not experienced.

These phenomena occur in people without mental illnesses. The most common medical condition associated with disturbances of experience is partial-complex (temporal lobe) epilepsy; schizophrenia is the most commonly associated psychiatric condition.

When disturbances of experience are frequent or severe, they are called **identifying paramnesias**, and can cause difficulty with the veracity of memory. Patients may not be able to accurately recall if an event occurred or not (as if it may have happened in a dream and the person can't be certain).

Time perception can also be altered. Patients experiencing *déjà vu* may think that little or no time has passed because experiences seem familiar to them.

An **autoscopic hallucination** is the experience of seeing oneself in a mirror image, or projected onto the external world. Recognition remains intact, and the image is correctly identified by the person. The opposite can also occur, called **negative autoscopy**. Here, the person looks in the mirror and sees nothing (which may make him a vampire). This condition is also called **heautoscopy**.

Disturbances of experience can be a feature of parietal lobe lesions, which can cause other abnormalities of perception:
• **Anosognosia** – lack of awareness of physical illness, or non-recognition of one side of the body (hemi-inattention)
• **Prosopagnosia** – the inability to recognize familiar faces

# Pseudohallucinations & Degree of Insight Into Perceptual Disorders

**Pseudohallucinations** retain the quality of a perception without a stimulus (hallucination), but the person recognizes that the event is not actually occurring. True hallucinations appear to be concrete, real, and happening apart from the patient (in their external or objective space). Pseudohallucinations occur in subjective, inner space. Patients refer to the "inner eye" or "inner ear" as perceiving the stimulus, which is usually auditory or visual. Pseudohallucinations can be vivid and formed. The "pseudo" part refers to the insight on the patient's part, not to poorly formed perceptions (called **elementary hallucinations**). In other words, these experiences are "pseudo" because there is an awareness of their false origin, not because the experience is any less vivid. In these situations, the patient's **reality perception** is impaired, but **reality testing** remains intact.

Pseudohallucinations are perceived as being distinctly different from fantasy/vivid imagery and true hallucinations. They are not indicative of any particular condition, and can occur in patients who have hallucinations (e.g. due to psychotic disorders) or those who have fleeting perceptual disturbances (e.g. personality disorders).

Othmer (1994) outlines five stages of insight into perceptual disturbances:
- Stage 1    no current disturbances; insight into their origin and that they are pathological
- Stage 2    no current disturbances; patient remains convinced that they were actually occurring
- Stage 3    recent experience of perceptual disturbances; unwilling to discuss them
- Stage 4    discusses perceptual experiences and still has them, but refrains from taking action
- Stage 5    acts on perceptual disturbance (e.g. command hallucinations)

# How Do I Ask About Perceptual Disturbances?

Perceptual disturbances, along with disorders of thought content, are usually the most difficult to ask about in interviews. There is a good understanding among the general population that having delusions and hallucinations make one "crazy," and some patients will become offended when they are asked questions about these areas.

In some cases, a patient's behavior is altered because he is responding to hallucinations. For example, a patient may look abruptly at an area of the room, or feel distracted by having to attend to both your voice and the hallucinations simultaneously. In other situations, patients simply choose not to share their experiences (some may have command hallucinations to say nothing to interviewers).

When asking about perceptual disturbances, indicate you know they occur and that you are prepared to discuss them: *"Mr. X, a lot of people with difficulties like yours have some other symptoms as well. In order to be thorough, I'd like to ask you about some of these things so I have a complete understanding of what's been happening."*

These questions are also good openers:
• *"Have you had any unusual experiences?*
• *"Have things been happening around you that seem puzzling, or that don't make sense?"*

One of the distinguishing factors of hallucinations is that they seem as real as, or are even more vivid than, actual experiences. A key point in establishing their presence is the *lack of corroboration* (i.e. others do not share their experiences).

After asking the above questions about perceptual disturbances, patients will either share their experiences, or will need you make your questions more specific:

- *"Have you heard a voice from someone not in the room?"*
- *"Have you seen something that others couldn't see?"*
- *"Have you had experiences such as . . . (example of a hallucination) that others didn't share?"*
- *"Have you ever heard something and not been sure where it was coming from?"*
- *"Did you ever hear something that sounded like a voice and not know who was talking?"*

If the presence of a perceptual abnormality can be established, treat this as you would any other symptom, and get as much detail as possible. The questions in this section are geared at exploring auditory hallucinations because they are the most common type encountered in psychiatric disorders. In general, questions should assess duration, quality, intensity, variation, associated events, etc.

- *"Did you recognize whose voice it was?"*
- *"Did the voice/voices tell you to do something?"*
- *"Did you comply? Why or why not?"*

The question of *"Did the voice seem to come from inside or outside your head?"* is often asked. The significance of this question is that true auditory hallucinations are considered to originate from outside the person (e.g. from radio towers). True hallucinations can also be deemed to arise from within the person as well. Another way of asking this question is to discern whether the experience felt like a product of the person's mind (i.e. obsessions or images) or whether it was a completely foreign experience. Questions about other hallucinations can be posed as follows:

- *"Have you ever experienced a taste that wasn't due to something you were eating?"*
- *"Have you smelled something that didn't fit with the situation you were in at the time?"*
- *"Have you ever experienced a strong/bad taste or smell that you couldn't account for?"*
- *"Have you had sensations in your body that felt like they were due to unseen forces?"* (e.g. being touched or moved by something; ants crawling on your skin; internal organs being shifted etc.)

# Perceptual Disorders in Substance Use

Perceptual disorders occur frequently during both the intoxication and withdrawal states of substance use syndromes. A summary is as follows:

## Substance Ingestion/Intoxication

• **Hallucinogens** consist of LSD, mescaline (peyote) and psilocybin (mushrooms). These substances act on serotonergic neurons to produce any or all of the possible disturbances in perception. Of note are the blending of senses (called **synesthesias**) where, for example, a color has an associated taste and smell. **Hallucinogen persisting perception disorder (flashbacks)** involves spontaneous, transient experiences of geometric shapes, micropsia, macropsia, spoken words, and false perceptions of movement. These substances can also cause a **trailing phenomenon**, where moving objects are seen as a series of disconnected images (as if lit by a strobe light).

• **Cannabis** use is frequently accompanied by a heightened awareness to external stimuli. Experiences are more vivid and new detail may appear to the user. Derealization and depersonalization can also occur. The perception of time passing appears to go more slowly.

• **Phencyclidine** (PCP) is chemically distinct from LSD and considered separately in substance disorder literature. This drug can cause very marked behavior disturbances due (in part) to the perceptual aberrations that occur. Depersonalization, auditory and visual hallucinations, tactile hallucinations of tingling and warmth, and distortions of time and space are commonly reported.

• **Amphetamines**, **MDMA**, and **cocaine** can cause psychotic episodes with visual hallucinations being predominant. Because other symptoms also occur, this psychotic state can be indistinguishable from paranoid schizophrenia.

## Substance Withdrawal

• **Alcohol hallucinosis** (called *alcohol-induced psychotic disorder with hallucinations* in the DSM-IV) occurs when the person stops drinking, and consists of auditory hallucinations that are critical, derogatory, and threatening. These hallucinations occur in a clear sensorium and are distinct from alcohol withdrawal delirium. They usually disappear within several days. The quality of the voices can be identical to Schneider's first-rank symptoms for schizophrenia.

• Alcohol withdrawal leading to **delirium tremens** (DTs) is most often accompanied by visual (e.g. lilliputian) and tactile (e.g. formication) hallucinations

• **Cocaine withdrawal** can also lead to the tactile hallucination of formication; visual hallucinations can also occur, but the most common psychotic disturbances are paranoid delusions

• **Benzodiazepine** and **barbiturate** withdrawal can lead to a state of delirium, which is indistinguishable from the DTs; usually the hallucinations are visual in nature, but can be tactile or auditory in nature

In practice, almost any substance of abuse can cause perceptual abnormalities as part of an intoxication effect/delirium, or withdrawal effect/delirium. The examples listed above were included to illustrate that distortions of perception are common in substance abuse syndromes. That various states of intoxication or withdrawal can be clinically indistinguishable from major psychiatric illnesses is a fascinating area for psychiatric research.

Prescription medication is also capable of causing such reactions in patients. This happens frequently in situations where patients are quite ill due to blood loss, dehydration, etc. Drug-drug interactions are also etiologically important causes of perceptual disturbances. Certain types of medications alone can affect perception, e.g. opioids, atropine, nitrous oxide anesthesia, anticholinergics, sympathomimetics, bromocriptine, L-dopa, etc.

# Psychodynamic Aspects of Perceptual Abnormalities

Hallucinations can be thought of as serving important psychological functions for patients. As with delusions, hallucinations represent projections onto the environment of a "voice" belonging either to patients or their caretakers (**introjected objects**). While psychotic disorders are being delineated as "brain diseases," important psychosocial contributions still need to be considered. Convincing evidence for this is that the concordance rate for schizophrenia in identical (monozygotic) twins is nearly 50%. Clearly, there are environmental factors influencing the expression and course of psychiatric disorders. A major area of psychosocial contribution is **expressed emotion (EE)**, defined as criticism, overinvolvement, or hostility on the part of caretakers (usually parents). Psychotic patients frequently experience auditory hallucinations of criticism, which appears to be a re-living of childhood. Frequently, the voices can be identified as those of parents or other significant figures from their past.

# Neurodynamic Aspects of Perceptual Abnormalities

CT scans showing lateral ventricular enlargement have been a consistent finding in schizophrenia. MRI scans have found reductions in temporal lobe size, and that specific temporal subcortical nuclei are affected (e.g. the limbic system, particularly the amygdala and hippocampus). It is of significance that these structures are adjacent to the body of the lateral ventricle. The terminal area for the auditory pathway is the transverse gyrus of Heschl (Brodmann area 41) in the temporal lobe. This provides a rudimentary explanation for the major perceptual disturbance in schizophrenia (auditory hallucinations) in that demonstrable pathology has been found in the auditory association area of the temporal lobe (which also contains visual association areas).

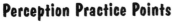

### Perception Practice Points

- Hallucinatory voices are sometimes called **phonemes**; the term is also used to denote the audible components (speech units) of words; **phonemic aphasias** were covered in the *Speech Chapter*
- Hallucinations that occur in conjunction with delusions are often difficult to differentiate; for example a somatic delusion and a haptic hallucination may be clinically indistinguishable because there is no way of determining the presence of hallucinations
- Hallucinations are one of the most easily faked symptoms in factitious disorder and malingering
- It is important to avoid corroborating hallucinatory experiences, regardless of how adamant patients are about the vividness of these phenomena; some patients ask about such things as a reality check and depend on your candor
- Mood congruent/incongruent hallucinations occur as a specifier for psychotic mood disturbances; as with delusions, the content of hallucinations congruent with depression have themes of punishment, nihilism, etc.
- Patients with histrionic personality disorder have a cognitive style which is impressionistic and diffuse; **hysterical misapperception** describes (sensory) perceptual disturbances stemming from patients being only vaguely aware of events occurring around them
- **Hypochondriasis** is the preoccupation of having a serious illness based on the misinterpretation or misperception of bodily signs or symptoms

# Summary

The human brain needs stimulation in order to develop properly and to maintain a coherent sense of self and the world. Perception provides new information, which changes a person's feelings, thoughts, and behavior.

Perceptual abnormalities occur in many psychiatric and medical illnesses, and are one of the hallmark symptoms of psychosis.

# References

## Books

American Psychiatric Association
**Diagnostic and Statistical Manual of Mental Disorders, 4th Ed.**
American Psychiatric Association, Washington D.C., 1994

M. Galanter, & H.D. Kleber, Editors
**The American Psychiatric Press Textbook of Substance Abuse Treatment, 2nd. Ed.**
American Psychiatric Press, Inc., Washington D.C., 1999

G. Asaad
**Hallucinations in Clinical Psychiatry**
Brunner/Mazel, New York, 1990

R. Campbell
**Psychiatric Dictionary, 7th Ed.**
Oxford University Press, New York, 1996

D.M. Kaufman
**Clinical Neurology for Psychiatrists, 5th Ed.**
W.B. Saunders, Philadelphia, 2001

L. Rolak
**Neurology Secrets**
Hanley & Belfus, Philadelphia, 1993

B.J. Sadock & V.A. Sadock, Editors
**Comprehensive Textbook of Psychiatry, 7th Ed.**
Lippincott, Williams & Wilkins, Philadelphia, 2000

A. Sims
**Symptoms in the Mind, 2nd Ed.**
Saunders, London, England, 1995

M.A. Taylor
**The Neuropsychiatric Mental Status Exam**
PMA Publishing Corp. New York, 1981

E.L. Zuckerman
**The Clinician's Thesaurus, 5th Ed.**
Clinician's Toolbox, The Guilford Press, New York, 2000

## Articles

B. Adityanjee
**Clinical Significance of Pseudohallucinations** (letter)
*General Hospital Psychiatry* 22(2): 124 – 126, 2000

J.L. Carter
**Visual, Somatosensory, Olfactory, and Gustatory Hallucinations**
*Psychiatric Clinics of North America* 15(2): 347 – 358, 1992

P. Cheung, I. Schweitzer, K. Crowley, & V. Tuckwell
**Violence in Schizophrenia: Role of Hallucinations and Delusions**
*Schizophrenia Research* 26(2–3): 181 – 190, 1997

G. Chouinard & R. Miller
**A Rating Scale for Psychotic Symptoms Part I: Theoretical Principles and Subscale 1: Perception Symptoms (Illusions and Hallucinations)**
*Schizophrenia Research* 38(2–3): 101 – 122, 1999

M.A. Cohen, C.A. Alfonso, & M.M. Haque
**Lilliputian Hallucinations and Medical Illness**
*General Hospital Psychiatry* 16(2): 141 – 143, 1994

D. Hellerstein, W. Frosch, & H.W. Koenigsberg
**The Clinical Significance of Command Hallucinations**
*American Journal of Psychiatry* 147(2): 245 – 247, 1990

T.R. Kwapil, J.P. Chapman, L.J. Chapman, & M.B. Miller
**Deviant Olfactory Experience as Indicators for Risk for Psychosis**
*Schizophrenia Bulletin* 22(2): 371 – 382, 1996

J. Mitchell & A.D. Vierkant
**Delusions and Hallucinations of Cocaine Abusers and Paranoid Schizophrenics: A Comparative Study**
*Journal of Psychology* 125(3): 301 – 310, 1991

K.N. Sokolski, J.L. Cummings, B.I. Abrams, E.M. DeMet, L. Katz, & J. Costa
**Effects of Substance Abuse on Hallucination Rates and Treatment Responses in Chronic Psychiatric Patients**
*Journal of Clinical Psychiatry* 55(9): 380 – 387, 1994

M. Stephane, M. Folstein, E. Matthew, & T.C. Hill
**Imaging Auditory Verbal Hallucinations During Their Occurrence**
*Journal of Neuropsychiatry and Clinical Neurosciences* 12(2): 286 – 287, 2000

H. Suzuki, C. Tsukamoto, Y. Nakano, S. Aoki, & S. Kuroda
**Delusions and Hallucinations in Patients With Borderline Personality Disorder**
*Psychiatry and Clinical Neurosciences* 52(6): 605 – 610, 1998

K. Takaota & T. Takata
**"Alice in Wonderland" Syndrome and Lilliputian Hallucinations in a Patient With a Substance-Related Disorder**
*Psychopathology* 32(1): 47 – 99, 1999

A.P. Weiss & S. Heckers
**Neuroimaging of Hallucinations: A Review of the Literature**
*Psychiatry Research* 92(2–3): 61 – 74, 1999

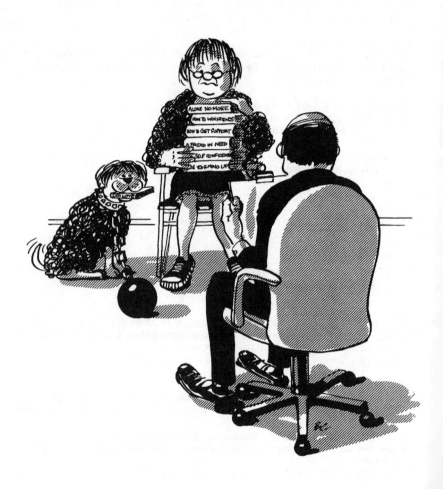

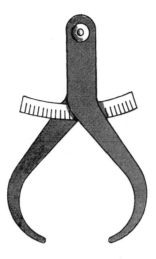

# Chapter 11

# Insight & Judgment

## How Are Insight & Judgment Assessed?

On a basic level, **insight** can be defined as having an aware-ness of one's illness. A more extensive definition is provided by Markova (1992a): *Insight is a form of self-knowledge which includes not only information on problems, but also an under-standing of their effect on the way in which the self interacts with the world.*

Insight is not a symptom, but a process or a continuum. Inferences are made about a patient's level of insight from other areas of the MSE (i.e. thought content and behavior). Methods for obtaining gauging level of insight in a more direct manner are presented in this chapter. While insight is usually recorded as *absent, partial,* or *intact,* it has important implications for evaluating areas such as: suicidal risk and dangerousness, severity of illness, predicting the response to treatment, and compliance. Other matters, such as obtaining valid informed consent or determining the need for involuntary committal, rely heavily on a patient's degree of insight. Lastly, the term "insight" is used in psychoanalytic literature to refer to the process of bringing into consciousness repressed impulses or emotions.

Insight is a cognitive awareness, and is technically a component of thought content. Within the limited time frame of the MSE, it may be practical to limit the assessment of insight to the following aspects:
• The awareness of having an illness
• An understanding of the factors contributing to the illness
• An appreciation that various signs and symptoms are part of a disease process
• The awareness that one's illness impacts on other people and society at large
• Acknowledgment of the *need* for treatment

Readers interested in an elegant and comprehensive discussion of insight are encouraged to read the articles by Markova et al listed in the reference section.

**Judgment** is defined as a process that involves the transformation of uncertainty into a preference. Kaplan (1988) outlines five stages in this process:
**1.** Appraising the challenge
**2.** Surveying alternatives
**3.** Weighing the alternatives
**4.** Deliberating about selection
**5.** Making a commitment to a choice

Judgment involves both a *cognitive awareness* (decision) and an *action* (behavior). Intact insight and judgment are the end result of many factors: intelligence, accurate perception (of both internal and external events), absence of significant mood changes, the ability to understand and communicate ideas, intact cognitive abilities, control over impulses, and the capacity for abstract thinking.

# What Is the Diagnostic Significance of Deficient Insight or Judgment?

Impaired insight (deficient awareness) and impaired judgment (poor decision making) are common to all illnesses, but are perhaps found more frequently with psychiatric conditions because the disease process affects brain function.

The DSM-IV contains severity and course specifiers for all conditions. Determination is based on:
• The current illness only
• The number and intensity of signs and symptoms
• The degree of social and occupational impairment

The severity specifiers are:
• Mild – few, if any symptoms in excess of those required to make the diagnosis, and result in no more than minor impairment in social or occupational functioning
• Moderate – between mild and severe
• Severe – many symptoms in excess of those required to make the diagnosis, or several symptoms that are particularly severe, or result in marked impairment in social or occupational functioning

Disorders including a "with poor insight" specifier are:
• Obsessive-compulsive disorder – if for most of the time during the current episode, the obsessions and compulsions are not seen as excessive or unreasonable
• Hypochondriasis – if for most of the time during the current episode, the individual does not recognize that the concern about having a serious illness is excessive or unreasonable

Diagnostic Criteria are from the DSM-IV.
© American Psychiatric Association, Washington, D.C. 1994
Reprinted with permission.

# What Are the Components of Insight?

Insight is a complex function requiring the integration of higher mental functions. The following components can be used to help determine the level of insight:
• Acknowledgment of the illness (knowing the diagnosis, subtype, course, features, etc.)
• Being able to describe the consequences and repercussions of being ill
• The awareness of one's own thoughts, feelings, motivations, etc.
• Being aware of the subtleties and the symbolic aspects of behavior
• Having the ability to see the effects one has on others
• Being able to ascribe abnormal experiences to an illness
• Understanding that treatment may be able to reduce, control, or alleviate symptoms (even if treatment is not accepted, which is more of a measure of judgment)

Insight is an important aspect of determining a patient's capacity for giving **informed consent**. An assessment of the capacity to consent to treatment focuses on many of the above issues. Insightful patients can appreciate the benefits of continuing with various forms of treatment, and are more likely to be compliant. Educating patients and families about psychiatric disorders helps to increase the level of insight. Insight varies with many factors: mood state, degree of thought disorder, drug intoxication, length of time since medication was taken, etc. Although in interviews an assessment is made of patients' awareness of being ill, their degree of insight into other aspects of their lives can show a considerable range.

# How Is the Degree of Insight Measured?

Gauging a patient's level of insight, and applying this determination to a treatment plan is virtually a daily occurrence for psychiatrists. Yet, despite the frequency and significance of evaluating insight, the clinician is left with few structured or objective approaches. Two rating scales are summarized here. McEvoy (1989a) developed the *Insight and Treatment Attitudes Questionnaire* (**ITAQ**), consisting of 11 questions scored from 0 (no insight) to 2 (good insight). He demonstrated that the ITAQ was able to predict compliance with treatment, and also the likelihood of relapse.

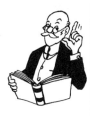

## Insight and Treatment Attitudes Questionnaire (ITAQ)

1. At the time of admission to this hospital, did you have mental (nerve, worry) problems that were different from most other people's? Explain.

2. At the time of admission, did you need to come to this hospital? Explain.

3. Do you have mental (nerve, worry) problems now? Explain.

4. Do you need to be in this hospital now? Explain.

5. After you are discharged, is it possible you will have mental (nerve, worry) problems again? Explain.

6. After you are discharged, will you need to be followed (looked after) by a psychiatrist (mental health center)? Explain.

7. At the time of admission, did you need to be treated with medications for mental problems (nerves or worries)? Explain.

8. Do you need to be treated with medications for mental problems (nerve or worries) now? Explain.

9. After you are discharged, will you need to take medications for mental problems (nerve or worries)? Explain.

10. Will you take the medications? Explain.

11. Do the medications do you any good? Explain.

From McEvoy et al, 1989a
© 1989 Lippincott, Williams and Wilkins
Reprinted with permission.

Markova (1992b) devised *The Insight Scale,* which contained 32 questions scored as 'yes,' 'no,' or 'don't know.' The questions were assigned to two groups: Group A, if answered positively, indicate greater insight; and Group B, indicating less insight if answered positively.

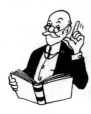

## The Insight Scale
### Group A
• My condition can be treated with medicines.
• I have come to the hospital because I am ill and need treatment.
• I have been having some silly thoughts.
• No one believes I am ill.
• Something very strange is happening to me.
• I feel my mind is going.
• I know that my thoughts are silly but I cannot help it.
• I cannot stop worrying about things.
• I feel different from my normal self.
• I am losing contact with my environment.
• I am losing contact with myself.
• I understand why I am in the hospital.
• I understand why other people think I should be in hospital.
• I want to know why I am feeling like this.

### Group B
• I have come into the hospital for a rest.
• Mental illness does not exist.
• Someone else should be here instead of me.
• Nothing is the matter with me.
• The mind cannot become ill, only the body.
• My neighbors are after me.
• Someone is controlling my mind.

Adapted from Markova, 1992b
© 1992 Munksgaard International Publishers, Ltd.
Copenhagen, Denmark
Reprinted with permission.

Markova deleted some of the original 32 questions from her statistical analysis because she deemed them to be ambiguous. Only the questions she deemed valid, and whose answers were used in her statistical analysis, were included in the previous table. Markova (1992b) found that insight scores improved with the duration of admission, and that more severely ill patients scored worse on the insight scale.

# Other Insight Scales

McEvoy (1993) employed another technique to try to get an objective measure of insight. He had patients read a series of vignettes that were based on the classical positive and negative signs of schizophrenia, including symptoms of:
• Conceptual disorganization
• Suspiciousness
• Unusual thought content
• Avolition/apathy
• Anhedonia/asociality
• Affective flattenting/blunting
• Alogia

He found that patients with diminished insight were unable to see the extent to which the symptoms in the vignettes described their situation (as judged by one of the authors). Secondly, impaired insight prevented patients from even acknowledging that the contents of the vignette described the symptoms of a serious mental illness.

Hayashi (1999) developed the *Awareness of Being a Patient Scale* (**ABPS**). The definition of insight in developing this scale was based on two factors: to what extent patients recognized their need for treatment, and to what extent they accepted the treatment. The ABPS is a 25-question instrument, with each question answered on a four-point scale: 4 for strongly agree, 3 for mildly agree, 2 for mildly disagree, and 1 for strongly disagree. Similar to Markova (1992b), this scale contains two groups, one with affirmative answers indicating awareness, the other with affirmative answers indicating a lack of awareness.

# How Do I Describe Insight?

Because insight occurs along a continuum, there are three levels or degrees that are typically used to describe the awareness patients have of their illnesses:

**Full Insight**
• Recognizes that signs and symptoms are part of an illness
• Able to modify behavior
• Fully cooperative with treatment

**Partial Insight**
• Recognizes that there are problems but does not attribute them to an illness
• May understand others (family, doctor) see them as ill
• Some ability to modify behavior
• Variable degree of cooperation with treatment

**Impaired/No Insight**
• Denial of illness or that there are problems
• Has no capacity to understand the concerns of others
• Poor compliance with treatment

# How Do I Ask About Insight?

Many of the aspects of insight are dealt with in the body of the interview. In situations where the degree of insight needs to be specifically addressed, the following questions can help introduce an assessment of insight:
• *"Is it your opinion that you have an illness?"*
• *"How do you account for the difficulties you were having?"*
• *"Have you had experiences that you think aren't normal?"*
• *"What does (name of condition) mean to you?"*
• *"What is important to help your recovery?"*
• *"What will happen if you don't follow through with the treatment proposed for this condition?"*
• *"What would help you feel better?"*

# How is the Degree of Judgment Determined?

Judgment is a process that leads to a decision or an action. In interview situations, it can be distilled down to an assessment of what the person did or didn't do with respect to his or her illness. Kaplan (1988) proposes the following approach to gauging judgment:
• What is the patient's understanding of the medical problem?
• What is the patient's understanding of the doctor's recommendations?
• What is the patient's understanding of the doctor's rationale?
• What is the patient's choice?
• What is the patient's rationale for his or her choice?
• What does the patient anticipate as the consequences of the choice being made?

This protocol contains many of the key elements a clinician would consider in determining if a patient is capable of providing informed consent. A fuller explanation of this process can be found in Wear-Finkle (2000).

Other factors assisting in determining judgment are:
• The ability to enumerate the pros and cons for a course of action
• The degree to which a patient's actions are in his or her best interests
• The extent to which insight is present
• The degree of contemplation prior to taking action

Poor judgment can be evidenced by the following actions:
• Impulsivity
• Engaging in actions with a high probability of damaging consequences (regardless of how impulsively they were carried out):
  · shoplifting          · sexual promiscuity
  · buying sprees        · reckless driving

· physical assault      · vandalism
· switching brands of cola

Although the most important factor leading to sound judgment is adequate insight, the terms are not synonymous. For example, personality-disordered patients may well have an awareness that their actions cause considerable distress to others, yet they do not change their behavior (despite having at least partial insight).

Similarly, some patients display good judgment despite having poor insight. For example, some patients take medication because others want them to, not because they are convinced they need it. Other patients visit emergency departments for social reasons when ill. While they are in need of help, their visit may well be coincidental to the need for treatment.

In the time constraints of the MSE, a practical approach to determining judgment focuses on how a patient came to medical attention. If it is not clear, ask about how he or she entered the mental health system:
• Did the person seek assistance of his or her own volition?
• To what extent were others (e.g. the police) needed to motivate or push the patient into getting assistance?
• How long did the person wait before seeking help?
• How bad did things get before help was sought?
• Were there associated medical problems?
• Did others suffer harm because of the patient's actions?
• What was the "final straw" before taking action?

## How Do I Ask About Judgment?

In situations where judgment needs to be directly assessed, the following questions may be useful:
• *"What are your plans for the future?"*
• *"What would you do if you became acutely suicidal?"*
• *"What are the first signs you are aware of when things are starting to go downhill? What do you do about them?"*

# "Traditional" Assessments of Judgment

Judgment has traditionally been assessed by asking patients how they would respond to either of these situations:
• Smelling smoke in a movie theater
• Finding a sealed, stamped envelope on the ground

Claypoole & Tucker, in the textbook *Psychiatry* (Tasman, Kay, & Lieberman, 1997), still advocate the use of these scenarios, and even suggest others, such as asking for an explanation of why laws are necessary, or why one should avoid bad company.

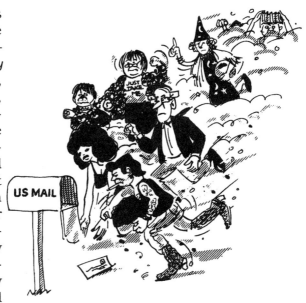

Kaplan (1988) points out that these scenarios are tests of intelligence, not judgment. In fact, these questions are from the verbal comprehension subtest of the **Wechsler Adult Intelligence Scale – Revised (WAIS-R)**. This subtest asks for explanations about day-to-day experiences (Why is land more expensive in the city? Why do we wash clothes?) and is a measure of a patient's ability to use practical information.

Manley, in the *Comprehensive Textbook of Psychiatry* (Sadock & Sadock, 2000), along with Kaplan (1988), points out the following deficiencies in using hypothetical situations:
• Valid tests of judgment should be specific to a patient's

situation; questions such as, *"Why did you stop taking your medication?"* provide more accurate assessments
• Smoky theaters and stamped envelopes are simplistic scenarios that require only a single correct response
• Patients can answer questions about hypothetical situations correctly, but still evidence deficient judgment in their own lives; intact judgment in one area is not a global test of decision-making ability
• Depending on a patient's circumstances, alternative answers need to be considered; for example, a destitute patient who opens an envelope to look for money is probably exercising good judgment

# Proverbs

Proverbs are distilled pieces of wisdom that describe universal human truths, tendencies, or concerns. Asking patients to interpret proverbs is another part of the verbal comprehension subtest of the **WAIS-R**.

Andreason (1977) points out that proverb interpretation in the MSE is a time-honored tradition, and that some clinicians are so fascinated with asking patients to interpret them that they omit other crucial sections.

Andreason (1977) conducted a study to try and establish the validity and reliability of proverb interpretation. Ten proverbs were rated on a three-point scale on five different aspects:
• Correctness
• Abstractness
• Concreteness
• Bizarreness
• Personalization

Additionally, Andreason (1977) investigated the diagnostic usefulness of using proverb interpretation to distinguish between patients with mania, depression, and schizophrenia. Her results were as follows:

Chapter 11 — Insight & Judgment

• Raters who were blind to the patient's diagnosis were unable to achieve adequate reliability
• Proverbs were most useful in distinguishing depression from mania; less so for depression from schizophrenia; and least useful in distinguishing mania from schizophrenia

Andreason (1977) summed up the results of her study as follows:
*"Thus at best proverb interpretation may have relatively good validity but poor reliability, and the greatest validity is obtained in those cases when differential diagnosis is not a problem. At worst, therefore, the validity of using proverbs in a clinical situation is somewhat questionable."*

A common criticism of proverbs has been that they are highly dependent on culture. Patients who grew up in other countries and whose native tongue is not English may miss the abstract meaning of a proverb, leading clinicians to incorrectly conclude that their thinking was concrete, and thus underestimating cognitive abilities.

Haynes (1993) conducted a study investigating (among other things) whether proverbs that are familiar or unfamiliar to patients were preferable for testing. Unfortunately, her results were inconclusive, and her recommendation was that a mixture of both should be used. Haynes notes that the advantages of using unfamiliar proverbs are that answers depend less on learned responses and memory, and do not exhibit the practice effect patients show after several interviews.

Haynes (1993) was able to generate a list of proverbs that did not appear to have racial or gender biases:
**Familiar Proverbs**
• The bigger they are, the harder they fall
• What goes around, comes around
• Don't judge a book by its cover
• Two wrongs don't make a right
• Don't count your chickens before they hatch

**Unfamiliar Proverbs**
• There is no rose without its thorns
• The dogs may bark, but the caravan moves on
• A man who chases two rabbits catches neither one
• When the elephants fight, the grass gets trampled

While proverb interpretation can provide some measure of judgment, it is more useful to look at the person's actions in reality instead of hypothetical situations. Questions of a similar nature assess **abstract thinking** (covered in the *Sensorium & Cognitive Functioning Chapter*).

# What Are Ego Defenses?

Ego defenses, also called **defense mechanisms**, serve to protect an individual from unpleasant thoughts or emotions. By definition, these are unconscious processes that result from interactions between the **id, ego**, and **superego** (explained below). Everyone uses ego defenses to some degree, and these mechanisms clearly have adaptive aspects. For example, some degree of denial of an illness often helps patients cope with stress and not feel completely overwhelmed. In many psychiatric disorders, ego defenses operate on a pathological level, with the end result being that patients have limited insight into their illnesses, relationships, need for treatment, etc.

## Where Do Ego Defenses Come From?

Their "headquarters" resides in Freud's **structural theory**, introduced with the publication of *The Ego and the Id* in 1923. This consisted of a *tripartite* structure containing the id, ego, and superego.

Present from birth, the id is completely unconscious and seeks gratification of instinctual (mainly sexual and aggressive) drives. The superego forms from an identification with the same sex parent at the resolution of the **oedipal conflict**. It suppresses instinctual aims, serves as the moral conscience in dictating what *should not* be done, and as the ego ideal, dictates what *should* be done. The superego is largely unconscious, but has a conscious element.

The ego is the mediator between two groups: i) the id and superego; and ii) the person and reality. The ego has both conscious and unconscious elements. The following are considered the conscious roles of the ego:
• Perception (sense of reality)
• Reality testing (adaptation to reality)
• Motor control
• Intuition
• Memory
• Affect
• Thinking and learning
• Control of instinctual drives (delay of immediate gratification)
• Synthetic functions (assimilation, creation, coordination)
• Language and comprehension

The fundamental concept in ego psychology is one of *conflict* amongst these three agencies. The id, ego, and superego battle for expression and discharge of sexual and aggressive drives. This conflict produces anxiety, specifically called **signal anxiety**. This anxiety alerts the ego that a defense mechanism is required, which is the unconscious role of the ego. The events can be conceptualized as follows:

The id seeks expression of an impulse
↓
The superego prohibits the impulse from being expressed
↓
This conflict produces signal anxiety
↓
An ego defense is unconsciously
recruited to decrease anxiety
↓
A character trait or psychiatric symptom is formed

An ego defense can be considered a compromise, which allows expression of the impulse in a disguised form. All defenses protect the ego from the instinctual drives of the id and are unconscious processes.

Freud directed most of his attention to **repression**, which he considered the primary ego defense. Repression is defined as expelling and withholding an idea or feeling from conscious awareness. He thought other defenses were used only when repression failed to diminish the anxiety. Anna Freud expanded the total to nine in her 1936 book, *The Ego and the Mechanisms of Defense*. Since then, many more defense mechanisms have been identified. Akin to the theories of **Life Cycle Development**, there is a progression in the use of ego defenses with maturity. George Vaillant catalogued defenses into four categories: **narcissistic, immature, neurotic**, and **mature**. These defenses are explained in standard reference texts.

**Narcissistic Defenses**
Denial
Distortion
Primitive Idealization
Projection
Projective Identification
Splitting

**Mature Defenses**
Altruism
Anticipation
Asceticism
Humor
Sublimation
Suppression

**Neurotic Defenses**
Controlling
Displacement
Dissociation
Externalization
Inhibition
Intellectualization
Isolation
Rationalization
Reaction Formation
Repression
Sexualization
Undoing

**Immature Defenses**
Acting Out
Blocking
Hypochondriasis
Identification
Introjection
Passive-Aggressive Behavior
Projection
Regression
Schizoid Fantasy
Somatization

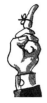

## Insight & Judgment Practice Points

• **Intellectual insight** refers to an awareness that a problem exists, but without substantial effort going into changing the situation; this is commonly referred to as "lip service" and is found most frequently in patients suffering from personality disorders and substance use disorders – they agree there is a problem, but the situation isn't serious enough to effect real change

• Emotional insight is a motivating influence that provides the fuel for patients to make real changes in their relationships, jobs, and even personality characteristics

• Mania and hypomania are common conditions where patients have impaired judgment; they can appear superficially reasonable in interviews but demonstrate an impaired ability to foresee the consequences of their actions

• Patients may be more capable of identifying emotional or behavioral problems than recognizing that their thinking (cognition) is disordered

• The frontal lobes are essential for higher reasoning and judgment; damage to this area causes disinhibition, impulsivity, loss of reasoning ability, and indifference

• Insight-oriented (also called expressive) psychotherapy seeks to help patients develop an awareness of their psychological functioning and personality; this type of therapy examines the dynamics of thoughts, feelings, and behavior with the aim of improving relationships through emotional insight

# Summary

Insight and judgment are complex processes that occur as a result of the integration of other aspects of functioning (emotional, cognitive, perceptual, etc.). Diminished insight and impaired judgment combine to cause the disruptions in social and occupational functioning that add to the severity of psychiatric conditions. Disturbed insight and judgment can occur with any psychiatric disorder, and are present at higher rates than in the majority of medically ill patients.

# Proverbs to Ponder . . .

• Remember, you are unique – just like everyone else

• It may be that your sole purpose in life is simply to serve as a warning to others

• It's always darkest before dawn – so if you're going to steal your neighbor's newspaper, that's the time to do it

• Never test the depth of the water with both feet

• Some days you are the bug, some days you are the windshield

• Good judgment comes from bad experience, and a lot of that comes from bad judgment

• A closed mouth gathers no foot

• Before you criticize someone, you should walk a mile in their shoes; that way, when you criticize them, you're a mile away and you have their shoes

• If you are going to rob Peter to pay Paul, you can at least count on Paul's support

• Two wrongs don't make a right, but three lefts do

• A memo is written not to inform the reader, but to protect the writer

• Even a stopped clock is right twice a day

• The only substitute for good manners is fast reflexes

• Give me ambiguity or give me something else

• All generalizations are false

# References

## Books

American Psychiatric Association
**Diagnostic and Statistical Manual of Mental Disorders, 4th Ed.**
American Psychiatric Association, Washington D.C., 1994

P.S. Appelbaum, Editor
**Informed Consent: Legal Theory and Clinical Practice, 2nd Ed.**
Oxford University Press, New York, 2000

R. Campbell
**Psychiatric Dictionary, 7th Ed.**
Oxford University Press, New York, 1996

T.G. Gutheil & P.S. Appelbaum
**Clinical Handbook of Psychiatry and the Law, 3rd Ed.**
Lippincott, Williams & Wilkins, Philadelphia, 2000

E. Othmer & S. Othmer
**The Clinical Interview Using DSM-IV**
American Psychiatric Press, Inc., Washington D.C., 1994

M.R.S. Manley
*Diagnosis and Psychiatry: Examination of the Psychiatric Patient*, in
B.J. Sadock & V.A. Sadock, Editors
**Comprehensive Textbook of Psychiatry, 7th Ed.**
Lippincott, Williams & Wilkins, Philadelphia, 2000

A. Sims
**Symptoms in the Mind, 2nd Ed.**
Saunders, London, England, 1995

K.H. Claypole & G.J. Tucker
*Consciousness, Orientation, and Memory*, in
A. Tasman, J. Kay, & J.A. Lieberman, Editors
**Psychiatry**
W.B. Saunders Co., Philadelphia, 1997

B.J. Winick
**The Right to Refuse Mental Health Treatment**
American Psychological Association, Washington D.C., 1997

G. Vaillant
**Ego Mechanisms of Defense**
American Psychiatric Press, Inc., Washington D.C., 1992

D.J. Wear-Finkle
**Medicolegal Issues in Clinical Practice: A Primer For the Legally Challenged**
Rapid Psychler Press, Port Huron, MI, 2000

# Articles

N.C. Andreason
**Reliability and Validity of Proverb Interpretation to Assess Mental Status**
*Comprehensive Psychiatry* 18(5): 465 – 472, 1977

A.S. David
**Insight and Psychosis**
*British Journal of Psychiatry* 156: 798 – 808, 1990

R.M. Haynes, P.J. Resnick, K.C. Dougherty, & S.E. Althof
**Proverb Familiarity and the Mental Status Examination**
*Bull. of the Menninger Clinic* 57(4): 523 – 528, 1993

N. Hayashi, M. Yamashina, & Y. Igarashi
**Awareness of Being a Patient and Its Relevance to Insight Into Illness in Patients With Schizophrenia**
*Compr. Psychiatry* 40(5): 377 – 385, 1999

J.R. Husted
**Insight In Severe Mental Illness: Implications for Treatment Decisions**
*J. Am. Acad. Psychiatry Law* 27(1): 33 – 49, 1999

S. Johnson & M. Orrell
**Insight, Psychosis, and Ethnicity: A Case-Note Study**
*Psychol. Med.* 26(5), 1081 – 1084, 1996

K.H. Kaplan
**Assessing Judgment**
*General Hospital Psychiatry* 10(3): 202 – 208, 1988

I.S. Markova & G.E. Berrios
**Insight in Clinical Psychiatry: A New Model**
*J. Nerv. Ment. Dis.* 183(12): 743 – 751, 1995a

I.S. Markova & G.E. Berrios
**Insight in Clinical Psychiatry Revisited**
*Compr. Psychiatry* 36(5): 367 – 376, 1995b

I.S. Markova & G.E. Berrios
**The Assessment of Insight in Psychiatry: A New Scale**
*Acta Psychiatr. Scand.* 86(2): 159 – 164, 1992a

I.S. Markova & G.E. Berrios
**The Meaning of Insight in Clinical Psychiatry**
*British Journal of Psychiatry* 160: 850 – 860, 1992b

J.P. McEvoy, N.R. Schooler, E. Friedman, S. Steingard, & M. Allen
**Use of Psychopathology Vignettes by Patients With Schizophrenia or Schizoaffective Disorder and by Mental Health Professionals to Judge Patient's Insight**
*American Journal of Psychiatry* 150(11): 1649 – 1653, 1993

J.P. McEvoy, P.S. Appelbaum, L.J. Apperson, J.L. Geller, & S. Freter
**Why Must Some Schizophrenic Patients be Involuntarily Committed? The Role of Insight**
*Compr. Psychiatry* 30(1): 13 – 17, 1989a

J.P. McEvoy, J.L. Apperson, P.S. Appelbaum, P. Ortlip, & J. Brecosky
**Insight in Schizophrenia: Its Relationship to Acute Psychopathology**
*J. Nerv. Mental Dis.* 177(1): 43 – 47, 1989b

J.H. Reich
**Proverbs and the Modern Mental Status Exam**
*Comprehensive Psychiatry* 22(5): 528 – 531, 1981

A.M. Shimkunas, M.D. Gynther, & K. Smith
**Schizophrenic Responses to the Proverbs Test: Abstract, Concrete, or Autistic?**
*J. Abn. Psychology* 72: 128 – 133, 1967

C.L. Swanson, O. Fruedenreich, J.P. McEvoy, & L. Nelson
**Insight in Schizophrenia and Mania**
*J. Nerv. Mental Dis.* 183(12): 752 – 755, 1995

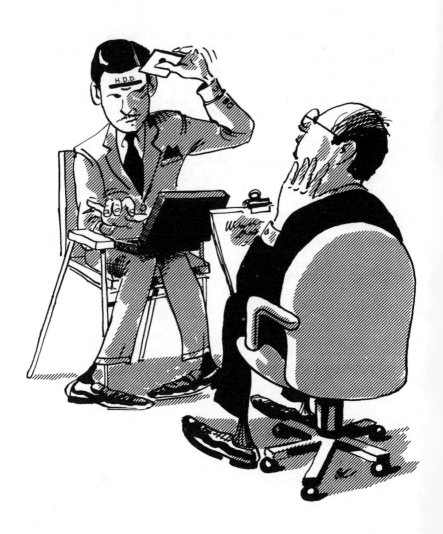

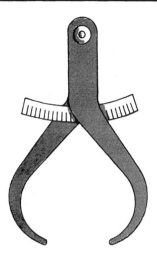

# Chapter 12

# Sensorium & Cognitive Functioning

## Which Aspects of Sensorium and Cognitive Functioning Are Tested?

- **Level of Consciousness/Alertness (Section I)**
(also covered in the *Cooperation & Reliability Chapter*)
- **Orientation (II)**
- **Attention and Concentration (III)**
- **Memory (IV)**
    Registration, Immediate, Recent, Remote

**333**

- **Estimation of Intelligence (V)**
- **Knowledge Base/Fund of Information (VI)**
- **Capacity to Read and Write (VII)**
- **Abstraction/Concrete Thinking (VIII)**
- **Visuospatial Ability (IX)**

Brief tests are employed to allow clinicians to rapidly screen for the presence of serious cognitive impairment. There is considerable diversity in the way cognitive screening is administered in the MSE. Some clinicians use many tests, rated by their own guidelines and observations, which form an important but unfortunately non-standardized contribution to assessing cognitive functions. What is most important is that some measure of a patient's cognitive function is made during the MSE, and that the same tests are administered in a consistent manner in interviews to monitor a patient's clinical course.

# What is the Diagnostic Significance of Deficits in Cognitive Function?

Cognitive impairments can occur in any psychiatric disorder. The findings are most prominent in the following disorders:

- **Delirium (of any etiology)** 293.0
A. Disturbance of consciousness with reduced ability to focus, sustain, or shift attention.
B. A change in cognition (such as memory deficit, disorientation, language disturbance) . . .

- **Dementia (of any etiology)** 290.X
A. The development of multiple cognitive deficits manifested by both:
(1) memory impairment (impaired ability to learn new information or recall previously learned information)
(2) one or more of the following cognitive disturbances:

- aphasia
- apraxia
- agnosia
- disturbance in executive functioning

• **Mental Retardation** 317/318.X
A. Significantly subaverage intellectual functioning: an IQ of approximately 70 or below on an individually adminis-tered IQ test
B. Concurrent deficits or impairments in present adaptive functioning in meeting the standards expected for his or her age in. . . communication, self-direction, functional aca-demic skills, work, etc.

• **Substance Intoxication**
B. Clinically significant maladaptive behavioral or psycho-logical changes that are due to the effect of a substance on the central nervous system (e.g. cognitive impairment, im-paired judgment, etc.)

• **Schizophrenia** 295.X
A. (5) negative symptoms – includes **attentional deficits**; social inattentiveness, inattention during testing on the MSE; and **alogia** – poverty of speech, poverty of speech content, increased latency of response

• **Major Depressive Episode** 296.X
A. (8) diminished ability to think or concentrate, or indeci-siveness, nearly every day (either by subjective account or as observed by others)

• **Manic/Hypomanic Episode** 296.X
B. distractibility (i.e. attention too easily drawn to unim-portant or irrelevant external stimuli)

• **Dysthymic Disorder** 300.4
B. (5) poor concentration or difficulty making decisions

• **Posttraumatic Stress Disorder** 309.81
D. (3) difficulty concentrating

• **Acute Stress Disorder** 308.3
B. (2) a reduction in awareness of the surroundings (e.g., "being in a daze")

• **Generalized Anxiety Disorder** 300.02
C. (3) difficulty concentrating or mind going blank

• **Dementia Syndrome of Depression**, also called **Depression-Related Cognitive Dysfunction**, or **Pseudo-dementia**
This is not a DSM-IV diagnosis, though this is often reported in patients with depression, particularly in severe cases or in geriatric populations (up to 15%). Deficits in attention are variable and memory is most impaired on free recall tests.
Diagnostic Criteria are from the DSM-IV.
© American Psychiatric Association, Washington, D.C. 1994
Reprinted with permission.

# Why Are Cognitive Functions Assessed?

Cognition refers to information processing. Cognitive functioning tests the patient's thinking and memory functions. Storage, retrieval, and the ability to manipulate information is assessed in this part of the MSE. Testing specific cognitive components reveals information about the function of cortical and subcortical structures.

Impairment in cognitive functioning is common in patients with psychiatric disorders, and has been estimated to be as high as 60% in some studies. Impairments in cognitive functions impact on the quality and reliability of information given by patients. In the mind/brain dimension, higher cortical functions ("mind") such as mood and perception cannot be adequately assessed if there is an organic ("brain") dysfunction.

Cognitive assessments also have three important functions:
• Rapidly determining if the patient is delirious or otherwise in need of urgent medical attention

• Gauging the severity of psychiatric illnesses; for example, prior to being called schizophrenia, the illness was called **dementia praecox** because of the early decline of mental abilities and deteriorating course
• Monitoring the effects of psychiatric medications; antipsychotics and mood stabilizers in particular can have a significant impact on cognitive abilities (though all psychotropic medications can cause negative effects)

Cognitive impairment can lead to inadvertent self-injury, and decreased compliance with treatment. It also calls into question the patient's ability to give informed consent for: treatment, financial matters (including the ability to make a will, called **testamentary capacity**), discretion over the release of medical information, ability to operate a motor vehicle or fly an airplane, etc.

Patients can appear cognitively intact for the balance of the interview and still have deficits when given specific tasks. Delirious patients have lucid moments, and if an interview is brief enough to occur during one of these periods, significant impairment can be missed. Repeated experiences of this phenomenon can be summarized as follows, *"The MSE always changes when the patient is reviewed by the consultant psychiatrist."*

Other situations where cognitive deficits can be masked are:
• Focal impairments and mild dementia are also unlikely to be picked up by the conversational manner of an interview or other parts of the MSE
• Patients who are hypomanic may seem charming and gregarious, and their deficits aren't highlighted until asked to perform structured tasks
• Psychotic patients often remain oriented and can appear intact as long as relatively straight forward questions are asked of them, and brief answers are accepted

It is not essential to completely test the cognitive functioning of every patient in every interview. While each task can be administered at the discretion of the interviewer, the fol-

lowing guidelines should be kept in mind:
• In examinations, be as thorough as possible in asking about cognitive functions (or have good reasons to justify why you didn't)
• When cognitive decline is suspected, test this early in the interview

The tests listed here do not provide a complete evaluation of a patient's cognitive abilities. As demonstrated in the first chapter, the interview and MSE delineate symptoms, generate a provisional diagnosis (along with differential diagnoses), and direct further testing. Following certain sections in this chapter, a list of standardized, neuropsychological tests is provided as a guide to ordering appropriate diagnostic investigations.

# I – Level of Consciousness/Alertness

It is essential that patients be alert for the MSE so that higher mental abilities can be tested. Alertness can be impaired in the following ways:
• Decreased level of consciousness
• Inability to screen out extraneous stimuli
• Disinterest in the interview (which can also be a matter of cooperation)

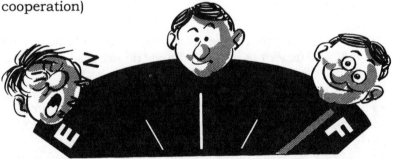

## Brain Areas Involved

Level of consciousness/degree of alertness and orientation involve many components: brainstem pathways, reticular activating system, cingulate gyrus, thalamic nuclei, the non-dominant parietal lobe, and frontal lobes.

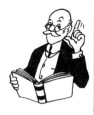

Many factors can diminish level of consciousness (which is almost always due to a medical cause):
• Delirium
• Substance intoxication (especially sedative-hypnotics, alcohol, opioids, etc.) or toxic levels of prescription medication (iatrogenic, deliberate, or unintentional)
• Drug-drug interactions, especially in the elderly
• Anticholinergic agents (used to treat parkinsonian side-effects) can be additive to the anticholinergic side-effects of most neuroleptic medications
• Strokes, infections, intracranial bleeding, etc.
• Post-ictal states
• Residents who are post-call

Level of consciousness doesn't generally require a formalized assessment. Tests for more subtle impairment have been developed and these are covered in the section on *Attention and Concentration.*

# II – Orientation

Orientation is tested with respect to the following parameters:
• Time (time of day, day of week, date, month, year, season)
• Place (hospital/clinic/office address and floor level, town or city, state, county)
• Person (identity of the person and recognition of family members, friends, health-care providers, etc.)

Orientation is usually lost in the sequence of:

**time (most common) > place > person (least common)**

## Disorientation to Time

Orientation to time can be asked about as follows:
*"Mr. XYY, I know you've been affected by this illness. Sometimes when people aren't feeling well, they lose track of some of the things happening around them. I'd like to ask you some questions as to how well you've been keeping track of time."*

Demented patients usually become disoriented to year first, so even if they get other parts correct, ask for the entire date. Some patients are clever enough to look at their watches, newspapers, or the calendar on the wall before answering questions about time. You can circumvent this by asking them not to look at anything first (and stand in their view of the wall calendar).

Inpatients frequently lose track of the day of the week and date, which doesn't itself indicate a pathological process. To be considered intact, patients should still know within a day or two what day of the week it is, and if it is closer to the beginning, middle or end of the month. Proximity to major holidays can also be inquired about if appropriate. Re-orienting patients to time is not only kind, it gives you the chance to test their short-term memory by repeating these questions a few minutes later.

## Disorientation to Place

Questions about orientation to place can be asked in an indirect manner, such as:
• *"Did you have any trouble finding the clinic today?"*
• *"Where did you. . . (park your car, get off the bus, etc.)?"*
• *"I've never heard of (patient's street), how would I get there from the hospital?"*
• *"Mr. Maple, if you were standing at the intersection of Cedar and Elm, how would (or wood) you get to Oak Street?"*
• *"What is the nearest main intersection to the hospital?"*

Delirium is the most common reason patients lose track of where they are, and why they are in the hospital. Delirious patients frequently misinterpret their location as being a hotel, jail, laboratory, or army barracks (which, at various times, seem to be the extended functions of a hospital).

If patients are unable to give adequate answers to questions like those above, ascertain where they think they are and what happens in the building:
• *"What type of building are you in now?"*

If they know it is a hospital/clinic/office, ask if they know the name. If they don't know this, try asking:
• *"What goes on in this building?"*
• *"Do you think this is a school, a library, a bank. . . ?"*

### Disorientation to Person

Disoriented patients rarely are so impaired that they lose track of their own identity. This occurs in severe delirium, head injuries (especially involving the frontal lobes), profound dementia, and in dissociative disorders. Orientation to person can be tested at the beginning of the interview by asking patients to state their full name (as if you needed to check that you were speaking to the right person or had a sudden interest in the person's middle name). Another approach is to have patients write their names and the date at the top of a piece of paper at the start of the interview.

# III – Attention & Concentration

**Attention** is the ability to direct mental energy when fully alert. It is a conscious, willful focusing of cognitive processes while excluding competing stimuli (such as mood state, thoughts, perceptions, etc.). **Concentration** is the sustained focus of attention for a period of time. While these terms are interrelated, they are still evaluated separately. For example, patients with mild-to-moderate dementia can attend to tasks but have deficits in their ability to concentrate.

Questions about attention and concentration are fairly easy to introduce in the MSE because patients frequently complain about difficulties in these areas. When complaints of this nature arise, you have the option of either performing tests of concentration at that time, or using the patient's expressed difficulties as a bridge later in the interview. For patients that do not specifically complain about diminished concentration, the topic can be introduced as follows: *"Ms. Nebular, it is common for people who have the kinds of problems with. . . (repeat presenting difficulties) to have difficulties with their concentration."*

If the patient agrees that she's had trouble, say that you would like to test this more formally. For patients that do not endorse such difficulties, you can say something like: *"Ms. Nebular, I would like to do as thorough an assessment as possible, and this involves some screening tests to check your level of concentration. Would you be agreeable to proceeding with this?"*

## Attention

Attention is assessed by administering the **digit span test**. This isn't the size of patients' fingers, but the string of numbers they can recall. Introduce this test by asking the patient to repeat a list of numbers. Once you've read the list, you can signal this by lowering the tone of your voice with the last digit. Another technique is to keep your head down, and make eye contact with the patient only at the end of the sequence. This gives you the advantage of being able to write the numbers down as you recite them (note: the patient is not allowed to write the numbers down).

Read off the numbers so that there are pauses of about one second between them. Avoid adding emphasis (prosody) to the numbers as you read them. Numbers that are grouped too closely together or with some rhythm can give the spurious impression of good recall. For example, many companies have developed a jingle so that their phone numbers are more memorable. Another consideration is to avoid using numbers in a sequence (5-6-7-8), or exclusively odd or even numbers.

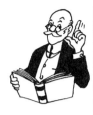

Digit span is impaired in patients with:
• Dementia
• Delirium
• Frontal lobe lesions
• Head injuries
• Marked medication side-effects
• Anxiety disorders
• Mania/hypomania

It is unusual to have a greater recall span for numbers backwards than forwards. If this happens, it should prompt an investigation for an organic cause.

Digit span testing is given for numbers both in a *forward* and *backward* direction. It may help to start with an example to illustrate what you're expecting. You can usually start by testing 4 numbers recited in a forward fashion. Most adults have digit recall spans of between 5 to 7 numbers forward and 4 to 6 numbers backward, without errors, and completed within 30 seconds.

## Concentration

Concentration is most frequently tested with **serial seven subtractions**. Again, patients are not allowed to use any aid in this test, including counting with their fingers. You can introduce this as follows: *I'd like you to start with the number 100 and subtract 7; then, from this number, subtract 7 and keep going as far as you can."*

It may be necessary to give the patient an example of what you want by doing the first subtraction, so that the first attempt he makes is 93 – 7. Alternative numerical tests have not been standardized. Some suggestions are:
• Subtracting serial 3's starting at 20
• Serial additions
• Starting at another number using a different interval of subtraction (e.g. 103 – 8)

It is a strength and weakness of the serial seven subtractions that both concentration and arithmetic ability are tested. For this reason, other tasks involving concentration over 30 – 60 seconds can be used. For patients who have had repeated admissions to hospital, the serial subtractions test becomes too familiar to be valid (some patients will even ask when you want them to do this test even if it isn't requested). For these patients, a different interval of subtraction is warranted. A more advanced test involves alternating between serial seven subtractions and reciting the months backwards (i.e. December, 93, November, 86, etc.).

While the serial sevens subtraction test is commonly employed, it suffers from a lack of standardization. As far as could be established, there are no guidelines regarding:
• Time allowed between subtractions
• Time allowed for the entire test
• How many subtractions should be recorded
• Number of errors that are considered in the normal range

The *Comprehensive Textbook of Psychiatry, Second Edition* (1975) suggests that 30 seconds should be allowed between successive subtractions. Smith (1967) conducted a study using subjects with an above-average level of education, and found the following:
• Only 42% made errorless subtractions
• 19% made one error, 14% made two errors

The serial sevens test is frequently abandoned by patients lacking at least high school education and by those with "math phobia" (in the DSM-IV, Mathematics Disorder 315.1).

Other tests that can be used in interviews involve reciting the months of the year in reverse order, or spelling five-to-six letter words backwards.

## Brain Areas Involved

Attention and concentration are also "global" brain functions and involve many of the same structures required to maintain alertness; the frontal lobes are of particular importance in concentration.

## Standardized Tests

Standardized tests include visual, verbal, and auditory tests of concentration. Common ones are:
• **Trailmaking Test Part A** (Trails A) is a pen-and-paper test that involves connecting 25 circled, randomly scattered, numbers in ascending order
• **Trailmaking Test Part B** (Trails B) is more complicated, and involves alternating between numbers and letters (e.g. 1 – A – 2 – B – 3 – C, etc.); because of the "shifting cognitive sets" between letters and numbers, this is a more sensitive test; both tests are unaffected by aphasias
• **Stroop Test** consists of four parts (i) reading the names of colors printed in black on white cards (ii) reading the names of colors printed in a different color, such as the word *red* printed in *green* ink (iii) naming the colors of dots, and (iv) reading the cards from part (ii) again, but this time naming the color of the ink
• **Concentration Endurance Test** requires the patient to mark a certain target letter which is surrounded by distracting letters and symbols; this particular test uses the letters *d* and *p* with single and double quotation marks above and below the letter; as an example, the letter d with two marks can be the target (which can be: one quotation mark above and one below; two above; or two below)
• Another test is the *Digit Symbol Subtest* of the **Wechsler Adult Intelligence Scale – Revised (WAIS-R)**; symbols are paired with digits and patients are asked to fill in blanks next to the symbols

# IV – Memory: General Principles

Memory is one of the key elements that define a person as an individual. Our memories are our library of knowledge and experience. Memories influence our interpretation of the present. Memory is essential for a vast array of functions ranging from basic motor skills to complex intellectual tasks. It has an integral function in perception, thought, feeling, and behavior.

The study of memory encompasses an extensive and detailed body of literature. A brief review is provided here for the purpose of being able to more accurately specify memory problems discovered on the MSE. Memory is at the center of higher cognitive functions:

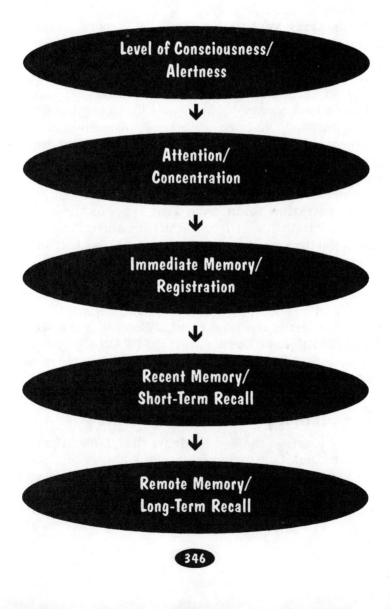

## Types of Memory

• **Registration** is the instantaneous recall of new information; this is also called **immediate memory**, and is dependent on alertness and adequate concentration

• **Short-term memory** generally has the capacity of around 7 items for a twenty-second time span, though this can be increased with training; **recent memory** is sometimes used as a synonymous term, but is also used to denote events that occurred in the past few hours; short term memory is either discarded or committed to long-term memory; for short-term memory to function, it is dependent on intact attentiveness, concentration, and registration

• **Long-term memory** has no demonstrable limits of storage and provides the **fund of knowledge** for patients; this is also called **remote memory** or **delayed recall**; this type of memory remains stable over time and is the type most affected by forms of amnesia; long-term memory has two subtypes:

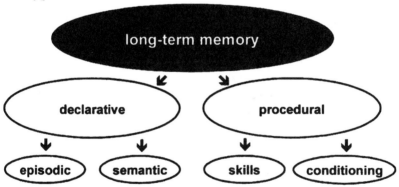

**Declarative memory** is factual and directly accessible to consciousness. It is also called "knowing that" or "knowing what" memory. This type of memory that can be acquired in a short time and is the form most impaired in amnesia.

**Procedural memory** refers to acquired skills and habits. It is also called "knowing how" memory. This type of memory evolves after many trials, and is largely intact in various forms of amnesia (for both learned and new tasks).

Other terms associated with these types of memory are:

| **Declarative** | **Procedural** |
| --- | --- |
| explicit | implicit |
| working | reference |
| elaboration | integration |
| conscious recollection | automatic skills or habits |

Declarative memory is further subdivided into:
• **Episodic memory**, which involves the recall of events and the context in which they occurred (where, when, etc.); this type of memory is personalized and also called *autobiographical*; an example of episodic memory would be a first beer, first kiss, or first driving lesson
• **Semantic memory**, which refers to general knowledge that is not remembered in a specific context; for example, many people know the colors that make up the spectrum of light but wouldn't know where and when this was learned

## Amnesia

**Amnesia** is the inability to recall learned material or past experiences in a person who has no impairment of attention. This is further divided into two types:
• **Retrograde amnesia** is the loss of memories that were made prior to an event (e.g. accident, ECT), this is also called **circumscribed** or **backward amnesia**
• **Anterograde amnesia** is the inability to make memories after the occurrence of an event; this is also called **continuous** or **forward amnesia**

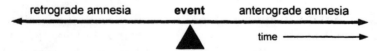

Memory can be impaired at the level of:
• **Encoding** – perceptions are not properly "encoded" by an inability to attend to the delivery of information
• **Storage** – after memories are encoded, they must be *consolidated* and *maintained* to allow retention
• **Retrieval** – deficits in recalling consolidated material

## Testing Memory in the MSE

The most common test of verbal memory involves word recall. This is used to test **immediate memory** (registration) and **short-term memory** (recent memory). The patient is given a list of between three to five words and asked to repeat them approximately five minutes later.

The words chosen should have the following characteristics:
• They should be unrelated to each other (e.g. don't use red, white & blue)
• They should not be something that is in the room or shown to the patient (e.g. a set of keys, coins, chairs, light bulbs)
• They should be unrelated to the person's vocation or interests (e.g. don't ask a mechanic to remember a lug nut, cam shaft, and exhaust manifold)

A popular combination involves a color, quality and item not in the room (e.g. green, honesty, postcard). This test is presented to the patient as follows:
*"Arnold, I'd like to formally test your memory now. I'm going to give you three items to remember. I'd like you to repeat them so I know you've heard me, and then I'm going to ask you to repeat them in a few minutes. The words are bench press, dumbbell fly, and arm curl. Can you please repeat them for me now?"*

Of course, if Arnold is a body-builder, these wouldn't be good choices of items for him to remember. If patients are not able to register these items, repeat them once. If they have trouble a second time, this may indicate a cognitive deficit and more formalized testing of concentration is warranted. Registration tests the same cognitive abilities as digit span. There is no clear rationale for why numbers are used in one area and words in another.

Some clinicians use four or five words for this test. Again, there is no standardization for what is considered average. Missing one item out of four or five is less significant than missing one out of three. You can vary the number of words to suit the educational status, degree of alertness, and level of cooperation of the patient being interviewed.

If a patient cannot remember all of the items, it is a common practice to prompt her. This can be done initially by stating the category of the missing item(s) (e.g. *Was it a color? . . . A brand of soap?*). If this doesn't work, present a list of other words which include the missing item(s). This provides patients with more help than listing the category, and may be useful when more serious impairment is present. Make sure you don't list the missing item too close to the beginning of the list, and don't add any inflection to your voice when giving the correct word.

Again, there is no established standard with which to compare performance of short-term memory. If the patient requires prompting or a word list, record this as such.

Keeping an eye on the time is important. Report the duration as accurately as possible between registration and testing. Typically, this is recorded as, "Mr. T was able to register all three items and recall two of three at around four minutes time. He was able to recall the third with prompting."

Patients with **Korsakoff's syndrome** have anterograde amnesia, but intact registration and a variable short-term memory. Testing such patients too quickly will miss this important deficit.

Verbal recall is often included at the beginning of the cognitive evaluation. In many interviews (such as the Psychiatry & Neurology Board Exams) there is only thirty minutes allotted for the whole exam, and five minutes for the entire MSE may be all that is available. Frequently, interviewers forget to ask patients to recall these items. It is prudent to get in the habit of writing these items down, because:
• This ensures you won't forget what they were
• You get a visual cue to ask the patient to repeat them

It is embarrassing when patients ask (invariably at the end of an exam) if you still want them to repeat the three items.

Other tests of verbal short-term memory involve:
• The name, address, and zip code of a fictitious person
• A short "story" of three-to-four sentences with about 25 points of information; an intact response involves remembering around 15 points of detail
• Word lists of 15 items which can be related or unrelated; intact recall is considered to be somewhere in the vicinity of 50% of the words, which declines as age increases; a standardized test assessing this is the **Rey Auditory-Verbal Learning Test (RAVLT)**.

Short-term memory can also be assessed with **visual design reproduction tests**. One such test involves copying a design from memory that was placed in front of the patient for up to 30 seconds. These designs are usually an amalgamation of several geometric shapes.

A variation on this is to give patients the chance to study a certain number of shapes, and then select them from a larger group presented for a fixed period of time (e.g. 30 seconds) later. A standardized assessment is the **Rey Visual Design Learning Test (RVDLT)**, which consists of two parts:
• Showing patients 15 geometric shapes, and then asking that they be drawn from memory (part one)
• Having patients select the 15 designs they have seen from a larger group of 30 (part two)
• The **Wechsler Memory Scale** has a **Visual Reproduction Subtest**

Auditory short-term memory can be tested with a rhythm tapped by the examiner and repeated by the patient. This assessment has been formalized, and is called the **Seashore Rhythm Test**, which is a component of the larger **Seashore Test of Musical Ability**.

**Long-term memory** can be assessed in terms of recent events (hours to days) or remote (years to decades). This

can be tested in a practical manner in interviews by having patients answer questions to which you can verify the answers. For example, the following information is usually readily available:
• Date of birth
• Address, zip code, and phone number
• Previous appointments or hospitalizations
• Medication type and dosage
• The recollection of your name (as long as you introduced yourself)

Remote memory can be distinguished from fund of knowledge by testing for personal details. Various other forms of personal information can be elicited, but need to be corroborated to exclude the possibility of **confabulation** (the falsification of memory in response to questions).

## Brain Areas Involved in Memory
• Verbal memory      dominant temporal lobe
• Visual memory      non-dominant temporal lobe
• Registration      frontal & temporal lobes
• Short-term memory      hippocampus (consolidation and retrieval); temporal lobe (storage); medial dorsal thalamic nuclei (storage)
• Long-term memory      association cortex of temporal lobe (medial temporal region)

Other structures involved in memory:
• **Hippocampus** – part of the limbic system; has connections to the thalamus and temporal lobe
• **Amygdala** – part of the limbic system; involved in the integration of memories and the recognition of faces
• **Mamillary bodies** – part of the hypothalamus, implicated in the pathology of Korsakoff's syndrome
• **Pulvinar** – part of the thalamus; needed for memory retrieval

# V – Estimation of Intelligence

Intelligence is a multi-faceted constellation of mental abilities involving:
• The assimilation and recall of factual information
• Logical reasoning
• Problem-solving skills
• The use of abstraction, generalization, and symbolization
• Integration of parts into a whole

Three distinctive types of intelligence have been described: mechanical, abstract, and social. Intelligence is usually reported as an **intelligence quotient (I.Q.)**

$$\textbf{I.Q.} = \frac{MENTAL\ AGE}{CHRONOLOGICAL\ AGE} \times 100$$

Mental age is a measure of intellectual level. The most widely used and best standardized intelligence test is the **Wechsler Adult Intelligence Scale (WAIS)**. The current version is the **WAIS-R** (for revised). Because chronological age has such a bearing on IQ, there are separate versions for children (ages 5 to 15) and preschoolers (ages 4 to 6). By definition, a normal IQ is 100. Mental retardation is defined as an IQ less than 70; superior intelligence is above 120.

The WAIS-R consists of six verbal subtests and five nonverbal subtests. The **Kent test** consists of four problem solving and six knowledge questions that can be given in interviews and yield an approximate level of intelligence.

Intelligence is one dimension of cognitive functioning. It can be gauged in interviews by:
• Degree of insight, judgment, and abstract thinking
• Fund of knowledge
• Vocabulary (considered the best single indicator)
• Level of education, vocation, interests, and hobbies

# VI — Knowledge Base/Fund of Information

Another component of assessing cognitive function is to test a patient's knowledge base. This can be something that is estimated by incidental factors that arise during the interview, or may need to be more fully explored if cognitive deficits are discovered in other areas of testing. Head injuries and dementia are the most common causes of permanent knowledge deficits. The pseudo-dementia of depression can give the appearance of impaired cognitive functioning because patients tend to answer with, *"I don't know"* responses. When pressed to respond, they often can if sufficient time is allowed.

Common questions involve:
• Naming political figures
• Significant dates (e.g. W.W.I, W.W.II, etc.)
• Naming capital cities, neighboring states, etc.

This information is "common knowledge" and doesn't involve the personal significance of the questions used to test remote memory.

# VII — Capacity to Read and Write

Assessment of these basic functions is often omitted in initial interviews. Illiteracy is present at an unfortunately high rate and can be masked by people with good verbal skills. It is common for illiterate patients to be able to sign their names, which is often all that is required in clinical settings. As described in the *Orientation Section*, having patients write down their names and the date and (later) follow a simple written command will screen for deficits in reading and writing. It is also useful to have patients write a sentence on a page. This is part of the **Folstein Mini-Mental Status Exam** (covered in the Chapter 14), and can provide information about patients as they often succinctly express their presenting problems when writing these sentences.

# VIII – Abstraction/Concrete Thinking

Abstract thinking is a complex mental ability. It requires a person to think in a multidimensional manner by keeping all the characteristics of a "mental set" in mind, and integrate the nuances into a new understanding. In interviews, patients demonstrate abstract thinking when they can understand all the meanings of a word, appreciate similarities and differences, use logical reasoning, and by moving from item to item, be able to integrate the "whole picture."

Abstract thinking is made possible by the integration of many brain structures. The main areas involved are:
• **Frontal lobes** – attention, executive functioning, organizing, integration of other brain areas
• **Temporal** & **parietal lobes** – association areas, language
• **Limbic system** – memory and emotional tone

The dominant hemisphere regulates the language aspect, while the non-dominant hemisphere provides an integration of other elements (e.g. spatial, emotional, graphic) into a global understanding.

The opposite of abstraction is **concrete thinking**. This is a literal, unimaginative, narrow-minded understanding of a concept. It is also called **one-dimensional thinking** and is often a feature of lower intelligence.

Examples are as follows:
• *Why is property downtown so expensive?*
*abstract thinking* – high demand, limited amount available
*concrete thinking* – because they charge a lot for it

• *Whiskey kills more people than bullets.*
*abstract* – alcohol is deadlier to more people than gunfire
*concrete* – bullets don't drink

• *She's got a head on her shoulders.*
*abstract* – she uses common sense and thinks before acting
*concrete* – she has no neck

Abstraction/concrete thinking can be tested in the following ways:
• Similarities & Differences
• Proverbs

The **similarities test** involves asking patients to compare two objects and list as many common qualities as they can. For example:
• *What are the similarities between a chair and a desk*
*abstract* – both furniture, things can be put on them, etc.
*concrete* – four legs, made of wood, touch the floor, etc.

Abstraction involves function instead of form, and the ability to see a generalization of the two objects. The **differences test** requires patients to consider similar objects and list their distinguishing features (e.g. apple vs. orange; wine goblet vs. coffee mug, etc.)

**Proverb interpretation** is another commonly used method to test abstraction. Proverbs are "common truths" or generalizations born of experience. A concrete interpretation misses the point or "spirit" of the message contained in the saying:
• *The golden hammer opens an iron door.*
*abstract* – the right touch is all that is needed
*concrete* – you'd have to hit it awfully hard!

Intact abstraction is dependent on:
• Intelligence
• Degree of insight and judgment
• Education

Abstracting ability is reported to be diminished in schizophrenia in particular. However, low intelligence, irrespective of disease process, has been suggested as the central cause.

Uncooperative patients can take words out of context to obscure pertinent issues or resist the assessment process.

# IX — Visuospatial Ability

The ability to perform visuospatial functions is tested by assessing **constructional ability**. Patients are asked to draw a figure (usually a geometric shape) on a piece of paper, which demonstrates the integration of several functions:
• Motor coordination
• Praxis (performing and action)
• Dominant hemisphere function (mainly parietal) for the details of the design; lesions in this area cause drawings to be correct spatially but lacking in detail
• Non-dominant hemisphere function (mainly parietal) for the overall integration of the design; lesions in this area affect the spatial orientation of the components, which become scattered, duplicated or fragmented

The **Mini-Mental State Examination (MMSE)** uses interlocking pentagons for this test. Scoring the drawing involves (i) preserving the sides, (ii) the angles, and (iii) interlocking corners. A simpler test involves having patients draw a cube showing correct three-dimensional orientation.

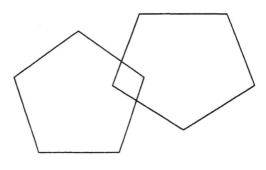

The **Rey-Osterreith Complex Figure Test** is appropriately named. This test has a Form A and B that involve the reproduction of a detailed geometric figure. This is done initially by copying the figure, and then having

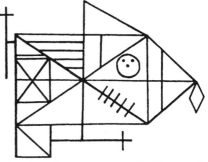

it reproduced from memory. Scoring keys are available and normative data has been established for this test.

## Clock Drawing

Clock drawing is used extensively to assess visuospatial ability and screen for cognitive impairment. Patients are usually given a blank sheet of paper, though some clinicians advocate using forms with pre-printed circles on them. If the circle is supplied, it should be about 4 in./10 cm. (the size of this circle) because patients may be able to spuriously fit numbers correctly into a smaller area.

The patient is asked to draw a complete clock face and indicate a specific time (the hands of the clock should not overlap – common times are 10 to 2, 20 to 4, and 10 after 10; unsuitable times are 6:30, 12:00, or 3:15). Different scoring schemes exist (see the reference section). Generally, clock drawings are scored for:
- Completeness (all the numbers)
- Correctness (numbers in the proper place and sequence)
- Orientation (numbers on both sides and evenly spaced).

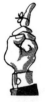

## Practice Points

- The **Rule of Ribot** states that the language one learns first is the one that is more automatic, and consequently is better preserved if one is rendered aphasic; **Pitres' law** states the language most recently learned and used is preserved in aphasia
- The most common early cognitive changes in dementia are diminished ability to concentrate, and impaired problem solving ability; later problems involve orientation, reasoning, perception, and memory
- Memory impairment in dementia is most prominent for recent events; as the illness progresses, this becomes marked and involves more distant memories

• **Acalculia** or **dyscalculia** is the inability to perform arithmetic operations

• **Agnosia** is the inability to recognize an object despite having intact sensory pathways

• **Asterognosis** is the inability to recognize an object when it is held in one's hand (with eyes closed)

• **Gerstmann's syndrome** involves the parietal lobes and consists of left-right disorientation, acalculia, agraphia, and an inability to localize fingers

• The **Klüver-Bucy syndrome** involves the temporal lobes and consists of visual and auditory agnosia, aphasia, dementia, apathy, and hypersexuality

# Summary

Testing of the sensorium and cognitive functioning is the last major area of evaluation in the MSE. These functions are of critical importance in a patient's ability to function autonomously in society. Posing questions to test sensorium and cognitive functioning can be a challenge to weave into the interview. However, many of the impairments are not evident in other parts of the interview or MSE, and need to be elicited specifically. Positive findings usually require further investigation.

# References

## Books

American Psychiatric Association
**Diagnostic and Statistical Manual of Mental Disorders, 4th Ed.**
American Psychiatric Association, Washington D.C., 1994

R. Campbell
**Psychiatric Dictionary, 7th Ed.**
Oxford University Press, New York, 1996

H. Kaplan & B. Sadock, Editors
**Comprehensive Textbook of Psychiatry, 2nd Ed.**
Williams & Wilkins, Baltimore, 1975

E. Othmer & S. Othmer
**The Clinical Interview Using DSM-IV**
American Psychiatric Press, Inc., Washington D.C., 1994

D. Reeves & D. Wedding
**The Clinical Assessment of Memory**
Williams & Wilkins, Baltimore, 1994

A. Sims
**Symptoms in the Mind, 2nd Ed.**
Saunders, London, England, 1995

O. Spreen & E. Strauss
**A Compendium of Neuropsychological Tests: Administration, Norms, and Commentary**
Oxford University Press, New York, 1991

## Clock Drawing

P. Manos & R. Wu
**The Ten Point Clock Test: A Quick Screen and Grading Method of Cognitive Impairment in Medical and Surgical Patients**
*Int. Journal of Psychiatry in Medicine* 24(3): 229 – 244, 1994

M.F. Mendez, T. Ala, & K.L. Underwood
**Scoring Criteria for the Clock Drawing Task in Alzheimer's Disease**
*Journal of the American Geriatric Society* 40: 1095 – 1099, 1992

D.R. Royall, J.A. Cordes, & M. Polk
**CLOX: An Executive Clock Drawing Task**
*J. Neurol. Neurosurg. Psychiatry* 64: 588 – 594, 1998

T. Sunderland, J.L. Hill, A.M. Mellow, & B.A. Lawlor
**Clock Drawing in Alzheimer's Disease: A Novel Measure of Severity**
*Journal of the American Geriatric Society* 37(8): 725 – 729, 1989

## Digit Span

J.P. Das
**Aspects of Digit-Span Performance: Naming Time and Order Memory**
*Am. J. Ment. Defic.* 89(6): 627 – 634, 1985

## Intelligence Estimation

M.G. Eppinger, P.L. Craig, R.L. Adams, & O.A. Parson
**The WAIS-R Index for Estimating Premorbid Intelligence: Cross-Validation and Clinical Utility**
*J. Consult. Clin. Psychol.* 55(1): 86 – 90, 1987

E. Grober & M. Sliwinski
**Development and Validation of a Model for Estimating Premorbid Verbal Intelligence in the Elderly**
*J. Clin. Exp. Neuropsychol.* 13(6): 933 – 949, 1991

# Memory

M. Albert
**Assessment of Memory Loss**
*Psychosomatics* 25(12 suppl.): 18 – 22, 1984

N. Butters, D.C. Delis, & J.A. Lucas
**Clinical Assessment of Memory Disorders in Amnesia and Dementia**
*Annual Rev. Psychol.* 46: 493 – 523, 1995

D.W. Loring & A.C. Papanicolaou
**Memory Assessment in Neuropsychology: Theoretical Considerations and Practical Utility**
*J. Clin. Exp. Neuropsyhology* 9(4): 340 – 358, 1987

D.E. Read
**Neuropsychological Assessment of Memory in the Elderly**
*Can. J. Psychology* 41(3): 158 – 174, 1987

A.F. Schwartz & T.M. McMillan
**Assessment of Everyday Memory After Severe Head Injury**
*Cortex* 25(4): 665 – 671, 1989

L.R. Squire, F. Haist, & A.P. Shimamura
**The Neurology of Memory: Quantitative Assessment of Retrograde Amnesia in Two Groups of Amnestic Patients**
*J. Neurosci.* 9(3): 828 – 839, 1989

E.M. Zelinski & M.J. Gilewski
**Assessment of Memory Complaints by Rating Scales and Questionnaires**
*Psychopharmacol. Bull.* 24(4): 523 – 529, 1988

# Serial Seven Subtractions

M. Ganguli, G. Ratcliff, F.J. Huff, S. Belle, M.J. Kancel, & L. Fischer
**Serial Sevens Versus World Backwards: A Comparison of Two Measures of Attention from the MMSE**
*J. Geriatric Psychiatry* 3(4): 203 – 207, 1990

R.T. Manning
**The Serial Sevens Test**
*Archives of Internal Medicine* 142(6): 1192, 1982

A. Smith
**The Serial Sevens Subtraction Test**
*Archives of Neurology* 17: 78 – 80, 1967

C.C. Young, B.A. Jacobs, K. Clavette, D.H. Mark, & C.E. Guse
**Serial Sevens: Not the Most Effective Test of Mental Status in High School Athletes**
*Clin. J. Sport Med.* 7(3): 196 – 198, 1997

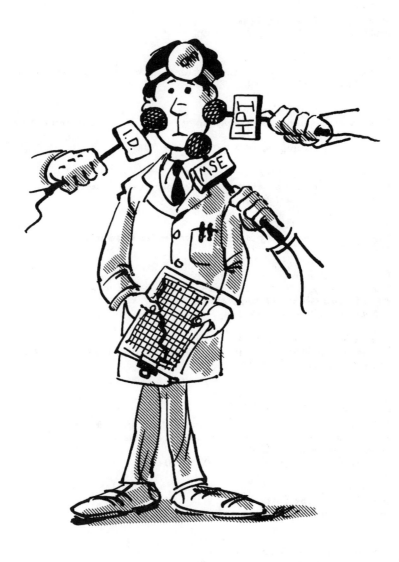

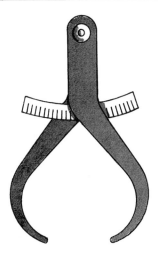

# Chapter 13

# Reporting the MSE

The general format of a verbal or written psychiatric report follows this outline:
• Identifying Data
• Presenting Complaint
• History of Present Illness
• Psychiatric History
• Medical History
• Substance Use History
• Personal History
• Family History
• Mental Status Examination
• Provisional Diagnosis & Differential Diagnoses
• Treatment Plan

The MSE is reported at the same point in the presentation as the physical exam would be in other areas of medicine. Depending on the number of findings, the MSE takes from one to three minutes to present.

Many clinicians make a demarcation from the history by using an introductory statement such as:
• *"The mental status exam revealed. . ."*
• *"Evaluation of the person's mental status showed. . ."*
• *"I will now describe this patient's mental status exam. . ."*

The presentation can be structured by introducing each section of the MSE before stating the findings. This may be especially important in examination settings as a means of demonstrating familiarity with the MSE. Another common practice is to provide a synopsis of the patient's problems at the beginning of the MSE. The following five examples contain sample MSE reports presented in various formats.

# Example 1

P.S. is a 33-year-old, single, unemployed male brought to the emergency department after accosting patrons for cigarettes outside of a shopping center.

• Appearance: tattered jeans, soiled sneakers and a sweater which seemed too heavy for the warm weather; unshaven with unwashed hair and had tobacco stains on his fingers
• Behavior: restless during the interview, stood up twice to look in the ashtray, but was able to be directed back to his seat; fidgeted constantly with his lighter and appeared to be easily distracted
• Cooperation: moderately interested in the interview; information limited but considered reliable; eye contact was continuous
• Speech: spontaneous and fluent, spoke in a low voice and had occasional difficulty naming people, places, and events
• Thought Content: answered questions grudgingly with little elaboration; spontaneously spoke about the injustices he'd suffered by "the system" and specified how today's events were part of a scheme to persecute him; this belief was strongly held throughout the interview and unwavering in its intensity
• Thought Process: his thoughts were logically connected with a restricted flow of ideas and one episode of thought derailment

• Affect & Mood: his emotional expression ranged from mildly sullen to moderately irritable; he became hostile when told he would have to remain in the hospital; he described his mood as "pissed off" and reported it as a one out of ten

• Perception: experienced continual, clearly formed auditory hallucinations throughout the interview which told him he was stupid to get detained at the hospital and he should find a way to get released immediately; he did not report perceptual disturbances in other sensory modalities

• Suicide/Homicide: no thoughts or plans for self-harm, he wishes to assault one of the officers who brought him to the hospital

• Insight & Judgment: impaired, denies he was bothering anyone or has any need for hospitalization or treatment

• Cognition
– alert and fully conscious throughout the interview
– oriented to person, day, date, month, year, season, and place
– able to register three objects on the second attempt and recall two of them four minutes later, (despite prompting, he couldn't recall the third); remote memory was impaired for historical details obtained from hospital record (dates and events)
– digit span five forward, four backward; attempted two serial seven subtractions (both were incorrect: 97, 87), then stopped this task
– declined to answer questions testing general knowledge, abstraction ability, proverb interpretation, or hypothetical situations

# Example 2

N.P. is a 50-year-old male real estate agent who presented to the clinic seeking counseling to deal with the loss of his dog, business, and mistress.

Mr. P is an immaculately groomed man who appears younger than his stated age. Of particular note were his gold rings, tailored suit, and manicured nails. He initially sat in the chair behind the desk (designated for the interviewer) and was unruffled when asked to move. He sat comfortably throughout the interview and spontaneously preened his hair and adjusted his tie on several occasions. He emphasized his speech with dramatic gestures of his hands.

He spoke spontaneously and made a special effort to enunciate his words clearly. As he talked about his losses, there were pauses of up to twenty seconds before he answered questions. There was a good deal of prosodic variation to his speech, and he had an engaging manner of speaking. He included a considerable amount of detail to emphasize a limited number of points. He seemed appreciative of the chance to speak and at times needed redirection to matters relevant to the interview. He focused principally on his losses and how he felt betrayed by everyone and everything in his life. In particular, he thought he had been too trusting and too generous with those around him. He denied thinking there was a conspiracy against him.

His emotions were intense – encompassing the range from tears to laughter, and were appropriate to the topic being discussed. His mood was predominantly described as "hopeless" and he thought this was one of the lowest times of his life. He had brief episodes of hearing his mistress whisper his name when she wasn't in the room, but denied other experiences consistent with hallucinations or illusions. There were no thoughts of harm to others, but he had fleeting suicidal wishes. He understood he wouldn't always feel this upset and had hope for his future. He was willing to attend weekly appointments and did not feel he would act on his thoughts of life not being worth living.

Orientation was not formally tested as Mr. P. found the clinic, had his watch set properly, and carried a newspaper. He related historical information in considerable detail. Despite his complaints of being unable to concentrate, he was able to register five items and recall them at about four minutes time. He could recall seven digits forward and five backward. Serial sevens were correct to five subtractions. He was able to read, write, and copy a diagram without difficulty. He had an overly personal interpretation of proverbs, and related them back to wisdom that he should have possessed. He had an in-depth knowledge of current events and historical information.

# Example 3

Ms. B.A. is an 88-year-old woman referred to the psychiatric consultation-liaison service due to recent behavioral problems after suffering from a stroke and suspected alcohol withdrawal.

**Appearance, Behavior, & Cooperation** – unkempt, slightly obese woman dressed in a hospital gown with food stains on the front, hair was dyed brown several weeks ago; prominent right facial droop and right hemipareisis; she looked at areas in the room where there was nothing occurring and she was talking out loud in that direction prior to the introduction of the interviewers; she picked at unseen objects in the air and then knocked over the items on her bedside table; she struggled continuously against her waist restraint; a wide-amplitude resting tremor was noticed; she was unable to focus on the interview and did not appear to comprehend the reason for the consult or that there was anything amiss; her level of consciousness varied from alert at the beginning of the interview to somnolent (but still rousable) at the end.

**Speech, Thought, & Perception** – non-fluent speech, did not appear to comprehend many of the statements made to her and could not repeat them when asked; expressed speech that was dysarthric, halting, and had an irregular rhythm; she spoke at times in stock phrases, examples of which were:

"Check's in the mail."

"No thanks."

"I'll see."

At other times, longer phrases were out of grammatical sequence and contained mainly verbs and nouns; she seemed impervious to the questions put to her and made replies that were not relevant to what was asked; she appeared to be experiencing perceptual disturbances that contained at least visual and auditory hallucinations (based on her reaction to non-existent stimuli); it was not possible to gather information about other abnormal experiences.

**Affect & Mood** – labile with considerable intensity; she was startled by the appearance of the interviewers and began to cry; later became terrified by the hallucinatory experiences, but after knocking her bedside items on the floor, she was calm enough to drift off to sleep.

**Insight & Judgment** – not testable at the time of the interview.

**Cognitive Functions** – not able to answer any questions regarding orientation despite wall calendar in clear view; responses to other questions were either non-sensical or too garbled to understand.

# Example 4

M.E. is a 29-year-old college student brought to the hospital by her roommate. Despite having final exams, M.E. had been busying herself with a wide number of activities unrelated to her studies.

Ms. M.E.'s **appearance** was that of a woman who looked her stated age and was dressed in mismatched clothes, consisting of a suit jacket, leotards, and hiking boots. In the interview, her **behavior** involved refusing to be seated, and speaking only if she was allowed to walk around the room. She rummaged through her purse at the beginning of the interview and then wrote out several lists for the remainder of the time. She was superficially **cooperative** with the assessment and said she'd talk as long as she could write her lists and if the interview didn't last more than ten minutes. She was considered **reliable**, but biased towards minimizing the significance of her activities.

Her **speech** was loud, rapid, and pressured, but remained understandable and had proper syntax. Prosody was exaggerated, regardless of the content. **Thought process** involved connections that were logical. On two occasions she was unable to repeat the questions posed to her or to relate the connection between them and what she was just saying. The **content** of her thoughts had to do with her plans to start at a senior management level of a Fortune 500 company of her choice after graduation. She has developed powerful insights into the business world and offered the interviewer an autographed copy of her term paper.

Her **affect** was forceful and exuberant, and remained consistently high for the interview. She described her mood as energetic and said she'd never felt better, giving herself a nine out of ten (she says she'll be a ten after graduation). She denied any **perceptual** problems. She stated she felt well and could not understand why her roommates were concerned. On this basis, her **insight** and **judgment** were both deemed to be impaired.

Testing of her **cognitive functions** revealed that she was completely oriented. She was able to **register** four items and **recalled** them at around five minutes time. However, she could not recall the interviewer's name nor her exam schedule, so her **long-term memory** was considered impaired. Her attention and concentration were intact for six numbers forward and four backward. She performed three **serial seven subtractions** correctly and then told a story about the number seventy-nine. She was able to enumerate a considerable list of **similarities and differences**, many of which demonstrated a high level of abstraction.

Her **knowledge base** was consistent with her level of education and her **intelligence** seemed above average.

# Example 5

Mrs. D.E. is a 47-year-old separated woman who is employed as a professional cello player. After missing her third rehearsal, she was brought to the clinic by her close friends after being found in the basement of her home.

• Her appearance is that of a woman appearing older than her age. She was dressed in a housecoat and slippers. She is thin, has an odor of poor hygiene, and has old scars on her left wrist and forearm.

• She sat throughout the interview in an immobile position with her hands at her sides and her head slumped forward on her chest. There were no spontaneous movements when she spoke.

• She was uncooperative with the interview and said she wanted to be left alone. The information she shared did not seem reliable.

• Her speech was fluent and syntactically correct. There was a latency of several seconds before replying to questions. She spoke in a monotonous manner with no variability of prosody.

• Her thought process showed intermittent loosening of associations with periods of rambling when asked open-ended questions.

• The content of her thought involved delusions of persecution and infestation. On a recent trip overseas, she inadvertently knocked over the display of a merchant who was selling rare cultural artifacts. This merchant put a "curse" on her, and the patient has been coping poorly and declining since that time. She is convinced she has a type of flesh-eating organism inside her.

• She had passive wishes to die, but denied that she'd do anything to harm herself. There were no thoughts of harm to others.

• Her affect was flat and showed no range during the interview. She felt doomed and hopeless and described her mood as depressed.

• She described perceptual abnormalities in the form of tactile (beetles crawling on her skin) and cenesthetic hallucinations (the lining of her intestine is being gnawed away). She was also constantly harassed by the voice of the merchant.

• Her insight and judgment were both considered impaired on the basis of her bizarre delusions, her inability to understand that she is ill, and because she needed others to bring her in for help

• Cognitive testing revealed that she was only oriented to person, month, year, and season. She knew that she was in a hospital, but not which one. She was able to register only one object after two tries, and was not able to recall this after three minutes time. Her digit span was intact only for three numbers forward and two numbers backward. She did not attempt the serial sevens test. She was able to follow a written command and wrote a sentence ("I am going to die for what I did."). In response to many questions she replied, "I don't know." Testing of similarities and differences revealed concrete thinking and highly idiosyncratic replies.

# References

## Books

J. Morrison & R.A. Muñoz
**Boarding Time, 2nd Ed.**
American Psychiatric Press, Inc., Washington D.C., 1996

B.J. Sadock & V.A. Sadock, Editors
**Comprehensive Textbook of Psychiatry, 7th Ed.**
Lippincott, Williams & Wilkins, Philadelphia, 2000

## Articles

J.G. Carroll & J. Monroe
**Teaching Medical Interviewing**
*Journal of Medical Education* 54: 498, 1979

G.G. Kent, P. Clarke, & D. Dalrymple-Smith
**The Patient is the Expert: A Technique for Teaching Interviewing Skills**
*Medical Education* 15: 38 – 42, 1981

J.D.E. Knox, D.W. Alexander, A.T. Morrison, & A. Bennett
**Communication Skills and Undergraduate Medical Education**
*Medical Education* 13: 345 – 348, 1979

C.R. Lake, K.M. Moriarty, & S.W. Alagna
**The Acute Psychiatric Diagnostic Interview**
*Psychiatric Clinics of North America* 7(4): 657 – 670, 1984

L.M. Lovett, A. Cox, & M. Abou-Saleh
**Teaching Psychiatric Interview Skills to Medical Students**
*Medical Education* 24: 243 – 250, 1990

G.P. Maguire & D.R. Rutter
**History Taking For Medical Students: Evaluation of a Training Program**
*Lancet* ii: 558 – 560, 1976

G.P. Maguire, P. Roe, & D. Goldberg
**The Value of Feedback in Teaching Interviewing Skills to Medical Students**
*Psychological Medicine* 8: 695 – 704, 1978

B. McConville
**Hints on Passing Post-Graduate Clinical and Oral Examinations in Psychiatry**
*Australian and New Zealand Journal of Psychiatry* 16: 73 – 78, 1982

J.R. McCready & E.M. Waring
**Interviewing Skills in Relation to Psychiatric Residency**
*Canadian Journal of Psychiatry* 31: 317 – 322, 1986

P. McGuire
**Psychiatrists Also Need Interview Training (comments)**
*British Journal of Psychiatry* 141: 423 – 424, 1982

D.C. Pollock, D.E. Shanley, & P.N. Byrne
**Psychiatric Interviewing and Clinical Skills**
*Canadian Journal of Psychiatry* 30: 64 – 68, 1985

M. Rutter & A. Cox
**Psychiatric Interviewing Techniques I. Methods and Measures**
*British Journal of Psychiatry* 138: 273 – 282, 1981

M. Saghir
**A Comparison of Some Aspects of Structured and Unstructured Psychiatric Interviews**
*American Journal of Psychiatry* 128: 180 – 184, 1971

N.C. Scott, M.D. Donnelly, & J.W. Hess
**Changes in Interviewing Styles of Medical Students**
*Journal of Medical Education* 50: 1124 – 1126, 1975

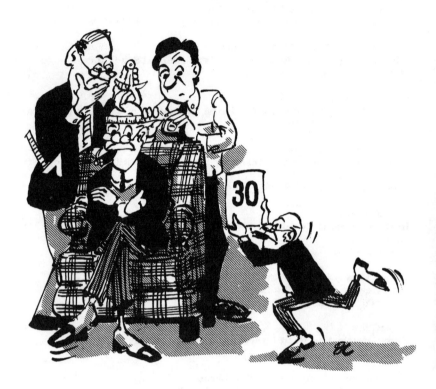

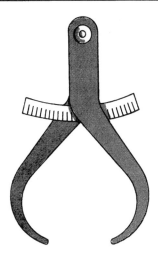

# Chapter 14

# The Mini-Mental State Exam

## What is the Mini-Mental State Exam?

**The Mini-Mental Status Exam (MMSE)** is a structured clinical assessment of cognitive functioning. It was published by Folstein et al in 1975 and has been referred to as "The Folstein Test" or the "Folstein MMSE." The MMSE provides a quantified assessment of various dimensions of cognitive functioning. The original article does not describe time limits for giving this test. The usual time required for administering this test is between three to five minutes. The test is scored out of a maximum thirty points. An average score for patients without cognitive impairment is twenty-eight. Scores of twenty-four or less indicate that an abnormality is present, which is usually dementia or delirium.

# The Folstein Mini-Mental State Exam

## Orientation
Score
- What is the – (day) (date) (month) (season) (year)?    **/ 5**
- Where are you now?  (building) (floor) (town)
                    (state) (country)    **/ 5**

## Registration
- List 3 objects at one-second intervals, then ask
the patient to repeat all 3; give one point for each
correct answer given on the first trial; repeat this
until the patient can recite all 3 items    **/ 3**

## Attention/Concentration
- Serial 7's Test up to 5 subtractions (starting with
100 – 7); alternatively ask the patient to spell
"WORLD" backwards (D - L - R - O - W)    **/ 5**

## Recall
- Ask the patient to recite the above 3 items    **/ 3**

## Language
- Show the patient a watch and a pen and ask the
patient to name these items    **/ 2**

- Ask the patient to repeat the following statement:
"No ifs, ands, or buts."    **/ 1**

- Ask the patient to follow these commands:
"Take a piece of paper in your right hand." (1 pt.)
"Fold it in half." (1 pt.)
"Place it on the floor." (1 pt.)    **/ 3**

- Read and follow this command:
"Close your eyes."    **/ 1**

**Score**

• Write a sentence:

/ 1

• Copy the following diagram:

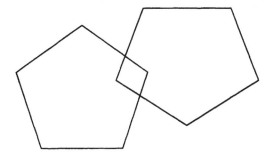

/ 1

## Total Score                                          / 30

* M. Folstein, S. Folstein & P. McHugh
**Mini-Mental State: A Practical Method for Grading the Cognitive State
of Patients for the Clinician**
*Journal of Psychiatric Research* 12:189 – 198, 1975
Reprinted with permission.

# Instructions for Administering the MMSE

## Orientation
• Ask for the date, then ask specifically for the parts omitted (e.g. season, year)
• Ask patients to tell you exactly where they are now, then ask for the parts omitted (state, country, etc.)

## Registration
• Ask if you may test memory, then list 3 unrelated objects in a clear voice with about 1 second between each item. After giving the list once, ask the patient to repeat this list and score 1 point for each item on this trial. Because you will be testing recall later, continue to give patients the list of objects until they can repeat them fully. If patients are unable to repeat these items after 6 trials, they cannot be meaningfully tested.

## Attention and Concentration
• Ask patients to begin with 100 and count backwards by 7. Stop after 5 subtractions (93, 86, 79, 72, 65 ). Score the total number of correct answers. If patients can't or won't perform this task, ask them to spell the word "world" backwards. The score is the number of letters in correct order, e.g., dlrow = 5, dlorw = 3, dolrw = 2, dolwr = 1, world = 0

## Recall
• Ask patients to recall the 3 words you previously asked them to remember. Score 0 – 3.

## Language
• Naming: Show patients a wrist watch and ask them to name it. Repeat for a pen or pencil. Score 0 – 2.
• Repetition: Ask the patient to repeat the sentence after you. Allow only one trial. Score 0 or 1.
• 3-Stage command: Use blank paper and repeat the command. Score 1 point for each part correctly executed.
• Reading: On a blank piece of paper print the sentence

"Close your eyes," in letters large enough for patients to see clearly. Ask them to read it and do what it says. Score 1 point only if the eyes are closed.

• Writing: Give patients a blank piece of paper and ask them to write a sentence for you. Do not dictate a sentence, it is to be written spontaneously. It must contain a subject and verb and be sensible. Correct grammar and punctuation aren't necessary.

## Copying

On a clean piece of paper, draw intersecting pentagons, each side about 1 in., and ask the patient to copy it exactly as it is. All 10 angles must be present and the pentagons must intersect to score 1 point. Tremor and rotation are ignored.

# Critique of the MMSE

The following scenario plays itself out over and over:

It is the first day of a rotation in psychiatry for a group of clinical clerks. A keen student grabs a chart to review the presenting history before seeing the patient. After having some idea what to ask about, she tries to recall the format of a psychiatric interview. "Not much different than a standard interview" she muses "except for this weird thing called the mental status exam." Somewhere, somehow she comes across a copy of the MMSE, and her confusion disappears. She presents the case thoroughly, and when it comes time to present the mental status, she smiles and says, "On the mental status exam, the patient scored 26."

The major pitfall of the MMSE is that it is NOT the same as a complete mental status exam. The similarity in names contributes to this confusion. The MMSE was designed to be a rapid screening instrument for cognitive impairment, and has three main clinical applications:

**1.** It tests features that are often omitted in traditional mental status exams, such as reading, writing, copying, repetition, following commands, and detailed orientation questions.

**2.** On the basis of the score from the initial test, it is useful for screening for dementia and delirium (e.g. a score less than 24 indicates impairment)

**3.** It provides a quantifiable score to follow the day-to-day progress of a patient in hospital

The MMSE does not include most of the features assessed by a thorough MSE. It is certainly a useful addition, but it is not a replacement. The MMSE is the most popular psychiatric screening assessment and has a large body of literature supporting its use. MMSE scores have been validated with performance on intelligence tests and deficits found on brain imaging.

The MMSE is more specific than it is sensitive. An abnormal score is highly suggestive of cognitive impairment, though patients with mild dementia or delirium often score higher than twenty-five on the test. Patients with little formal education may have spuriously low scores. Another pitfall involves patients who develop dementia but had a superior level of intelligence. Such patients continue to have normal scores on the MMSE despite their worsening deficits.

Extensive clinical use has shown the MMSE to have a high reliability both between interviewers, and on successive days with the same interviewer.

Molloy (1991) points out several factors that affect the reliability of scores from the MMSE:
• Brief scoring guidelines allow variation between raters
• Questions require different wording when testing outpatients, which may affect responses
• Scoring of the interlocking pentagons is subjective
• A patient's level of education affects the results
• The lack of a time limit may have a bearing on scoring
• Spelling 'world' backwards has been found to be easier to perform than serial 7's, despite the equivalence in scoring
• There are no guidelines for scoring near misses, e.g. being wrong by one day, especially at the beginning of a new month

# Other Versions of the MMSE

Molloy (1991)developed the **Standardized Mini-Mental Status Exam (SMMSE)** and has made two books (Molloy 199a, Molloy & Clarnette, 1999b) available with detailed instructions for administering and scoring. Molloy refers to the original as the **Traditional MMSE**. The SMMSE has been shown to have both greater inter-rater and intra-rater reliability. It was also found to be faster to administer.

Teng & Chui (1987) also developed an alternative version, called the **Modified Mini-Mental State Exam (MMMS or 3MS)**. In developing their version, they hoped to improve the ability of the test to distinguish between dementia and other types of cognitive disorders.

The 3M differs from the Folstein MMSE in the following ways:
• The score is out of 100, thus extending the floor and ceiling of the test
• Sampling a wider variety of cognitive abilities
• Enhancing reliability and validity by standardizing the testing procedure and scoring

The scoring range in the 3MS for many of the subtests was increased by allowing points for near misses. In other subtests the number of scoreable items was increased (e.g. from naming two items to five).

Four new subtests were added:
• Asking patients for their date and place of birth, which is scored for: year, month, day, town/city, and state/province
• Naming as many four-legged animals in thirty seconds as possible (to a maximum score of 10)
• Asking for similarities between: an arm and leg; laughing and crying; and eating and sleeping
• Second recall – after the patient registers three items, he is asked to recall them two times, the second time occurring at the end of the exam; this is administered even if the patient was unable to recall any items on the first recall

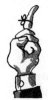

## MMSE Practice Points

• Scores on the MMSE are affected by a number of factors; Frisoni (1993) found the following variables to be of statistical significance: financial dissatisfaction, loss of independent function, number of diagnoses and medications, and degree of social activity

• Frisoni (1993) also found that the level of education affected MMSE scores: white collar workers scored an average of 2.33 points higher than farmers, which was also of statistical significance

• Heeren (1990) found that MMSE scores in elderly people remained high for those unaffected by psychiatric or neurologic illness: the median score in 85 – 95 year olds was 28; he suggests that when a 90-year-old patient scores less that 25 points, a neuropsychiatric evaluation is warranted

• Beckett (1997) developed a simplified algorithm for scoring the 'WORLD' backwards subtest, which she noted was insufficiently specified in the instructions accompanying the Folstein MMSE; Molloy (1999a) also provides a comprehensive scoring chart

# References

## Books

D.W. Molloy
**Standardized Mini-Mental State Examination**
Newgrange Press, Troy, Ontario, Canada, 1999a

D.W. Molloy & R. Clarnette
**Standardized Mini-Mental State Examination: A User's Guide**
Newgrange Press, Troy, Ontario, Canada, 1999b

## Articles

L.A. Beckett, R.S. Wilson, D.A. Bennett, & M.C. Morris
**Around the WORLD Backward: An Algorithm for Scoring the MMSE WORLD Item**
*Neurology* 48(6): 1733 – 1734, 1997

J.R. Cockrell & M.F. Folstein
**Mini-Mental State Examination (MMSE)**
*Psychopharmacol. Bull.* 24(4): 689 – 692, 1988

M.F. Folstein, S. Folstein, & P. McHugh
**Mini-Mental State: A Practical Method for Grading the Cognitive State of Patients for the Clinician**
*Journal of Psychiatric Research* 12:189 – 198, 1975

G.B. Frisoni, R. Rozzini, A. Bianchetti, & A. Trabucchi
**Principal Lifetime Occupation and MMSE Score in Elderly Persons**
*J. Gerontol.* 48(6): S310 – 314, 1993

M. Ganguli, G. Ratcliff, F.J. Huff, S. Belle, M.J. Kancel, & L. Fischer
**Serial Sevens Versus World Backwards: A Comparison of the Two Measures of Attention from the MMSE**
*J. Geriatr. Psychiatry Neurol.* 3(4): 203 – 207, 1990

R. Ganguli, J.S. Brar, H. Vermulapalli, H. Jafar, & R. Ahuja
**Mini-Mental State Exam Performance of Partially Remitted Community-Dwelling Patients With Schizophrenia**
*Schizophr. Res.* 33(1–2): 45 – 52, 1998

T.J. Heeren, A.M. Lagaay, W.C. von Beek, H.G. Rooymans, & W. Hijmans
**Reference Values for the Mini-Mental State Examination in Octo- and Nonagenarians**
*Journal of the American Geriatric Society* 38(10): 1093 – 1096, 1991

L. Kurlowica & M. Wallace
**The Mini-Mental State Exam**
*J. Gerontol. Nurs.* 25(5): 8 – 9, 1999

D.M. MacKenzie, P. Copp, R.J. Shaw, & G.M. Goodwin
**Brief Cognitive Screening of the Elderly: A Comparison of the Mini-Mental State Examination, Abbreviated Mental Test, and Mental Status Questionnaire**
*Psychol. Med.* 26(2): 427 – 430, 1996

D.W. Molloy & T.I. Standish
**A Guide to the Standardized Mini-Mental State Examination**
*Int. Psychogeriatr.* 9(suppl. 1): 87 – 94, 1997

D.W. Molloy, E. Alemayehu, & R. Roberts
**Reliability of a Standard Mini-Mental State Examination Compared With the Traditional Mini-Mental State Examination**
*American Journal of Psychiatry* 148 (1): 102 – 105, 1991

E.L. Teng & H.C. Chui
**The Modified Mini-Mental State Exam**
*J. Clin. Psychiatry* 48(8): 314 – 318, 1987

Z. Zlotogorski, L. Lurie, & G. Oppenheim
**Memory Versus Intelligence in Dementia Screening – MMSE**
*Isr. J. Psychiatry Rel. Sci.* 36(1): 18 – 22, 1999

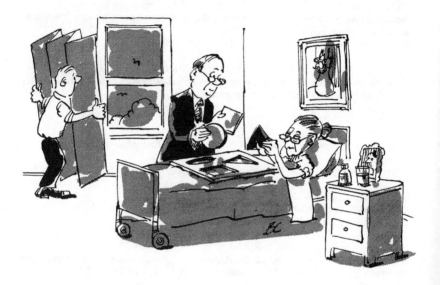

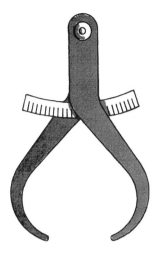

# Chapter 15

# Bedside Screening Instruments

Rating scales are used in psychiatry to standardize the information collected by different interviewers, or by the same interviewer on different occasions. Rating scales facilitate the process of obtaining specific information, and are formalized as questionnaires, checklists, or structured interviews. Some are self-assessments that patients complete, others need to be administered by an interviewer. Rating scales, when used appropriately, are useful for establishing a patient's baseline function, and then the response to treatment. Many research efforts rely on the quantifiable results provided by these instruments.

# What Do Psychiatric Rating Scales Measure?

Rating scales have been developed for these areas:
• Anxiety Disorders
• Cognitive Disorders
• Dissociative Disorders
• Eating Disorders
• Functional Status
• Mood Disorders
• Personality Disorders
• Psychiatric Diagnosis
• Psychotic Disorders
• Side Effects of Psychiatric Medication
• Substance Use Disorders

This chapter provides an overview of screening tests for cognitive disorders.

## What Makes a Scale Reliable?

Reliability is the repeatability, or test-to-test consistency of a particular instrument. A test is considered to be reliable if it is easy to agree on the score that should be given to a patient's performance. Reliability is enhanced with scales that have clearly worded instructions and questions, and that have a format for scoring that is easily applied. For example, if 10 raters independently assessed a patient using the MMSE and all agreed on the score, then this test would be considered valid.

## What Makes a Scale Valid?

Validity is the degree to which a test actually measures what it is supposed to measure. For example, if patients who scored twenty-five or less on the MMSE were subjected to further observation and neuropsychiatric evaluation and a high percentage of them actually had a delirium or dementia, then this test would be considered valid.

McDougall (1990), in an excellent review of cognitive screening instruments, notes that while rating scales for mental status, cognitive function, and dementia share an overlap, they also test a distinct constellation of functions.

# Domains Assessed in MSE, Cognitive Function, and Dementia Testing

|  | MSE | Cognitive Function | Dementia |
|---|---|---|---|
| Abstraction | ☑ |  | ☑ |
| Affect | ☑ |  |  |
| Appearance | ☑ |  |  |
| Attention Span | ☑ | ☑ | ☑ |
| Concentration | ☑ | ☑ |  |
| General Knowledge | ☑ | ☑ | ☑ |
| Hobbies |  | ☑ |  |
| Intelligence | ☑ | ☑ | ☑ |
| Judgment | ☑ | ☑ | ☑ |
| Language/Speech | ☑ |  | ☑ |
| Learning Ability |  | ☑ |  |
| Level of Consciousness | ☑ |  | ☑ |
| Memory | ☑ | ☑ | ☑ |
| Orientation | ☑ | ☑ | ☑ |
| Perception | ☑ | ☑ | ☑ |
| Personality Changes |  |  | ☑ |
| Problem Solving |  | ☑ |  |
| Psychomotor Ability | ☑ | ☑ | ☑ |
| Reaction Time |  | ☑ |  |
| Self Care | ☑ |  | ☑ |
| Social Intactness |  | ☑ |  |
| Thought Content | ☑ |  |  |

Adapted from McDougall, 1990
© Lippincott, Williams & Wilkins
Reprinted with permission.

A number of scales assess cognition and screen for dementia. Six will be detailed here: **Brief Cognitive Rating Scale (BCRS)**; **Blessed Dementia Scale (BDS)**; **Cognitive Capacity Screening Examination (CCSE)**; **Global Deterioration Scale (GDS)**; **Mental Status Questionnaire (MSQ)**; and the **Short Portable Mental Status Questionnaire (SPMSQ)**.

# Domains Assessed by the BCRS, BDS, and CCSE

| | BCRS | BDS | CCSE |
|---|---|---|---|
| Abstraction | | | ☑ |
| Affect | | ☑ | |
| Attention Span | | ☑ | ☑ |
| Concentration | ☑ | ☑ | |
| Consciousness | ☑ | ☑ | ☑ |
| Constructional Ability | | | |
| Functional Ability | ☑ | ☑ | |
| General Knowledge | ☑ | ☑ | ☑ |
| Hobbies | | | |
| Intelligence | | ☑ | |
| Judgment | | ☑ | ☑ |
| Language/Speech | ☑ | ☑ | ☑ |
| Learning Ability | | ☑ | |
| Memory | ☑ | ☑ | ☑ |
| Orientation | ☑ | ☑ | ☑ |
| Perception | | ☑ | ☑ |
| Problem Solving | | ☑ | |
| Psychomotor Ability | | ☑ | |
| Reaction Time | | | |
| Self Care | ☑ | ☑ | |
| Social Intactness | | ☑ | |
| Thought Content | | ☑ | ☑ |

From McDougall, 1990
© Lippincott, Williams & Wilkins
Reprinted with permission.

## BCRS & GDS

The BCRS and GDS were developed as companion scales to stage the cognitive and functional status of patients with dementia. Both of these scales are scored on a seven-point basis ranging from normal (scored as 1) to profound deficits

# Domains Assessed by the GDS, MSQ, and SPMSQ

| | GDS | MSQ | SPMSQ |
|---|---|---|---|
| Abstraction | ☑ | | |
| Affect | ☑ | | |
| Attention Span | ☑ | | ☑ |
| Concentration | ☑ | | |
| Consciousness | ☑ | | ☑ |
| Constructional Ability | ☑ | | |
| Functional Ability | ☑ | | |
| General Knowledge | ☑ | ☑ | ☑ |
| Hobbies | | | |
| Intelligence | ☑ | | |
| Judgment | ☑ | | |
| Language/Speech | ☑ | | |
| Learning Ability | ☑ | | |
| Memory | ☑ | ☑ | ☑ |
| Orientation | ☑ | ☑ | ☑ |
| Perception | ☑ | | |
| Problem Solving | ☑ | | |
| Psychomotor Ability | ☑ | | |
| Reaction Time | | | |
| Self Care | ☑ | | |
| Social Intactness | ☑ | | |
| Thought Content | ☑ | | ☑ |

From McDougall, 1990
© Lippincott, Williams & Wilkins
Reprinted with permission.

(scored as 7), and were designed to be administered by a mental health professional or trained rater. The BCRS focuses specifically on five domains (called axes): concentration; recent memory; remote memory; orientation; and self-care. Each test typically takes between 30 – 45 minutes (each) to administer.

## BDS

The BDS was designed to screen for dementia, and contains 17 items that measure changes in a variety of functions: everyday activities; eating and dressing habits; personality; interests and drive; information; memory; and concentration. The BDS, sometimes called the **Blessed Dementia Inventory (BDI)**, was one of the first scales developed.

## CCSE

The CCSE consists of 30 items, and was designed to diagnose organic mental syndromes (i.e. delirium) in non-psychiatric patients. It takes approximately 10 – 15 minutes to administer. The CCSE measures areas that are not assessed in other tests, such as abstraction and language abilities. This test is not specific enough to differentiate among the dementias. Foreman (1987) compared the CCSE with the SPMSQ and MMSE, and found it to be the superior test.

## MSQ

The MSQ consists of ten items, and can be administered in minutes. It has been used to assess the capacity for self-care, and to screen for post-op delirium after hip fractures. It is a good predictor of the need for institutionalization.

## SPMSQ

The SPMSQ was developed and tested on community-dwelling and institutionalized elderly patients. It also consists of ten items. It has not been found to accurately predict the capacity for self-care, nor is it able to predict clinical course.

# Clock Drawing

Clock drawing was introduced in the *Sensorium & Cognitive Screening Chapter* as a means of testing visuospatial ability, as well as cognitive functioning. Some of the reported clinical applications of clock drawing are:

• Tuokko (1992) used three clock subtests – clock drawing, clock setting (putting in the time), and clock reading; it was determined that clock tests are a sensitive measure in differentiating normal elderly from those with Alzheimer's disease

• Esteban-Santillan (1998) found that individuals who made two or more errors in clock drawing warranted further investigation; elderly participants who made no errors were unlikely to have even mild Alzheimer's disease

• Hermann (1999) noted that patients with schizophrenia made significantly more errors than normal controls in placing and spacing numbers on freehand and pre-drawn clocks, despite similar MMSE score in both groups

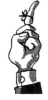

### Practice Points

Brief, portable tests of mental status and cognitive function hold a tremendous appeal for clinicians. O'Neill (1993) has termed such assessments "brain stethoscopes" and considers them to be perhaps the innovation in the twentieth century that the stethoscope itself was in the nineteenth century. Judging by the number of screening instruments available, as well as the substantial literature supporting their reliability and validity, it appears that many researchers share O'Neill's opinion.

Unfortunately, no instrument has won acclaim as the single best test. Contradictory studies about the usefulness of each test can be found in the literature. The qualities that make a screening test appealing (e.g. brevity and simple scoring guidelines) decrease its accuracy. The MSQ consists of only ten items, and may well be used as a screening test to determine if more detailed screening tests are necessary.

It is important to be familiar with the conditions under which various tests were developed. Some considerations are:
• Was the test used only on inpatients?
• Are alterations recommended (i.e. different cut-off scores) for patients living in the community?
• Was the test meant to detect subtle or significant impairment
• Has a different sensitivity and specificity been developed for different populations?
• To what degree does the test rely on the level of education, age, and cultural background?
• How clear are the scoring guidelines?

Clinicians are best served by becoming familiar with a small number of cognitive screening tests, and using the scores they provide in context with the rest of the MSE, history, and patient's level of function.

# References

## Books

E.W. Busse & D.G. Blazer, Editors
**Textbook of Geriatric Psychiatry, 2nd Ed.**
American Psychiatric Press Inc., Washington D.C., 1996

B.J. Sadock & V.A. Sadock, Editors
**Comprehensive Textbook of Psychiatry, 7th Ed.**
Lippincott, Williams & Wilkins, Philadelphia, 2000

## Articles

G. Blessed, B. Tomlinson, & M. Roth
**The Association Between Quantitative Measures of Dementia and of Senile Changes in the Cerebral Gray Matter of Elderly Subjects**
*British Journal of Psychiatry* 114: 797 – 811, 1968

D.L. Cresswell & R.I. Lanyon
**Validation of a Screening Battery for Psychogeriatric Assessment**
*Journal of Gerontology* 36(4): 435 – 440, 1981

J.L. Cummings & D.F. Benson
**Dementia of the Alzheimer Type: An Inventory of Diagnostic Clinical Features**
*Journal of the American Geriatrics Society* 34(1): 12 – 19, 1986

J. Curtis
**Mental Status Questionnaire**
*Home Healthcare Nurse* 7(1): 45 – 48, 1989

J.E. Dalton, S.L. Pederson, B.E. Blom, & N.R. Holmes
**Diagnostic Errors Using the Short Portable Mental Status Questionnaire With a Mixed Clinical Population**
*J. Gerontol.* 42(5): 512 – 514, 1987

T. Erkinjuntti, R. Sulkava, J. Wikstrom, & L. Autio
**Short Portable Mental Status Questionnaire as a Screening Test for Dementia and Delirium Among the Elderly**
*Journal of the American Geriatrics Society* 35(5): 412 – 416, 1987

C. Esteban-Santillan, R. Praditsuwan, H. Ueda, & D.S. Geldmacher
**Clock Drawing Test in Very Mild Alzheimer's Disease**
*Journal of the American Geriatrics Society* 46(10): 1266 – 1269, 1998

G.G. Fillenbaum, L.R. Landerman, & E.M. Simonsick
**Equivalence of Two Screens of Cognitive Functioning: The Short Portable Mental Status Questionnaire and the Orientation-Memory-Concentration Test**
*Journal of the American Geriatrics Society* 46(12): 1512 – 1518, 1998

G.G. Fillenbaum
**Comparison of Two Brief Tests of Organic Brain Impairment: The MSQ and the SPMSQ**
*Journal of the American Geriatrics Society* 33(8): 381 – 384, 1979

M.D. Foreman
**Reliability and Validity of Mental Status Questionnaires in Elderly Hospitalized Patients**
*Nursing Research* 36(4): 216 – 220, 1987

K.K. Gnanalingham, E.J. Byrne, & A. Thornton
**Clock-Face Drawing to Differentiate Lewy Body Dementia and Alzheimer Type Dementia Syndromes (letter)**
*The Lancet* 347: 696 – 697, 1996

N.P. Gruber, R.V. Varner, Y.W. Chen, & J.M. Lesser
**A Comparison of the Clock Drawing Test and the Pfeiffer Short Portable Mental Status Questionnaire in a Geropsychiatry Clinic**
*Int. J. Geriatr. Psychiatry* 12(5): 526 – 532, 1997

N. Hermann, D. Kidron, K.I. Shulman, E. Kaplan, M. Binns, & J. Soni
**The Use of Clock Tests in Schizophrenia**
*General Hospital Psychiatry* 21: 70 – 73, 1999

J.W. Jacobs, M.R. Bernhard, A. Delgado, & J.J. Strain
**Screening for Organic Mental Syndromes in the Medically Ill**
*Annals of Internal Medicine* 86: 40 – 46, 1977

R.L. Kahn, A.I. Goldfarb, M. Pollack, & A. Peck
**Brief Objective Measures for the Determination of Mental Status**
*American Journal of Psychiatry* 117: 326, 1960

D. Kaufman & L. Zun
**A Quantifiable, Brief Mental Status Examination for Emergency Patients**
*Journal of Emergency Medicine* 13(4): 449 – 456, 1995

D.M. Kaufman, M. Weinberger, J.J. Strain, & J.W. Jacobs
**Detection of Cognitive Deficits by a Brief Mental Status Examination: The Cognitive Capacity Screening Examination – A Reappraisal and a Review**
*General Hospital Psychiatry* 1(3): 247 – 255, 1979

D.M. MacKenzie, P. Copp, R.J. Shaw, & G.M. Goodwin
**Brief Cognitive Screening of the Elderly: A Comparison of the Mini-Mental State Examination (MMSE), Abbreviated Mental Test (AMT), and Mental Status Questionnaire (MSQ)**
*Psychological Medicine* 26(2): 427 – 430, 1996

G.J. McDougall
**A Review of Screening Instruments for Assessing Cognition and Mental Status in Older Adults**
*Nurse Practitioner* 15(11): 18 – 28, 1990

J. Morris, A. Heyman, R. Mohs, J.P. Hughes, G. van Belle, & G Fillenbaum
**The Consortium to Establish a Registry for Alzheimer's Disease (CERAD): Part 1 – Clinical/Neuropsychological Assessment of Alzheimer's Disease**
*Neurology* 39(9): 1159 – 1165, 1989

D. O'Neill
**Brain Stethoscopes: The Use and Abuse of Brief Mental Status Schedules**
*Postgraduate Medical Journal* 69(814): 599 – 601, 1993

E. Pfeiffer
**A Short Portable Mental Status Questionnaire for the Assessment of Organic Brain Deficit in Elderly Patients**
*Journal of the American Geriatrics Society* 23(10): 433 – 441, 1975

B. Reisberg, S.H. Ferris, M.J. De Leon, & T. Crook
**Global Deterioration Scale (GDS)**
*Psychopharmacol. Bull.* 24(4): 661 – 663, 1988

B. Reisberg & S.H. Ferris
**Brief Cognitive Rating Scale (BCRS)**
*Psychopharmacol. Bull.* 24(4): 629 – 636, 1988

B. Reisberg
**The Brief Cognitive Rating Scale (BCRS): Findings in Primary Degenerative Dementia (PDD)**
*Psychopharmacol. Bull.* 19(1): 47 – 50, 1983

B. Reisberg
**The Brief Cognitive Rating Scale (BCRS): Language, Motoric, and Mood Concomitants in Primary Degenerative Dementia**
*Psychopharmacol. Bull.* 19(4): 702 – 708, 1983

B. Reisberg, S.H. Ferris, M.J. De Leon, & T. Crook
**The Global Deterioration Scale (GDS) for Assessment of Primary Degenerative Dementia**
*American Journal of Psychiatry* 139(9): 1136 – 1139, 1982

H. Reisberg, S.H. Ferris, & S.G. Sclan
**Empirical Evaluation of the Global Deterioration Scale for Staging Alzheimer's Disease**
*American Journal of Psychiatry* 150(4): 680 – 682, 1993

W.G Rosen, R.C. Mohs, & K.L. Davis
**A New Rating Scale for Alzheimer's Disease**
*American Journal of Psychiatry* 141(11): 1356 – 1364, 1984

R.I. Shader, J.S. Harmatz, & C. Salzman
**A New Scale for Clinical Assessment in Geriatric Populations: Sandoz Clinical Assessment – Geriatric (SCAG)**
*Journal of the American Geriatrics Society* 22(3): 107 – 113, 1974

M.A. Smyer, B.F. Hofland, & E.A. Jonas
**Validity Study of the Short Portable Mental Status Questionnaire for the Elderly**
*Journal of the American Geriatrics Society* 27(6): 263 – 269, 1979

D. Towle, G. Wilcox & D. Surmon
**The Kew Test – A Study of Reliability and Validity**
*Journal of Experimental Gerontology* 9(4): 245 – 256, 1987

H. Tuokko, T. Hadjistavropoulous, J.A. Miller, & B.L. Beattie
**The Clock Test: A Sensitive Measure to Differentiate Normal Elderly From Those With Alzheimer's Disease**
*Journal of the American Geriatrics Society* 40(6): 579 – 584, 1992

L.A. Wilson & W. Brass
**Brief Assessment of the Mental State in Geriatric Domiciliary Practice: The Usefulness of the Mental Status Questionnaire**
*Age and Ageing* 2: 92 – 101, 1973

M. Zaudig, J. Mittelhammer, W. Hiller, A. Pauls, C. Thora, & A. Moringo
**SIDAM – A Structured Interview for the Diagnosis of Dementia of the Alzheimer Type, Multi-Infarct Dementia, and Dementias of Other Etiology According to ICD-10 and DSM-111-R**
*Psychological Medicine* 21(1): 225 – 236, 1991

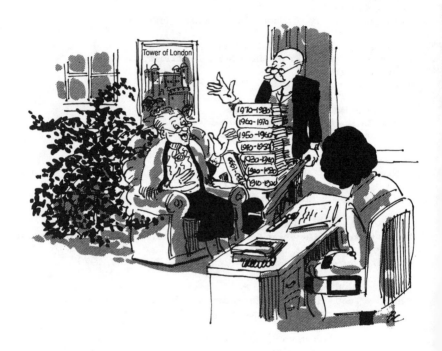

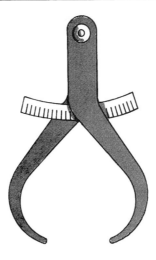

# Chapter 16

# The MSE and the Elderly

The MSE in interviews with elderly patients deserves special mention. Psychiatric disorders of at least moderate severity are relatively common in the elderly, leading to many positive findings on the MSE. In many cases, the MSE will be the principal part of the interview. Many authors have suggested that the MSE be included early in the interview, and not left to be tackled at the end of the interview. A point of technique is to make the MSE, particularly tests of cognitive function, blend in as naturally as possible. The use of pre-printed forms can help the tests of cognition seem like standard questions, and help patients avoid feeling self-conscious. It may not be possible to get all the information required from patients, necessitating that collateral history be obtained. It may also take more than one session or interview with patients to complete a thorough MSE.

# General Interviewing Techniques

Interviews with elderly patients often proceed at a slow pace. It is common for interviewees to give over-inclusive and circumstantial answers. Spontaneous digressions, tactfully called reminiscences, occur frequently. It is incumbent on interviewers to monitor the effect that the assessment is having on their patients. Should patients become frustrated or upset, it is suggested that digressions be allowed, or even encouraged, in order to preserve rapport. The opportunity for a break can be offered at the beginning of the interview, or scheduled at a certain point in time (e.g. at 30 minutes). Modifications in interview style are necessary. Opportunities for secondary education and beyond were far more limited in past decades, and questions should be phrased without the use of "high falutin'" words. Interviewers need to speak more slowly, and may need to ask the patient if she is hard of hearing. Mental illness is still stigmatized by society. Elderly patients, particularly if they are being assessed for the first time, can become quite anxious during the interview. Performance in all aspects of the interview can be affected (particularly cognitive functioning), leading to spurious concerns (e.g. dementia, anxiety disorders, etc.). A few minutes spent explaining your qualifications and intent for the interview will be most welcome.

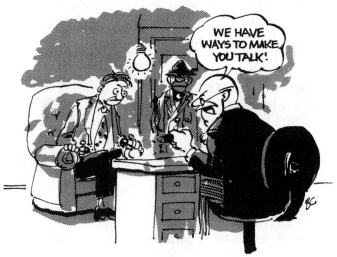

# Appearance

Many features of appearance can indicate the presence of serious psychiatric or medical conditions. Findings on the MSE are confirmed on physical exam and/or with investigations.

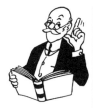

Features to look for in elderly patients (and their significance) are as follows:
• Poor nutrition – depression, incapacity to manage independently, medical illness (e.g. diabetes), etc.
• Hygeine – lack of motivation, inattentiveness (e.g. following a stroke), etc.
• Incontinence – substance intoxication or withdrawal, new neurologic problems
• Skin – jaundice, bruises, cuts, burns, signs of abuse

# Behavior

Blazer (1996) notes the following about behavior changes:
• Under-activity is characteristic for depression, severe schizophreniform illness, and some types of dementia
• Mild-to-moderately demented patients are notably distractible, and will walk around the room, or even leave
• Many elderly patients pace to relieve anxiety

# Thought Form

Moderate circumstantial speech, or **circumlocution**, is a common finding among the elderly. It is marked in patients with dementia, and often is used as a smoke screen to deflect attention from their cognitive deficits.

# Thought Content

Blazer (1989) reports abnormalities in thought content as being the most common disturbances in cognition in the elderly. Demented patients exhibit poverty of content and evasiveness.

Many elderly patients emphasize alterations in their bodily functions during interviews. Depression is frequently complicated by thoughts of defective body parts or aberrant functions.

The elderly are a high-risk group for suicide. During the interview or MSE, questions about death should be asked:
• What are the patient's thoughts about death?
• How prepared is he for death?
• What is his philosophy about death?

# Affect & Mood

Geriatric patients can suffer from depression but not complain of having a low mood. Often, somatic complaints dominate over vegetative ones. A more useful approach is to ask about:
• Lack of enjoyment of activities
• A sense of hope for the future
• The presence of guilty feelings

# Perception

Hypnagogic and hypnopompic hallucinations are more common in the elderly, but are not of themselves indicative of psychiatric illness. Problems in peripheral sense organs (eyes and ears especially) can affect perception.

# Insight & Judgment

Many elderly patients simply defer to their doctors for medical decisions because this was the tradition in decades past. Some patients do so because they feel their conditions or treatment options are too complicated to understand.

Irrespective of the methods used in interviews to assess insight and judgment, it is crucial to offer patients structured assessments in real-life situations when assessing their ability to live independently. For example, patients can be asked to prepare meals in kitchens, or be taken to banks to demonstrate their ability to manage money. Many patients can function at a higher level at home than when assessed in the hospital.

## Activities of Daily Living (ADLs) and Instrumental Activities of Daily Living (IADLs)

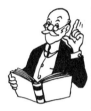

> ADLs are basic day-to-day functions:
> • Bathing/grooming
> • Dressing
> • Toileting/continence
> • Feeding
> • Ambulation/transfer (into and out of bed, bathtubs, etc.)

> IADLs involve the ability of the person to cope with her environment in terms of the following adaptive tasks:
> • Telephone          • Shopping
> • Food preparation    • Housekeeping
> • Laundry             • Transportation
> • Medication          • Finances

# Cognitive Assessment

Many clinicians suggest that interviewers make cognitive testing as interesting and light-hearted as possible for patients. By giving some feedback, positive wherever possible, interviewers can encourage patients to continue with the tasks they are asked to perform.

The use of structured instruments can be helpful in documenting a patient's performance and allows progress to be quantified. Some individual questions or subtests from various instruments are highly valid screens. For example, McDougall (1990) notes that the MSQ contains questions about the patient's date of birth and the previous president, both of which are good discriminators for assessing the presence of cognitive impairment.

Note that patterns of loss are at least as important as the total score derived from screening tests (i.e. the types of errors are as important as their presence).

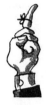

### Practice Points
• Perceptual, cognitive, and motor skills typically begin a slow decline when people are in their 40's
• General knowledge and verbal fluency remain virtually identical to the level people have when they are in their 20's
• The **Wechsler Adult Intelligence Scale – Revised (WAIS-R)** makes only slight allowances for age; most of the subtests are the same for all adults
• In contrast to verbal IQ, performance IQ shows a considerable decline with time
• The **digit symbol subtest** shows the most change with age; here, geometric symbols are substituted for numbers, and the task is to translate a random list of numbers with the substituted symbols
• **Benign senescent forgetfulness** refers to mild memory problems and some organizational difficulties; this does not appear to be a prognostic indicator for future dementia

# References
## Books

E.W. Busse & D.G. Blazer, Editors
**Textbook of Geriatric Psychiatry, 2nd Ed.**
American Psychiatric Press, Inc., Washington D.C., 1996

R. Butler & B. Pitt, Editors
**Seminars in Old Age Psychiatry**
Royal College of Psychiatrists/Gaskell, London, England, 1998

C.E. Coffey & J.L. Cummings, Editors
**Textbook of Geriatric Neuropsychiatry, 2nd Ed.**
American Psychiatric Press, Inc., Washington D.C., 2000

C. Oppenheimer & R. Jacoby
*The Psychiatric Examination,* in
**Psychiatry in the Elderly**
Oxford University Press, New York, 1997

J. Sadavoy, L.W. Lazarus, L.F. Jarvik, & G.T. Grossberg
**Comprehensive Review of Geriatric Psychiatry – II, 2nd Ed.**
American Psychiatric Press, Inc., Washington D.C., 1996

# Articles

C. Dellasega & E. Cuzeto
**Strategies Used by Home Health Nurses to Assess the Mental Status of Homebound Elders**
*J. Community Health Nursing* 11(3): 129 – 138, 1994

S. Katz
**Assessing Self-Maintenance: Activities of Daily Living, Mobility, and Instrumental Activities of Daily Living**
*Journal of the American Geriatrics Society* 31(12): 721 – 727, 1983

V.A. Kral
**Some Trends in Geriatric Psychiatry**
*Canadian Psychiatric Association Journal* 15(6): 605 – 614, 1970

M.P. Lawton & E.M. Brody
**Assessment of Older People: Self-Maintaining and Instrumental Activities of Daily Living**
*Gerontologist* 9(3): 179 – 186, 1969

G.J. McDougall
**A Review of Screening Instruments for Assessing Cognition and Mental Status in Older Adults**
*Nurse Practitioner* 15(11): 18 – 28, 1990

B.S. Meyers & R. Greenberg
**Late Life Delusional Depression**
*J. Affective Disorders* 11(2): 133 – 137, 1986

K.P. O'Keefe & T.G. Sanson
**Elderly Patients with Altered Mental Status**
*Emergency Medical Clinics of North America* 16(4): 701 – 715, 1998

J.D. Nadler, N.R. Relkin, M.S. Cohen, R.A. Hodder, J. Reingold, & F. Plum
**Mental Status Testing in the Elderly Nursing Home Population**
*J. Geriatr. Psychiatry Neurol.* 8(3): 177 – 183, 1995

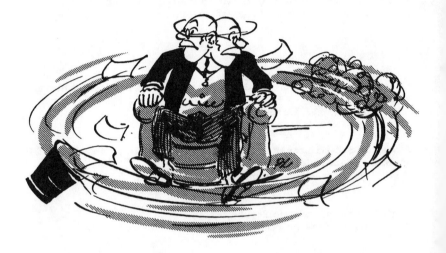

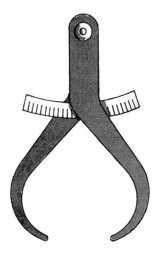

# Chapter 17

# The Child Mental Status Exam

The child mental status exam differs markedly from the adult version described in this text. Further complicating this matter is that most clinicians who evaluate and treat adults do not routinely assess children. For the purposes of a complete presentation of the MSE, a skeletal outline will be presented here, with a list of references for interested readers.

Because children cannot provide all of the information needed by clinicians, Goodman & Sours (1998) outline a three-stage assessment:

**1.** Developing an understanding the child's family and social milieu, as well as the history of the presenting problem

**2.** Constructing a developmental biological profile that contains information about physical growth, developmental history, and the primary care physician's input

**3.** The phenomenological assessment of the child, which also can include neurological and psychological testing

# Developmental Frame of Reference

Clinicians assessing children require at least a working knowledge of developmental stages and age norms to be able to ascertain what constitutes an abnormal finding. A child's language, perceptual, and motor development needs to be gauged with expected norms for her age. Many theorists have proposed sequences for social development, notably Bowlby, Erikson, Freud, Mahler, and Piaget. A child's cognitive development will dictate the content of the MSE. For example:

• Age 12 to 18 months – knows animal sounds
• Age 2 years – knows some body parts
• Age 3 years – knows colors and age
• Age 4 years – have object permanence
• Age 5 years – understand right and wrong
• Age 7 years – develop problem solving skills

Description of normal development and age-appropriate skills can be found in standard reference texts.

# Diagnostic Classification

The DSM-IV contains a separate section called *Disorders Usually First Diagnosed in Infancy, Childhood, or Adolescence.* The **American Psychiatric Association (APA)** suggests that there should be no clear distinction between childhood and adult disorders. The APA indicates that if an adult meets the criteria for a diagnosis (e.g. pica), it should be applied even though this condition is described in the childhood disorders section. With few exceptions, there are no age limits incorporated into the diagnostic criteria listed in the adult section of the DSM-IV. However, there is some debate about when certain disorders (e.g. schizophrenia) can be reliably diagnosed in children.

# Challenges in Assessing Children

• Children's responses are rarely offered directly, but are transformed into an activity, usually play

• **Primary process thinking** is not bound by logic, permits contradictions to coexist, contains no negatives, has no regard for time, and is highly symbolized; this type of thinking is seen in dreams, psychosis, and children's thinking

• In children, the significance of certain findings is disputed as to whether it is a sign of illness, normal development, or a reaction to the environment

• Some clinicians start the interview by allowing children to explore their offices, however a balance between flexibility and enforcing boundaries is recommended

• Hallucinations rarely occur in children

• Direct questions are often not successful with children

• The MSE requires clinicians to actively participate in play and to encourage cooperation

• The MSE is observational with younger children, based on interaction with older children

Goodman & Sours (1998) suggested preparing children for the interview, and made a list of recommendations for posing questions, arranging an office, and what toys to have available.

# MSE for Children

• Appearance
• Mobility & coordination
• Self-regulation
• Preferred mode of communication
• Speech & language
• Intellectual function
• Modes of thinking and perception
• Emotional reactions
• Relatedness to the interviewer and parents
• Coping mechanisms
• Dreams & fantasies
• Play

# The Role of Play in the MSE

Of all the components in child MSE, the role of play is most foreign to adult psychiatrists. Play and talking enhance one another. Play acts as a projective test, as children will act out their fears, fantasies, etc. The objects used for play can be kept relatively simple. Items such as paper, crayons, blocks, puppets, pencils, and play dough allow a child to express his imagination and creative abilities. More sophisticated toys tend to detract from the examination and instead only provide an opportunity for recreational play.

Goodman and Sours (1998) list six different aspects of play that can be recorded:
• Initiative
• Goal-directedness
• Sex-appropriateness
• Ingenuity
• Age-appropriateness
• Intensity/aggression

These aspects of play provide many clues as to the structure and dynamics of a child's personality. Additionally, play offers the opportunity to assess many features of the MSE:
• Motor coordination
• Intelligence
• Mobility
• Speech
• Fantasy
• Self-regulation

Goodman and Sours (1998) also detailed a neurological play examination that tests for the following:
• Cerebral function
• Reflexes
• Cerebellar function
• Cranial nerves
• Motor function
• Sensory function

# References

## Books

American Psychiatric Association
**Diagnostic and Statistical Manual of Mental Disorders, 4th Ed.**
American Psychiatric Association, Washington D.C., 1994

J.D. Goodman & J.A. Sours
**The Child Mental Status Examination – Expanded Edition**
Jason Aronson, Inc., Northvale, New Jersey, 1998

S.I. Greenspan & N.T. Greenspan
**The Clinical Interview of the Child, 2nd Ed.**
American Psychiatric Press, Inc., 1991

L. Hechtman, Editor
**Do They Grow Out of It?**
American Psychiatric Press, Inc., Washington D.C., 1996

M. Lewis, Editor
**Textbook of Child and Adolescent Psychiatry: A Comprehensive Textbook**
Lippincott, Williams & Wilkins, Philadelphia, 1996

J. Morrison & T.F. Anders
**Interviewing Children and Adolescents**
The Guilford Press, New York, 1999

J. Noshpitz
**Handbook of Child and Adolescent Psychiatry**
John Wiley & Sons, New York, 1998

J. Wiener
**Textbook of Child and Adolescent Psychiatry, 2nd Ed.**
American Psychiatric Press, Inc., Washington D.C., 1997

## Articles

American Academy of Child and Adolescent Psychiatry
**Practice Parameter of Psychiatric Assessment of Infants and Toddlers**
*J. Am. Acad. Adolesc. Psychiatry* 36(Suppl.): 21S, 1997

R. Nass
**Rapid Assessment of Mental Status in the Infant and Young Child**
*Emerg. Med. Clin. North Am.* 5(4): 739 – 750, 1987

I.I. Riddle
**The Florence H. Erickson Inaugural Lectureship: Reflections on Children's Play**
*Matern. Child. Nurs. J.* 19(4): 271 – 279, 1990

# Index

## A

A's (Bleuler's cardinal symptoms of schizophrenia)  159

Abnormal Involuntary Movement Scale (**AIMS**)  77 – 78

Abstract Thinking  15, 322, 355 – 356, 385, 386, 387

Abstraction – see Abstract Thinking

Abulia  57, 129

Abuse  38

Acalculia  359

Accent  133

Acetylcholine  73 – 75

Activities of Daily Living (**ADLs**)  399

Activity  53 – 58

Acute Stress Disorder  259, 285, 336

Adaptation  185

Adiposity  38

Adjustment Disorder  268, 272

Advertence  65

Aerophagia  77

Affect  11, 15, 17, 54, 85, 104, 257, 261 – 267, 269, 270, 271, 272, 317, 325, 385, 386, 387, 398

Affect, Types of  261

Age  35 – 36, 222 – 223

Agitation  54

Agnosia  124, 359

Agrammatism  127

Agoraphobia  205, 206, 298

Agraphia  124

AIDS  34

Akathisia  56, 58, 78, 90, 231

Akinesia  56, 72

Akinetic Mutism  64

Alcohol  33, 34, 35, 55, 60, 72, 83, 138, 155, 156, 193, 223 – 224, 240, 305

Alcoholic Hallucinosis  305

Alexia  124

Alexithymia  279

Alogia  161

Altruistic Suicide  233

Amantadine  78, 84

Ambitendency  65

Ambivalence  200

American Psychiatric Association (**APA**)  8, 246, 404

Amnesia  348

Amnestic Aphasia  131

Amoxapine  71

Amphetamines  78, 81, 83, 223, 304

Amygdala  352

Anabolic Steroid Use  34, 38

Anal Phase  200

Anal Triad  200

Angst  208

Angular Gyrus Aphasia  131

Anhedonia

# I

# P

# T

## The Author

Dave Robinson is a psychiatrist practicing in London, Ontario, Canada. His particular interests are consultation-liaison psychiatry, undergraduate and postgraduate education. A graduate of the University of Toronto Medical School, he completed a Residency in Family Practice before entering the Psychiatry Residency Program. He is a Lecturer in the Department of Psychiatry at the University of Western Ontario in London, Canada.

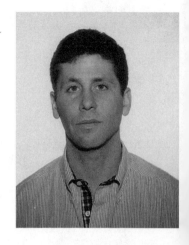

## The Artist

Brian Chapman is a resident of Oakville, Ontario, Canada. He was born in Sussex, England and moved to Canada in 1957. His first commercial work took place during W.W. II when he traded drawings for cigarettes while serving in the British Navy. Now retired, Brian was formerly a Creative Director at Mediacom. He continues to freelance and is versatile in a wide range of media. He is a master of the caricature, and his talents are constantly in demand. He doesn't smoke anymore. Brian is an avid trumpeter, and per-

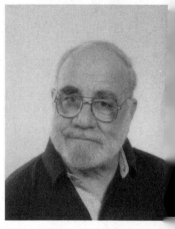

forms regularly in the Toronto area as a member of several bands. He is married to Fanny, a cook, bridge player, and crossword puzzle solver extraordinaire.

Rapid Psychler Press was founded in 1994 with the aim of producing textbooks and resource materials that further the use of humor in mental health education. In addition to textbooks, Rapid Psychler specializes in producing 35mm slides, overhead transparencies, and digital graphics for presentations.

**Rapid Psychler Press**